Series in Laboratory Medicine

Leo P. Cawley, M.D., Series Editor

Clinical Laboratory Statistics, Second Edition
Roy N. Barnett, M.D.

Laboratory Diagnostic Procedures in the Rheumatic Diseases, Second Edition
Alan S. Cohen, M.D.

Renal Function Tests:
Clinical Laboratory Procedures and Diagnosis
Cristobal G. Duarte, M.D.

Practical Blood Transfusion, Second Edition
Douglas W. Huestis, M.D., Joseph R. Bove, M.D.,
Shirley Busch, M.P.H., SBB (ASCP)

Exfoliative Cytopathology, Second Edition
Zuher M. Naib, M.D.

Immunopathology: Clinical Laboratory Concepts and Methods
Robert M. Nakamura, M.D.

Laboratory Management
Jack E. Newell, M.D.

The Diagnosis of Bleeding Disorders, Second Edition
Charles A. Owen, Jr., M.D., Ph.D., E. J. Walter Bowie, M.A., BM., F.A.C.P.,
John H. Thompson, Jr., Ph.D.

Urinary Cytology
Duane N. Tweeddale, M.D.

Serum Protein Abnormalities: Diagnostic and Clinical Aspects
Stephan E. Ritzmann, M.D., Jerry C. Daniels, M.D., Ph.D.

Histopathology of the Bone Marrow
Arkadi M. Rywlin, M.D.

Laboratory Procedures in Clinical Microbiology
John A. Washington II, M.D.

Renal Function Tests

Renal Function Tests
Clinical Laboratory Procedures and Diagnosis

Edited by
Cristobal G. Duarte, M.D.
Associate Professor of Medicine, Uniformed Services
University of the Health Sciences, Bethesda;
Lieutenant Colonel, United States Army Medical Corps,
Division of Medicine, Department of Nephrology, Walter
Reed Army Institute of Research, Washington, D.C.
Formerly Director of the Laboratory of Renal Function,
Mayo Clinic and Mayo Foundation, Rochester, Minnesota

Foreword by James C. Hunt, M.D.
Dean, College of Medicine, The University of Tennessee, Memphis
Formerly Chairman, Department of Medicine, Mayo Clinic
and Mayo Foundation, Rochester, Minnesota

Little, Brown and Company
Boston

First Edition

Library of Congress Catalog Card No. 79-91500

ISBN 0-316-19398-4

Printed in the United States of America

HAL

Contents

Foreword

A variety of excellent publications have become available during recent years with respect to renal pathophysiology, renal physiology, and the clinical aspects of renal disease. However, most have not emphasized methods of evaluating renal function in health and disease. In my judgment, this book is an excellent treatise on laboratory nephrology.

Physicians who do renal function tests will find in this book technical information that enables them to develop diagnostic procedures that can be adapted to almost any clinical laboratory. This book will be helpful not only to the nephrologist but to all clinicians who consider it necessary to understand the complex interaction of the kidney with other organ systems. Furthermore, medical students will find this book an excellent guide to indications for laboratory procedures needed to evaluate kidney malfunctions as well as a guide to the interpretation of the results of laboratory assessment.

There have been significant advances during the last few years in the interpretation of the pathological processes that mediate renal disease, and now more patients than ever survive far-advanced impairment of kidney function through renal dialysis and transplantation. However, the commonly employed laboratory procedures for assessing renal function in the patient with renal disease have remained relatively unchanged.

Most physicians are now aware that a measurement of the blood urea nitrogen (BUN) tells little about the degree of impairment of renal function, particularly as contrasted with the serum creatinine. An abnormal serum creatinine is an important indicator of impaired renal function. When the creatinine value is abnormal, it may be advisable to undertake a more specific assessment of the renal disorder either through a determination of the creatinine clearance or through the use of even more quantitative assessments, including standard clearance studies. The modern adaptation of radiolabeled compounds as a means of measuring glomerular and tubular function is well outlined in this excellent book.

The single most valuable test of renal function is the complete analysis of the urine and the microscopic examination of the urine sediment. The patient who has an abnormal urinalysis or an elevation in serum creatinine deserves a more complete assessment through quantitation of glomerular or tubular function, or both. This is especially important because renal function may be seriously impaired even when one or both of these two procedures yield normal results.

It is imperative that the student of medicine appreciate the fact that the intravenous urogram measures only renal mass (size) and serves little purpose in the quantitative assessment of renal function. However, functional capacity of the individual kidneys should probably be evaluated in any patient who has abnormal urinalysis, serum creatinine, or intravenous urogram.

No laboratory assessment of renal function, individually or in combination, should replace a careful study of the patient by a complete medical history and physical examination. The extent of diagnostic evaluation needed for the patient with hypertension, seriously impaired renal function, or genitourinary symptoms should be determined in accordance with the findings of the history and physical examination. Furthermore, renal histopathology, renal angiography, renal venous renin activity measurements, and studies of aldosterone metabolism can be interpreted with accuracy only in light of all clinical information.

This book stimulates a greater awareness of the need for and value of an accurate assessment of renal function by methods that are more informative than those employed by most physicians. I congratulate the editor and the authors of the individual chapters on their contributions to clinical nephrology.

James C. Hunt

Preface

It was with hesitation but with a deep sense of humility that I accepted the task of organizing the writing of this book on diagnostic nephrology, now being added to the excellent Series in Laboratory Medicine published through the years by Little, Brown and Company.

I believe that I was selected as editor of this book at least in part because at the time I was director of the Laboratory of Renal Function at Mayo Clinic. Therefore, due credit is given to those who have been instrumental in creating this laboratory and in maintaining its high standards of excellence: Doctors Frank T. Maher, James C. Hunt, Cameron G. Strong and David M. Wilson.

Included in the first two chapters are some results of original studies on renal function. This research could not have been completed without the able assistance of Mr. Robert R. Liedtke, Supervisor of Laboratory Nephrology.

C. G. D.

Contributing Authors

Tomas Berl, M.D.
Associate Professor of Medicine, Division of Renal Diseases, University of Colorado Medical Center; Attending Nephrologist, Medicine Department, Colorado General Hospital, Denver

Claudio Bianchi, M.D.
Professor of Diagnostic Nephrology, Department of Internal Medicine and Nephrology, University of Pisa; Chief, Renal Services, Clinica Medica Generale 2, Ospedale S. Chiara, Pisa, Italy

Ronald D. Brown, M.D.
Associate Professor of Medicine, Mayo Medical School; Consultant, Endocrine Research Unit, Mayo Clinic and Mayo Foundation, Rochester, Minnesota

James C. M. Chan, M.D.
Professor of Pediatrics, Division of Health Sciences, Medical College of Virginia of Virginia Commonwealth University School of Medicine; Attending Physician and Director, Pediatric Nephrology Section, Medical College of Virginia Hospitals and Clinics, Richmond, Virginia

Cristobal G. Duarte, M.D.
Associate Professor of Medicine, Uniformed Services University of the Health Sciences, Bethesda; Lieutenant Colonel, United States Army Medical Corps, Division of Medicine, Department of Nephrology, Walter Reed Army Institute of Research, Washington, D.C.

Lila R. Elveback, Ph.D.
Professor of Biostatistics, Mayo Medical School; Consultant, Section of Medical Research Statistics, Mayo Clinic and Mayo Foundation, Rochester, Minnesota

William L. Henrich, M.D.
Assistant Professor of Medicine, University of Texas Southwestern Medical School; Attending Nephrologist, Medicine Department, Veterans Administration Hospital, Dallas

Keith E. Holley, M.D.
Associate Professor of Pathology and Medicine, Mayo Medical School; Consultant, Department of Pathology and Anatomy, Mayo Clinic and Mayo Foundation, Rochester, Minnesota

William J. Johnson, M.D.
Professor of Medicine, Mayo Medical School; Director, Artificial Kidney Center, Mayo Clinic and Mayo Foundation, Rochester, Minnesota

Robert A. Kyle, M.D.
Professor of Medicine, Mayo Medical School; Consultant, Division of Hematology and Internal Medicine, Mayo Clinic and Mayo Foundation, Rochester, Minnesota

Robert R. Liedtke, B.S.
Supervisor, Renal Laboratory, Department of Laboratory Medicine, Mayo Clinic and Mayo Foundation, Rochester, Minnesota

David C. Manahan, B.S.
Technologist, Renin Laboratory, Division of Nephrology, Mayo Clinic and Mayo Foundation, Rochester, Minnesota

John T. McCall, Ph.D.
Associate Professor of Biochemistry and Laboratory Medicine, Mayo Medical School; Consultant, Section of Clinical Chemistry, Mayo Clinic and Mayo Foundation, Rochester, Minnesota

James S. Robertson, M.D., Ph.D.
Professor of Laboratory Medicine, Mayo Medical School; Consultant, Diagnostic Nuclear Medicine, Mayo Clinic and Mayo Foundation, Rochester, Minnesota

Michael S. Rohrbach, Ph.D.
Assistant Professor of Biochemistry, Mayo Medical School; Senior Research Fellow, Thoracic Disease Research Unit, Mayo Clinic and Mayo Foundation, Rochester, Minnesota

J. Carlos Romero, M.D.
Associate Professor of Medicine, Mayo Medical School; Head, Hypertension Research Laboratory, Division of Nephrology and Internal Medicine, Mayo Clinic and Mayo Foundation, Rochester, Minnesota

Lynwood H. Smith, M.D.
Professor of Medicine, Mayo Medical School; Consultant, Division of Nephrology and Internal Medicine, Mayo Clinic and Mayo Foundation, Rochester, Minnesota

Cameron G. Strong, M.D.
Professor of Medicine, Mayo Medical School; Director, Multidisciplinary Hypertension Clinic, Mayo Clinic and Mayo Foundation, Rochester, Minnesota

Ross M. Tucker, M.D.
Associate Professor of Medicine, Mayo Medical School; Consultant, Division of Nephrology and Internal Medicine, Mayo Clinic and Mayo Foundation, Rochester, Minnesota

Jorge A. Velosa, M.D.
Assistant Professor of Medicine, Mayo Medical School; Consultant, Division of Nephrology and Internal Medicine, Mayo Clinic and Mayo Foundation, Rochester, Minnesota

John A. Washington II, M.D.
Professor of Microbiology and Laboratory Medicine, Mayo Medical School; Head, Section of Clinical Microbiology, Mayo Clinic and Mayo Foundation, Rochester, Minnesota

Peter G. Werness, Ph.D.
Instructor in Biochemistry, Mayo Medical School; Research Fellow, Division of Nephrology and Internal Medicine, Mayo Clinic and Mayo Foundation, Rochester, Minnesota

Max Wisgerhof, M.D.
Assistant Professor of Medicine, Wayne State University School of Medicine; Staff Physician, Department of Medicine, Hutzel Hospital, Detroit

Notice

The indications and dosages of all drugs in this book have been recommended in the medical literature and conform to the practices of the general medical community. The medications described do not necessarily have specific approval by the Food and Drug Administration for use in the diseases and dosages for which they are recommended. The package insert for each drug should be consulted for use and dosage as approved by the FDA. Because standards for usage change, it is advisable to keep abreast of revised recommendations, particularly those concerning new drugs.

1. Creatinine

Cristobal G. Duarte, Lila R. Elveback, and Robert R. Liedtke

A correct understanding of the concept of renal clearance is essential to the proper interpretation and evaluation of the results of studies of renal function. Renal clearance has been defined as the volume of plasma, expressed in milliliters, cleared of a determined substance in its passage through the kidneys in a unit time, usually 1 minute. The function of the kidneys in general, and of its physiological unit, the nephron, in particular, can be divided into the two main processes of glomerular filtration and tubular transport. This chapter and the first part of the next chapter will be concerned with concepts related to the glomerular filtration rate (GFR).

Homer Smith [65] was the first to propose that in order to be accepted as valid for the measurement of GFR, a substance must fulfill the following requirements: it must be metabolically inert and nontoxic; it must have no intrinsic effect on renal function; and after being filtered freely at the glomerulus, it must be neither reabsorbed nor secreted by the renal tubules. In addition, its clearance rate must not be affected by any other substance; it must remain constant regardless of variations in plasma levels and urine flow; and it must be possible to measure its concentration in plasma and urine by simple, reliable, and precise laboratory methods.

The clearance of inulin, a polysaccharide of molecular weight of approximately 5000, fulfills all these requirements and thus is the standard method for the measurement of GFR. Inulin, however, is not in endogenous concentration in the body. Studies of renal clearance of inulin require the intravenous administration of a priming dose followed by a constant infusion in order to maintain the plasma concentration of inulin constant during the determination of GFR. This procedure must be performed by specialized technical personnel; it requires that urine and blood samples be collected at constant, well-timed intervals, that the bladder be empty at the beginning and end of each clearance period, and that the specimens collected be processed chemically to obtain values for the calculation of the clearance. Because of these difficulties, simpler alternative methods have been sought for the measurement of GFR (for a detailed discussion of inulin and the use of radioisotopes for the measurement of GFR, see Chapter 2; for technical information on measurement of the clearance of creatinine, see Chapter 3).

The finding that creatinine is concentrated in the urine more than most other endogenous substances eliminated by the kidneys [53] led to the use of creatinine as a test of renal function. Creatinine is an amino-acid product of protein

This work was done while Dr. Duarte was Director of Laboratory Nephrology, Mayo Clinic Foundation, Rochester, Minn.

metabolism that is derived from creatine [6, 8, 22]. The main sites of creatine synthesis are the liver, the pancreas, and the kidney [8], but the bulk of creatine is contained in muscle, where creatine is stored as creatine and phosphocreatine before it is further metabolized and released into the circulation as creatinine [33], which is then excreted in the urine. Creatinine, therefore, is in endogenous concentration in the body and does not need to be infused for studies of renal function.

Technical Considerations

Three methods have been used for the determination of creatinine in blood, plasma, serum, and urine. The first method, based on the Jaffe reaction [3, 4, 7], measures, in addition to true creatinine chromogens, noncreatinine chromogens that do not appear in the urine since they are not filtered at the glomerulus [26]. Noncreatinine chromogens are acetone, pyruvic and ascorbic acid, proteins, barbiturates, phenolsulfonphthalein, sodium sulfobromophthalein, and other unknown substances [20, 34]. Another method for the determination of creatinine is based on the Folin-Wu reaction [34] and measures only true creatinine chromogens. A significant improvement in the precision of the determination of creatinine over the two manual methods has been achieved by the adaptation of the Jaffe reaction to an automatic chemical analyzer (the Technicon AutoAnalyzer). True serum creatinine concentration [11] is overestimated by 21 percent for values lower than 1 mg/dl by the AutoAnalyzer method and by 90 percent by the method that measures total creatinine concentration (the Jaffe reaction). For values of true serum creatinine higher than 1 mg/dl [11], the readings are 10 percent higher with the AutoAnalyzer and 21 percent higher with the Jaffe reaction.

Of the three methods used to measure the clearance of creatinine [51], the AutoAnalyzer gives the best correlation with the clearance of inulin. The extra amount of noncreatinine chromogens measured in plasma by the AutoAnalyzer method neutralizes the creatinine appearing in the urine by tubular secretion according to the mathematical calculation used to determine the clearance of endogenous creatinine:

$$\text{Creatinine clearance (ml/min)} = \frac{\text{Urine creatinine (filtered + secreted) mg/dl} \times V \text{ ml/min}}{\text{Plasma creatinine (True creatinine chromogens + Noncreatinine chromogens) mg/dl}}$$

Simultaneous measurements of inulin clearance, the clearance of true creatinine, and the clearance of creatinine by the AutoAnalyzer [1] demonstrated that at normal levels of GFR, true creatinine clearance overestimated GFR by a mean of 46 percent and creatinine clearance by the AutoAnalyzer by a mean of 8 percent. As there is a moderate to significant reduction in renal function

[1], the clearance ratios of creatinine/inulin (measured by the AutoAnalyzer) increase and this can be explained by two factors: first, as the plasma concentration of creatinine rises, the tubular secretion of creatinine is enhanced; and second, at these levels of renal dysfunction the plasma concentration of true creatinine increases in greater proportion than plasma noncreatinine chromogens. At a GFR lower than 20 ml/min [44], as a maximal secretory rate of creatinine is reached, the clearance of creatinine decreases toward the clearance of inulin. Some studies reported that the clearance of creatinine was significantly higher than that of inulin in nephrotic patients than in nonnephrotic controls [4], but such results have not been corroborated by others [1].

It is generally recognized [1, 43, 45, 46] that the clearance of endogenous creatinine consistently exceeds simultaneous values of inulin clearance, thus indicating that there is a secretory mechanism for creatinine at all levels of renal function. The existence of an active secretory process for creatinine has been further substantiated by results demonstrating that endogenous creatinine/inulin clearance ratios decline toward unity during the administration of iodopyracet (Diodrast) and para-aminohippurate [14], phlorhizin [61], and caronamide [9], substances that block the secretion of creatinine. Occasional findings of endogenous creatinine/inulin ratios of less than one [17] in patients with peritonitis or congestive heart failure suggest that there may also be a reabsorptive process for creatinine.

Two main procedures are usually followed for the measurement of the clearance of creatinine: the urine may be collected for a period of 1 or 2 hours (short creatinine clearance) or over a period of 24 hours (long creatinine clearance). Blood samples are usually drawn at the beginning and end of the study for plasma creatinine determination. The long creatinine clearance has been considered to be a more physiological index of renal function [9] because factors that are known to influence the GFR (e.g., physical activity, the effects of drugs and medications, emotional tensions, dietary intake, and changes in intra-abdominal and venous pressure) are included in the clearance determination. A complete 24-hour urine collection, however, is extremely difficult to obtain. The following mistakes, which invalidate the test, have been noted in the course of a 24-hour urine collection [17, 69]: the first voiding, instead of being discarded, may be included in the collection; one or more specimens may be lost because of forgetfulness or because of the patient's micturating in the toilet in the course of defecation; the patient may turn over a sample of each voiding at the end of the study instead of pooling all the urine; the urine container may become full before the end of the study and subsequent voidings may be discarded; or the last specimen, instead of being added to the collection, may be discarded. The advantages of the short creatinine clearance are that the study can be performed under good technical control and that a complete urine collection can be successfully obtained over a short period of time.

It is important, therefore, to determine the degree of correlation between the short and the long creatinine clearance. In a study performed in 10 volunteers (five male and five female laboratory personnel), we compared both clearances. Blood samples were drawn at hours 0, 1, and 24 under fasting conditions. The protocols that were followed for these studies are given in Chapter 3. The subjects were hydrated by the oral administration of water a half hour before the first blood sample was drawn at hour 0 and in the course of the first 1-hour collection. After the second blood sample was drawn at hour 1, the subjects resumed their usual activities, all the urine was collected for the following 23 hours, and another blood sample was drawn at hour 24. The results of the first 1-hour clearance and the total 24-hour clearance were compared; they are illustrated in Table 1–1. Because the results did not differ between the sexes, they were studied together statistically. The significantly higher urine flow and creatinine clearance and the lower plasma creatinine found in the short clearance studies were probably the result of the hydration. Others have demonstrated that the 1-hour and 24-hour creatinine clearances are similar [18, 54] but that this good correlation can be disrupted as a result of heavy hydration.

Normal Values and Factors Affecting Plasma Concentration and Clearance of Creatinine

The clearance of creatinine is increased and the plasma concentration of creatinine is reduced throughout pregnancy [63]. The clearance of creatinine determined in infants during the first week of life [16] was in the range of 12.8 to 57 ml/min/1.73 m^2 and increased progressively [70] to a mean of 113 ml/min/1.73 m^2 at age 3, when creatinine clearance acquired adult characteristics. Mean creatinine clearance in children 3 years old or younger [70] was 88 ml/min/1.73 m^2. During the third decade of life [41], creatinine clearance starts to decline from a mean of 110 ml/min/1.73 m^2 for men and 95 ml/min/1.73 m^2 for women to a mean of 37 ml/min/1.73 m^2 for males and 39 ml/min/1.73 m^2 for females in the ninth decade of life. Another study [56] reported that creatinine clearance remains constant until the fourth decade of life, when it starts to decline at a rate of 6.5 ml/min/1.73 m^2/decade. With the reduction of creatinine clearance with aging [29, 57] there also occurs a decrease in the urinary excretion of creatinine, which has been interpreted as being indicative of a reduction in muscle mass; however, the serum creatinine concentration remains constant. The higher values for creatinine clearance in men have been related to the larger muscle mass in this sex [18, 23, 24, 25].

Initially, values of creatinine clearance were expressed as a function of body weight [35], but since the basis for this correlation is the size of the muscular mass, such correction did not take into consideration the effects of obesity. At present, values for creatinine clearance are usually corrected for body surface area (1.73 m^2) using the empirical formula of Dubois [35] which, by taking into consideration height and weight, adjusts the results of creatinine clearance for obesity and crude total weight. When the results for creatinine clearance were corrected for lean body mass as determined by anthropometric measure-

Table 1–1. Comparison of 1-Hour and 24-Hour Creatinine Clearances

		Volume (ml/min)		Plasma Creatinine (mg/dl)		Creatinine Clearance (ml/min/1.73 m^2)	
Subject	Sex and Age	1 hour	24 hours	1 hour *	24 hours *	1 hour	24 hours
1	F, 31	8.19	1.81	0.95	0.99	93	99
2	F, 34	11.25	1.64	1.01	1.04	106	97
3	F, 22	9.86	2.57	1.05	1.11	104	101
4	F, 57	10.23	1.96	1.00	1.08	95	88
5	F, 26	5.71	1.35	0.69	0.72	158	151
6	M, 47	4.34	1.65	1.33	1.38	81	81
7	M, 26	5.30	1.50	1.05	1.08	139	128
8	M, 34	1.03	2.78	0.90	0.93	122	121
9	M, 29	3.53	1.17	1.25	1.26	108	99
10	M, 34	10.18	2.92	1.05	1.08	105	106
Mean ± SE	—	6.96 ± 1.09	1.90 ± 0.21 †	1.03 ± 0.05	1.06 ± 0.05 †	111 ± 7.24	107 ± 6.56 ‡

* One-hour plasma creatinine: Mean of samples taken at hours 0 and 1; 24-hour plasma creatinine: mean of samples taken at hours 0 and 24. Significantly different from 1-hour collection: † $P < 0.001$; ‡ $P < 0.05$.

ments [18], it was possible to eliminate the statistical difference between the sexes. A better relationship was obtained by correlating creatinine to body content of potassium [35], either by the administration of an isotope of potassium or by natural potassium-40 activity, as measured in a whole-body counter. The usefulness of this expression, as applied to creatinine clearance, is based on the fact that two-thirds of total body potassium is in skeletal muscle, and since the content of potassium in body fat and bone is small, total body potassium is not affected by changes induced by obesity or fasting [35].

Normal values for plasma concentration of creatinine are in the range of 0.8 to 1.2 mg/dl in males and 0.6 to 0.9 mg/dl in females. Serial measurements taken throughout the day in adults [64] revealed that the clearance of creatinine decreases in the hours of deepest sleep (between 12:00 P.M. and 4:00 A.M.), but this variation was not observed in patients with congestive heart failure [3]. In samples taken at 4-hour intervals [64], a 5- to 17-percent variation in plasma concentration of creatinine was detected, and these fluctuations were not related to changes in creatinine clearance. Plasma concentration of creatinine was higher by 11 percent in the afternoon [18, 48, 49], and the urinary excretion of creatinine was elevated in the evening hours [49]. Fasting eliminated or minimized these variations [49] in plasma concentration and urinary excretion of creatinine. Determinations of creatinine clearance in the same subject over a period of years [68] demonstrated significant fluctuations in values, probably as a result of biological variations. Because of the significant fluctuations in plasma concentration of creatinine throughout the day, the time when a blood sample is drawn can have a significant influence on the results of the clearance [54]. It is recommended, therefore, that blood samples for plasma creatinine determinations be drawn in the morning under fasting conditions.

In studies conducted on normal kidney donors [48] it was found that after nephrectomy, hypertrophy and hyperplasia of the remaining kidney occur and that a functional response is already in evidence 24 hours after the operation. Seven days after the removal of the kidney [48], the function in the remaining organ was found to be 70 percent of the total preoperative creatinine clearance. Two to six years after the uninephrectomy, the clearance of creatinine in the remaining kidney varied from 71 percent [48] to 85 percent in females and 87 percent in males [15] of the values that were obtained before the operation. Measurements of several parameters of renal function in one study [15] indicated that the functional recovery in normal kidney donors was significantly better in males and that this sex difference was related to the stimulatory effect of testosterone on renal growth as well as the parenchymal damage resulting from urinary tract infections, which females are prone to develop.

The plasma concentration and urinary excretion of creatinine may be affected significantly by the content of creatine and creatinine in the food. The administration of a diet free from creatine and creatinine [5] causes a parallel decrease in the plasma concentration and urinary excretion of creatinine, although the clearance of endogenous creatinine does not change. Raw meat is high in creatine and has little creatinine [9], but the content of creatinine increases progressively with the temperature as the meat is subjected to heat. Canned meat also has large amounts of creatinine [35], since creatine is converted to creatinine in the process of thermal sterilization. The consumption of a well-cooked steak (which is high in creatinine) causes a significant increase in the clearance of creatinine [9].

In view of the fact that it is in muscle where creatine is metabolized to creatinine [61], it is not surprising that the production of creatinine is related to muscle mass. Males have a larger muscle mass, and thus more creatinine is excreted in the urine of men than in that of women; infants have low urinary excretion rates of creatinine that increase with age [35]. Professional athletes, either males or females [35], have a higher rate of excretion of creatinine in the urine than do controls. In clinical myopathies, in which the muscular mass is diminished [10, 55], the urinary excretion of creatine increases because the muscles are unable to metabolize fully the creatine released from the liver, pancreas, kidneys, and other organs, and since the endogenous production of creatinine is diminished [66], the urinary excretion and plasma concentration of creatinine are low [32], the plasma concentration of creatinine does not increase appropriately in relation to the impairment in renal function [32], and creatinine clearance must be calculated in order to obtain a better estimate of renal function [32]. In diseases such as tetanus, in which there is increased muscular activity [66], there may be an increase in the urinary excretion of creatinine. During heavy exercise, the urinary excretion of creatinine increases significantly [52, 67] and there is a decrease in creatinine clearance [52]. The urinary excretion of creatinine is increased in pyrexia [60].

The significantly low plasma concentration of creatinine and the high urinary excretion and clearance of creatinine in juvenile diabetics before the onset of renal disease [2] are probably related to the high levels of renal function in these patients resulting from high growth hormone activity [47]. Therefore, normal levels of plasma creatinine and creatinine clearance in diabetics [2] may be indicative of renal disease. With the onset of proteinuria [28], the values of creatinine clearance are lower in diabetics than in nondiabetic controls.

Creatinine and the Kidney: Theoretical Considerations

The validity of creatinine as a test of renal function is based on the assumption [42] that in a normal subject under steady-state conditions, as creatinine is released from muscle stores at a constant rate throughout the day, accumulation in the body is prevented by a renal excretory mechanism. Plasma concentration of creatinine, therefore [42], must be maintained at constant normal levels in a subject with a normal renal function, since the filtered load and urinary excretion of creatinine equal the amount of creatinine released from muscle. The dynamic changes in creatinine metabolism that have been postulated to take place as a result of variations in renal function [42] are demonstrated schematically in Figure 1–1. If creatinine is excreted exclusively by the kidneys by a process of glomerular filtration [42], a 50 percent reduction in renal function

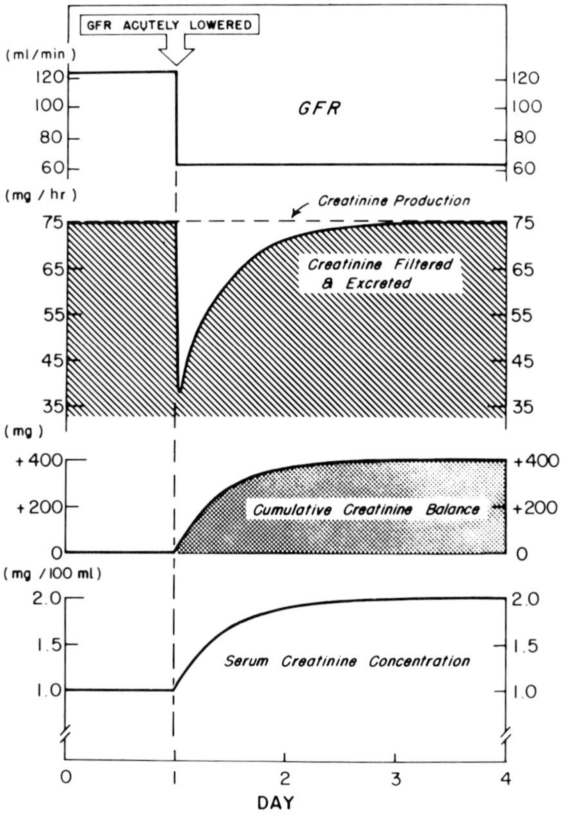

Figure 1–1
Postulated changes in the plasma concentration of creatinine in response to a reduction in GFR. At normal levels of renal function (between days 0 and 1), all the creatinine released into the circulation is excreted by the kidneys by the mechanism of glomerular filtration, and plasma levels of creatinine remain constant at a normal level. On day 1, after an acute reduction in GFR, there is a temporary fall in the filtered load of creatinine, but since the release of creatinine from muscle stores remains unchanged, the plasma creatinine rises until the filtered load of creatinine and the urinary excretion of creatinine again equal the amount of creatinine released into the circulation. A steady state is then reached in which, in response to a 50-percent reduction in GFR, the filtered load and the urinary excretion of creatinine equal control levels at the expense of a doubling in plasma creatinine. (Reprinted with permission, from J. P. Kassirer, Clinical evaluation of kidney function, *N. Engl. J. Med.* 285:386, 1971.)

in a person with a previously normal plasma concentration of creatinine of 1 mg/dl in the presence of unchanged release of creatinine from muscle will be expected to cause an accumulation of creatinine in the body and an increase in the plasma concentration of creatinine to 2 mg/dl. When this new steady state is achieved, the filtered load and urinary excretion of creatinine will rise to control levels at the expense of the 100 percent increase in plasma creatinine and will equal the amount of creatinine released from muscle [42] (Fig. 1–1). A further deterioration in renal function to a level that is 25 percent of the normal GFR will be expected to cause an increase in the plasma concentration of creatinine to a level of 4 mg/dl and, at a steady state, the filtered load and urinary excretion of creatinine will again rise to values equal to those of controls [42].

From pharmacodynamic studies of creatinine metabolism [12], it has been estimated that the biological half-life of creatinine in a normal young adult is 3.85 hours and is expected to be prolonged to 7.7 hours with a 50 percent reduction in GFR when a steady state is reached 24 hours after the onset of renal disease. With a progressive deterioration in renal function, prolongation of the half-life of creatinine is expected to occur [12] and will be expected to measure 38.5 and 77 hours at 10 and 5 percent of remaining renal function, respectively. Therefore, it should take 6.7 and 13.6 days to achieve 95 percent of a steady state for the corresponding plasma concentration levels of creatinine of 10.6 and 21.1 mg/dl [12].

In order to validate these postulates further [12, 42], it must be demonstrated that a proportional inverse relationship does indeed exist between plasma concentration of creatinine and GFR at different levels of renal function; that the urinary excretion of creatinine remains constant in the presence of a progressive decrease in GFR; that there is not a significant secretion of creatinine by the renal tubules; and that creatinine is excreted exclusively by the kidneys and is not further metabolized in the body.

Variability in the Urinary Excretion of Creatinine

Folin [27] was the first to report that the urinary excretion of creatinine remains strikingly constant in the same individual from day to day. The constancy in the urinary excretion of creatinine has been used to validate the completeness of a 24-hour collection of urine in patients in whom the daily excretory rate of steroids in the urine is being investigated [35].

The constancy in the urinary excretion of creatinine was evaluated in seven subjects who collected 24-hour urine specimens daily for 31 days. The volunteers for this study were laboratory personnel who, being directly involved in studies of renal function, were well aware of the importance of obtaining a complete urine collection. The subjects pursued their usual physical activities and normal diets throughout the study. The urinary flow and the urinary concentration of creatinine (see Chap. 3) were determined in each urine collection. The

Table 1–2. Mean Daily Urinary Creatinine Excretion (for 31 days)

			Creatinine					
			Urine					
Subject	Sex and Age	Urine Protein (mg/ 24 hours)	mg/kg/ 24 hours	CV %	$\bar{x}$ range	$\bar{x}$ % range	Plasma (mg/dl)	Clearance (ml/min/1.73 m^2)
1	M, 33	206	22.1	5.2	20–25	90–113	1.15	101
2	M, 46	134	22.4	11.0	20–29	89–129	1.15	81
3	M, 26	145	26.5	15.0	17–35	64–132	0.95	119
4	M, 28	112	22.8	7.7	19–27	83–118	1.20	100
5	F, 21	54	25.6	13.1	15–32	59–125	1.00	87
6	F, 23	68	23.6	8.6	21–29	89–123	0.90	90
7	F, 25	108	27.3	8.6	24–33	88–121	0.95	139
Range	—	54–206	22–27	5–15	—	—	0.9–1.2	81–139

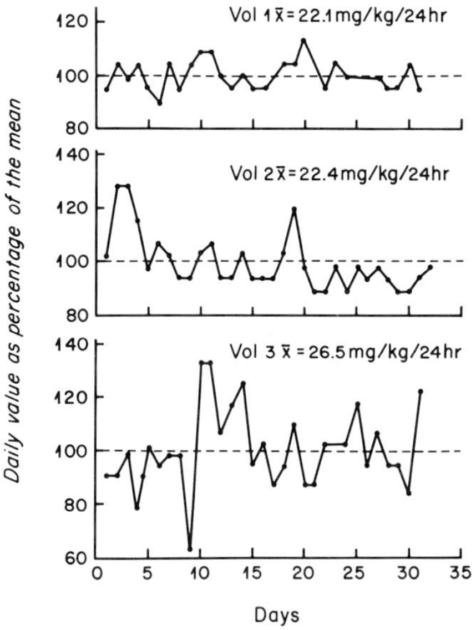

Figure 1–2
Daily urinary excretion of creatinine in three representative volunteers. *Top:* subject with the smallest variation (CV = 5.2%); *middle:* subject with the average variation (CV = 11%); *bottom:* subject with the greatest variation (CV = 15%).

excretion of proteins [58] was measured in one of the urine collections, and a blood sample was drawn for the determination of plasma creatinine in order to calculate the clearance of creatinine. The normal value for the excretion of protein in our laboratory is $\leqslant$ 270 mg/day. None of the subjects was proteinuric, and the plasma concentration and clearance of creatinine were within normal limits (Table 1–2). The mean coefficient of variance [CV = (standard deviation/mean) × 100] for the daily urinary excretion of creatinine, however, varied significantly (Table 1–2). To illustrate these results better, the daily urinary excretion rates of creatinine (expressed as a percentage of the mean) of the subject who showed the greatest variation (volunteer 3, Table 1–2), of the subject with the smallest variation (volunteer 1, Table 1–2), and of the subject who, having results between these two extremes, was considered to be representative of the rest of the group (volunteer 2, Table 1–2) are represented graphically in Figure 1–2. As illustrated in the lower portion of Figure 1–2, the volunteer who showed the greatest variation (CV = 15%) had 64 percent of the mean daily creatinine excretion on the ninth day and 132 percent on the tenth day. The subject with the smallest variation (CV = 5%), represented in the upper portion of Figure 1–2, excreted 90 percent of the mean on the sixth day and 113 percent on the twentieth day. Shown in the middle portion of Figure 1–2 is the subject with the average variation (CV = 11%), who excreted 129 percent of the mean on the second day and 81 percent on the twenty-first day.

This study indicates that the daily urinary excretion of creatinine can vary significantly not only among different subjects but also in the same subject from one day to another. Identical results [31, 50] have been reported by others, and they indicate that the daily urinary excretion of creatinine cannot be used as a reliable index of the completeness of urine collection.

Creatinine in Uremia and Creatinine Deficit

In acute renal failure [38], the plasma concentration of creatinine increases at a daily rate of 2 to 3 mg/dl in direct proportion to the amount of creatinine that is retained in the body and to the reduction in renal function. In chronic renal failure, on the contrary [30], the urinary excretion of creatinine decreases as plasma concentration rises, and the rate of daily increase in plasma concentration of creatinine [38] is only one-half to one-third of what is expected from the creatinine retained as a result of the fall in GFR. This creatinine deficit becomes apparent at plasma concentrations of creatinine higher than 6 mg/dl and cannot be accounted for entirely by a reduction in endogenous production [30]. It has been estimated that 16 to 66 percent of the creatinine formed in uremia is metabolized or excreted extrarenally [30]. The existence of routes of creatinine excretion and metabolism other than the kidneys have been investigated in uremic patients.

Creatinine is uniformly distributed throughout body water [59] and, like urea and uric acid [39], diffuses into the gut. At a normal plasma concentration the amount of creatinine entering the gut is negligible, but in uremia it becomes significant [38]. The bacterial proliferation (streptococci and enterococci) [62] that develops in the upper gastrointestinal tract of chronically uremic patients [40] plays an important role in the induction of a creatininase system that is related to the degradation of creatinine. Metabolites of creatinine [40] have been identified in the lumen of the gut, plasma, urine, and expired air in uremic patients, thus providing evidence that creatinine is metabolized in the gut and recycled. The recognition of this important secondary route of metabolism and excretion of creatinine in uremic patients explains the significant variations in urinary excretion, plasma concentration, and clearance of creatinine in some patients with renal disease and gives reason to question seriously the validity of creatinine as a reliable test of renal function in uremia [40].

If the release of creatinine from muscle stores continues unchanged after the onset of renal failure, and if creatinine is a specific and sensitive method for the estimation of GFR, it is to be expected that plasma creatinine will rise in proportion to the decrease in creatinine clearance. However, as previously demonstrated by others [18, 25] and as shown in Figure 1–3, when different levels of plasma creatinine concentration are related to their corresponding creatinine clearance, a linear relationship fails to develop. The results of studies correlating plasma concentration with creatinine clearance in 253 males are shown in Figure 1–3A; the results for 223 females are given in Figure 1–3B. The protocols that were followed for these studies of 1-hour creatinine clearance and the methods that were used for the analytical determinations of the samples are described in Chapter 3. In agreement with studies reported by others [18, 25], the following observations can be made by examining Figures 1–3A and 1–3B from right to left: First, in the region in which results consistent with marked reductions in renal function (as indicated by significant elevations in plasma concentration of creatinine and decreases in creatinine clearance) are plotted, with small fluctuations in creatinine clearance there are correspondingly large variations in plasma creatinine concentrations. Next, in the intermediate area of Figures 1–3A and 1–3B, where plasma creatinine levels range from 6 to 2 mg/dl, there is a transitional zone in which a linear relationship between plasma concentration and clearance of creatinine becomes apparent. Finally, as shown in the left portion of Figures 1–3A and 1–3B and corresponding to values consistent with normal levels of renal function, the linear relationship is again lost, and in this area small variations in plasma creatinine relate to significantly wide changes in creatinine clearance.

To determine the adequacy of the changes in plasma concentration of creatinine as they relate to creatinine clearance, a scattergram was constructed by separating the values illustrated in Figures 1–3A and 1–3B into four main categories. The results are illustrated in Figures 1–4A and 1–4B. If values of 1.2 mg/dl and 0.9 mg/dl are taken as the highest normal plasma concentration of creatinine for males and females, respectively, and 80 ml/min as the lowest normal clearance of creatinine for both sexes, it can be appreciated that in approximately 76 percent of the values in the male population and in 74 percent of the females there was an adequate correlation between plasma concentration and clearance of creatinine, that is, either normal levels of plasma creatinine corresponded to normal levels of creatinine clearance (left upper quadrant in Figures 1–4A and 1–4B), or abnormally elevated levels of plasma creatinine were related to reduced levels of creatinine clearance (right lower quadrant in Figures 1–4A and 1–4B). In approximately 23 percent of males and 25 percent of females, however, plasma creatinine levels were not appropriate when related to creatinine clearance, that is, either normal levels of plasma creatinine corresponded to decreased creatinine clearance (left lower quadrant in Figures 1–4A and 1–4B), or elevated levels of plasma creatinine were related to normal values of creatinine clearance (right upper quadrant in Figures 1–4A and 1–4B).

Several attempts have been made to develop reliable methods that will allow

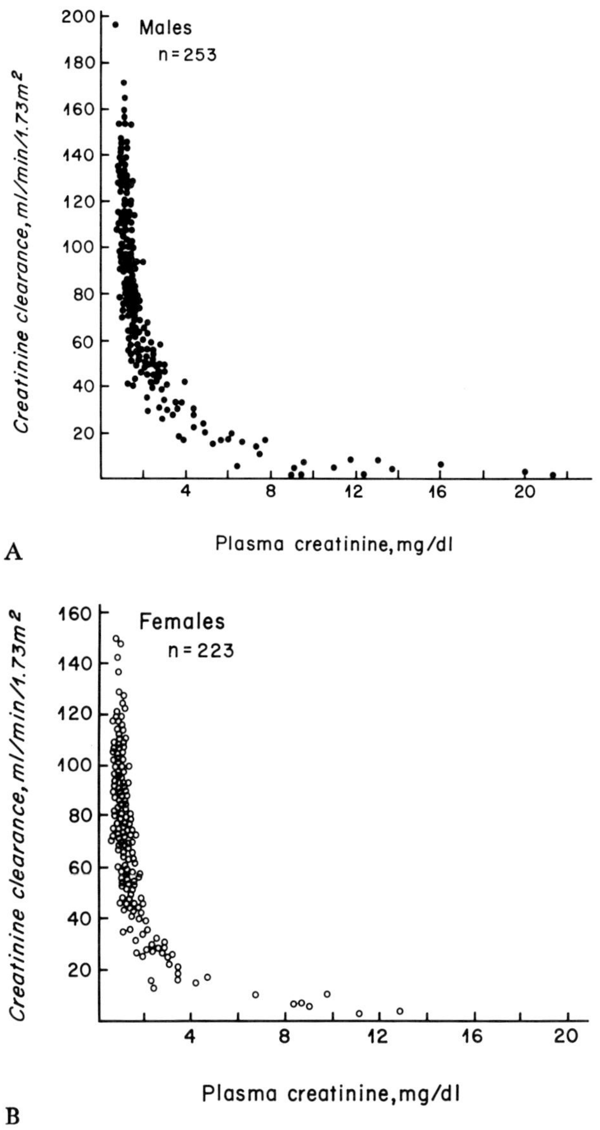

Figure 1–3
Correlation between a 1-hour creatinine clearance and plasma concentration of creatinine in males (A) and females (B).

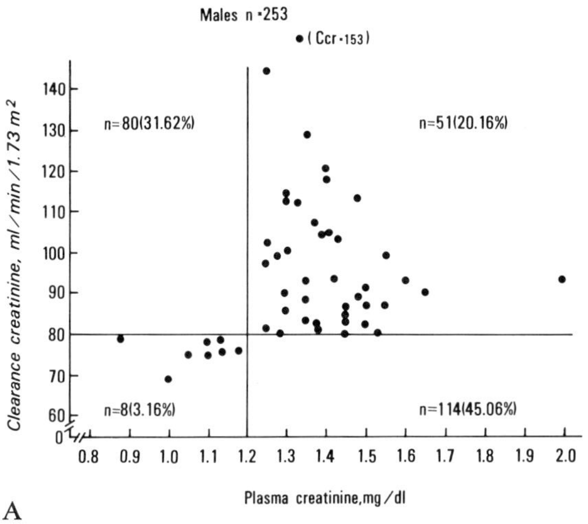

A

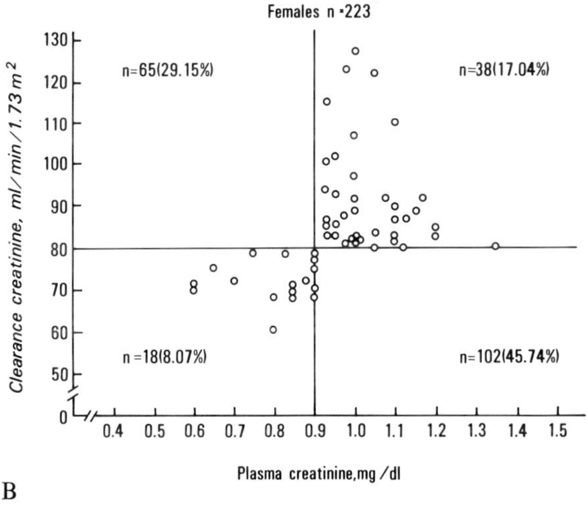

B

Figure 1–4
Analysis of the adequacy of changes between plasma concentration and clearance of creatinine in males (A) and females (B), based on the results shown in Figure 1–3.

a correct estimation of creatinine clearance as an index of renal function based on plasma creatinine concentration [13, 23, 36, 37, 56, 57], thus obviating the need for complete urine collections. Such mathematical calculations are of value when urine cannot be collected, or as a bedside guide in order to adjust the dosage of drugs administered to uremic patients that are eliminated by the kidneys. When the values shown in Figures 1–3A and 1–3B were processed according to some of the calculations proposed by others [13, 23, 36, 37] and by us, which took into consideration, in addition to plasma creatinine concentration and sex, other factors such as age, body weight, height, and surface area (Table 1–3), and when these results were compared with methods developed in our laboratory that included in the calculations only the factors of sex and plasma creatinine concentration, our mathematical formulations yielded similar or better results (Table 1–3).

Since it is evident that a linear relationship does not exist between the plasma concentration and the clearance of creatinine [12, 23, 24, 25] (Fig. 1–3), several mathematical transformations have been attempted to elicit a better correlation between both functions. It has been reported [18, 23, 25] that when the reciprocal of the plasma concentration of creatinine is related to the clearance of creatinine, a linear relationship with a positive slope develops. As previously shown by others [24] and as demonstrated in Figures 1–5A and 1–5B, when the results illustrated in Figures 1–3A and 1–3B are processed logarithmically, a significant linear correlation with a negative slope becomes apparent.

Because the clearance of inulin is the standard method for the determination of GFR, it is more relevant to explore a relationship between the clearance of inulin, on the one hand, and the plasma concentration or the clearance of creatinine, on the other. We carried out such studies in 149 males and in 127 females with normal and reduced renal function. The protocols that were followed, which correspond to the standard methods of study of renal clearance, are detailed in Chapter 3, where the methods that were used for the chemical analysis of the samples are also given. Creatinine and inulin concentrations were determined in each sample that was collected. The results of a correlation between the plasma concentration of creatinine and the clearance of inulin are given in Figure 1–6A for males and in Figure 1–6B for females; the correlation between the clearance of creatinine and that of inulin is shown in Figure 1–7. Each point in Figures 1–6 and 1–7 represents the mean value of three clearance periods. After these results were subjected to several statistical calculations, it was decided to express them logarithmically because by this method the significance of the correlation was enhanced and the scatter of the values was reduced.

When the plasma concentration of creatinine was related to the clearance of inulin, the correlation was linear and significant and the slope was negative (Figs. 1–6A and 1–6B); when the clearances of creatinine and inulin were correlated, the slope was positive and the correlation was more significant (Fig.

Table 1-3. Prediction of Creatinine Clearance from Plasma Creatinine

Regression Equation*	r_{xy}	$s_{y \cdot x}$	Reference
MALES			
$\left(\frac{100}{S_{cr}} - 12\right)\frac{1.73}{SA}$	0.834	24	Jeliffe [36]
$\left[\frac{98 - 16\left(\frac{\text{age} - 20}{20}\right)}{S_{cr}}\right]\frac{1.73}{SA}$	0.795	21.2	Jeliffe [37]
$\left(\frac{94.3}{S_{cr}} - 1.8\right)\frac{1.73}{SA}$	0.815	20.3	Edwards and Whyte [23]
$\frac{(140 - \text{age}) \cdot \text{weight (kg)}}{72\ S_{cr}}$	0.873	17.1	Cockcroft and Gault [13]
e^{f_M}†§	0.90	15.3	This study
$\frac{109.8}{P_{cr}} - 1.8$	0.905	14.9	This study
FEMALES			
$\frac{77.65}{P_{cr}} + 2.2$	0.833	16.8	This study
e^{f_F}‡§	0.86	15.7	This study

* SA = surface area; S_{cr} and P_{cr} = serum and plasma creatinine.
† $f_M = 2.938 - 0.15\ P_{cr} + (3.239/P_{cr}) - (1.354/P_{cr^2})$.
‡ $f_F = 2.622 - 0.121\ P_{cr} + (2.911/P_{cr}) - (1.008/P_{cr^2})$.
§ From stepwise regression in ln C_{cr} on height, (height)^2, weight, (weight)^2, 1/weight, 1/(weight)^2, ponderal index (PI), SA, P_{cr}, $1/P_{cr}$, and $1/(P_{cr})^2$.

1–7). Different levels of mean plasma creatinine and their corresponding inulin clearance together with the residual standard deviation around the regression line are shown in Table 1–4. If one accepts 1.2 mg/dl for males and 0.9 mg/dl for females as the highest normal plasma concentration of creatinine and 80 ml/min as the lowest normal inulin clearance for both sexes, it can be appreciated that at normal plasma levels of creatinine between 0.8 and 1.2 mg/dl for males and between 0.7 and 0.9 mg/dl for females, the clearance of inulin can be overestimated. Abnormally elevated levels of plasma creatinine ranging from 1.3 to 1.6 mg/dl for males and from 0.9 to 1.2 mg/dl for females can underestimate the clearance of inulin. Only at abnormally elevated plasma levels of creatinine of 1.6 mg/dl for males and 1.3 mg/dl for females are all ranges of estimated inulin clearance abnormally low.

Different levels of mean creatinine clearance and its corresponding estimated inulin clearance as well as the variation around the mean are given in Table 1–5. For any given value of mean creatinine clearance the estimated inulin clearance was always lower, and the variation around the regression line ($s_{y \cdot x}$) was

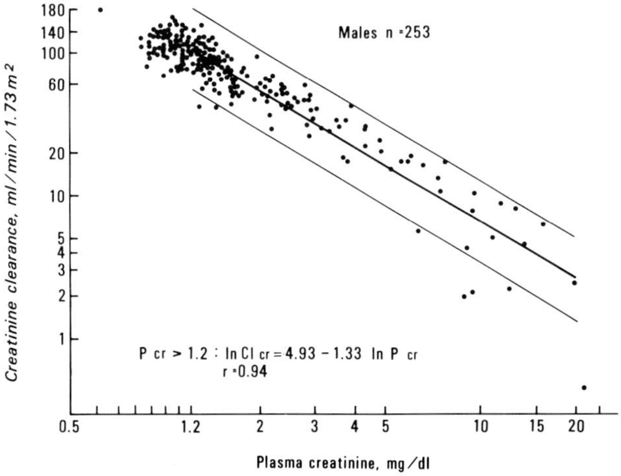

A

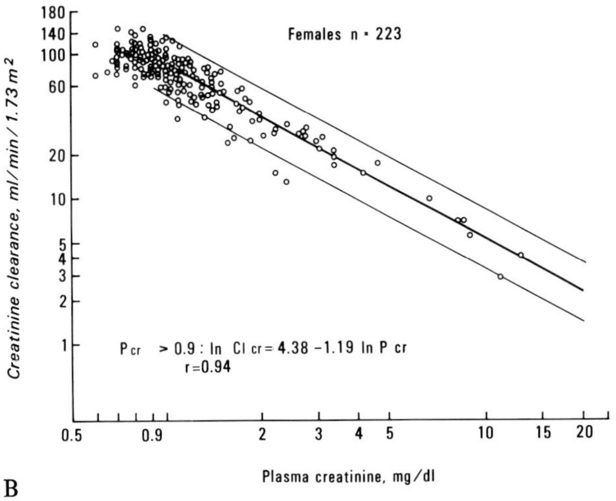

B

Figure 1–5
Logarithmic transformation of results shown in Figure 1–3. Regression line $\hat{y}$ (middle line) and confidence intervals ($\hat{y} \pm 1.96\text{SE}\ \hat{y}$) (outer lines) are shown, in which:

$$\text{SE}^2_{\hat{y}} = \frac{s^2 y \cdot x}{n}\left[1 + \left(\frac{x - \bar{x}}{s_x}\right)^2\right].$$

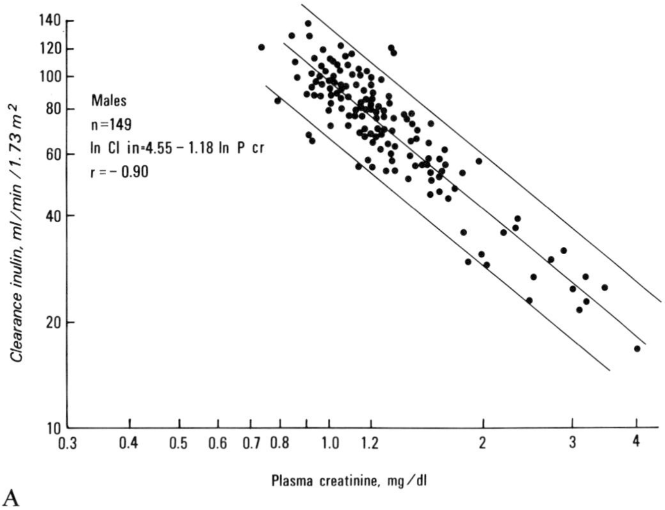

A

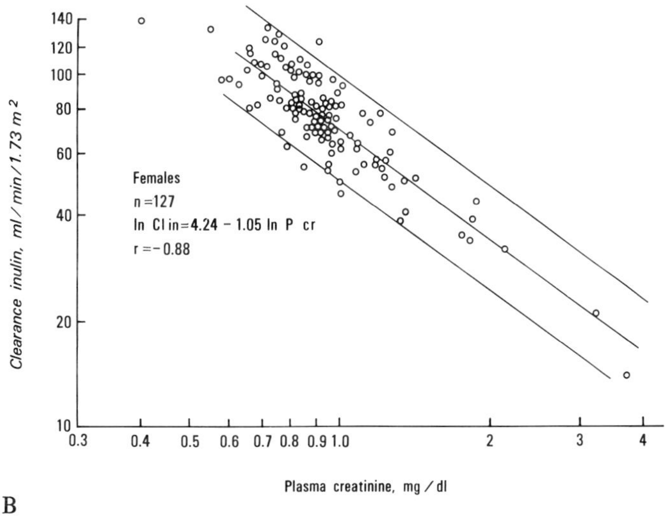

B

Figure 1–6
Correlation between the natural logarithms of plasma creatinine and inulin clearance in studies performed simultaneously in males (A) and females (B). Each point represents the mean of three clearance periods. The lines and symbols are as indicated in Figure 1–5.

Table 1–4. Relationship Between Inulin Clearance and Plasma Creatinine

Plasma Creatinine	Males *		Females †	
	Inulin Clearance Estimate		Inulin Clearance Estimate	
Mean	Mean	Interval	Mean	Interval
0.6	—	—	119	84–169
0.7	—	—	102	72–144
0.8	124	86–178	88	62–125
0.9	108	75–155	78	55–110
1.0	95	66–137	70	49–99
1.1	85	59–122	63	45–89
1.2	77	53–111	58	41–81
1.3	70	48–101	53	37–75
1.4	64	44–92	49	35–69
1.5	59	41–85	46	32–64
1.6	55	38–79	43	30–60
1.7	51	35–73	40	28–56
1.8	47	33–68	38	27–53
1.9	45	31–64	36	25–50
2.0	42	29–60	37	24–48
2.5	32	22–46	27	19–38
3.0	26	18–37	22	16–31
3.5	22	15–31	19	13–26
4.0	18	13–27	16	11–23
5	14	10–20	13	9–18
10	6	4–9	6	4–9
15	4	3–6	4	3–6
20	3	2–4	3	2–4

* Males: $\ln Cl_{in} = 4.55 - 1.18 \ln P_{cr}$; $s_{y \cdot x} = 0.18$.
† Females: $\ln Cl_{in} = 4.24 - 1.05 \ln P_{cr}$; $s_{y \cdot x} = 0.17$.

broader in the plasma creatinine-inulin clearance correlation (Table 1–4) than in the creatinine clearance-inulin clearance correlation (Table 1–5). When a scattergram was drawn in order to investigate the appropriateness of the changes between plasma creatinine and the clearances of both creatinine and inulin (as taken from values given in Figure 1–6), it became evident that in those instances in which there was a lack of correlation (normal values of plasma creatinine corresponding to abnormal values of creatinine or inulin clearance, or abnormally high values of plasma creatinine with corresponding normal clearances), plasma creatinine tended in most instances to overestimate inulin clearance and to underestimate creatinine clearance (Fig. 1–8). Likewise, when the appropriateness of changes between the clearance of inulin and that of creatinine was examined, it was evident that in those instances in which there was a lack of proper correlation (normal creatinine clearance with abnormal inulin clearance, or abnormal creatinine clearance corresponding to normal inulin clearance), in 14 percent of all subjects normal levels of creatinine clearance

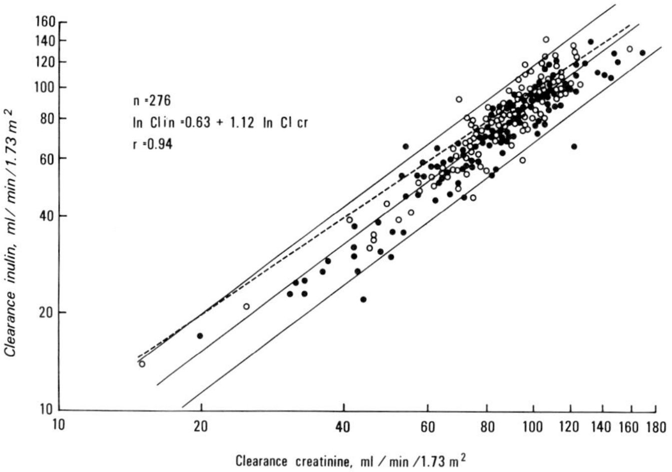

Figure 1–7
Correlation between the clearances of inulin and creatinine. The broken line denotes equality; other lines and symbols are the same as in Figure 1–5.

Table 1–5. Relationship Between ln Inulin Clearance and ln Creatinine Clearance

Creatinine Clearance	Inulin Clearance Estimate *	
(mean)	Mean	Interval
30	24	18–31
40	33	25–43
50	42	32–55
60	51	39–67
70	61	47–80
80	71	54–92
85	76	58–99
90	81	62–105
95	86	65–112
100	91	69–119
105	96	73–125
110	101	77–132
115	106	81–139
120	111	85–145
130	122	93–159
140	132	101–173
150	143	109–186

* $\ln \mathrm{Cl}_{\mathrm{in}} = -0.63 + 1.12 \ln \mathrm{Cl}_{\mathrm{cr}}$; $s_{y \cdot x} = 0.13$.

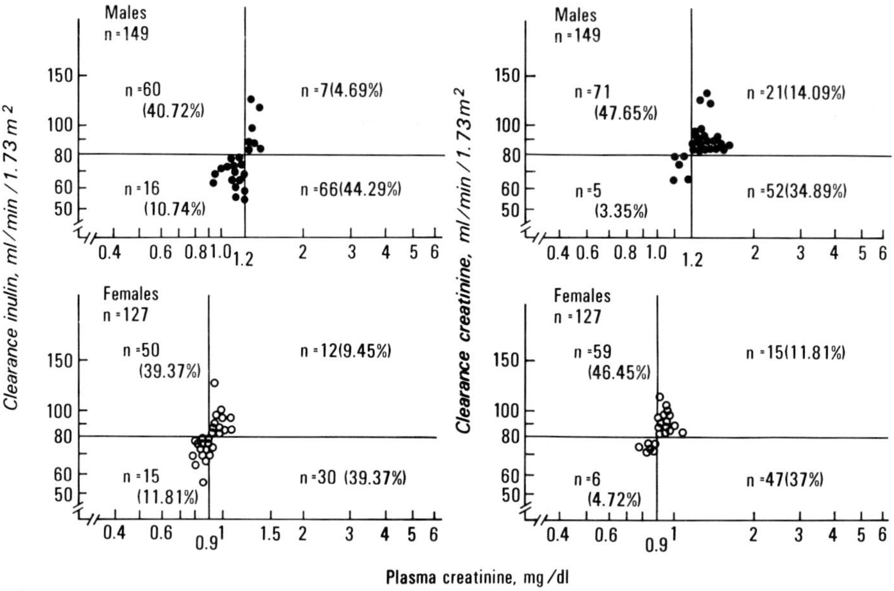

Figure 1–8
Analysis of the predictive value of plasma creatinine in the studies shown in Figure 1–6 reveals that in approximately 15 percent of males and 21 percent of females there were discrepancies between plasma creatinine and inulin clearance, and that in 17 percent of males and 16 percent of females there were discrepancies between plasma concentration and clearance of creatinine.

corresponded to reduced levels of inulin clearance (Fig. 1–9). In summary, these studies demonstrate that creatinine clearance is a better indicator than plasma creatinine concentration for the estimation of inulin clearance.

Other studies [43] have shown that creatinine clearance may be normal in 42 percent of patients with a definite reduction in GFR (clearance of inulin ranging from 61 to 70 ml/min), in 23 percent of patients with a moderate reduction in GFR (clearance of inulin ranging from 51 to 60 ml/min), and in 1 percent of patients with a severe reduction in GFR (clearance of inulin $\leqslant$ 50 ml/min). Studies of serum creatinine [43] have shown that in 50 percent of subjects with a concentration between 1.0 and 1.2 mg/dl, the GFR was $\leqslant$ 90 ml/min, and in 10 percent of subjects the GFR was $\leqslant$ 45 ml/min. In 10 percent of subjects with a serum creatinine concentration between 0.6 and 0.8 mg/dl [43], the GFR was $\leqslant$ 60 ml/min; in 90 percent of subjects with serum creatinine higher than 1.4 mg/dl, the GFR was lower than 100 ml/min. These findings emphasize the concept that a single determination of plasma concentration or clearance of creatinine in one subject may be misleading in assessing GFR [43]. Serial measurements in the same patient during the course of the

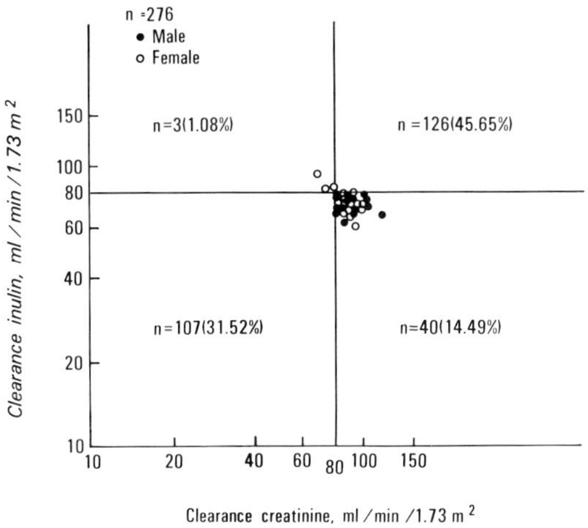

Figure 1–9
Analysis of the predictive value of creatinine clearance in the results shown in Figure 1–7 indicates that in 14 percent of subjects, normal levels of creatinine clearance corresponded to abnormally reduced levels of inulin clearance.

disease [43], however, may provide a better indication of the direction of the changes in renal function. As a result of starvation and reduction in muscle mass, the plasma concentration of creatinine may fall in progressive renal failure [43, 68], thus erroneously suggesting an improvement in renal function; in all cases creatinine clearance is a better indirect indicator of changes in GFR than is plasma creatinine.

Creatinine and Urea

In renal disease, as the GFR decreases the concentration of urea in blood rises, and renal function can be evaluated by relating the concentration of urea in the urine to the blood urea nitrogen (BUN) [21]. Although urea may be filtered at the glomerulus by a mechanism similar to that which filters inulin and creatinine, urea is highly diffusible and, depending on the concentration gradient, may diffuse passively between the tubular lumen and the renal interstitium at different levels of the nephron [17]; the clearance of urea is always lower than the GFR [17]. Furthermore, the clearance of urea is highly dependent on the urine flow [17]. At urinary flows greater than 2 ml/min, the clearance of urea (maximum urea clearance) is about three-fifths of the GFR, and at lower levels of urinary flows, the clearance of urea (standard urea clearance) is less than three-fifths of the GFR. In addition, the metabolism of urea [17] is influenced significantly by factors such as the intake of proteins, the catabolic state of the individual, the hepatic function, and so forth. Clinically, the clearance of urea as a single test of renal function has only historical interest, but significant information may be obtained by relating the BUN to the plasma concentration of creatinine or the clearance of urea to the clearance of creatinine.

The normal BUN-plasma creatinine concentration ratio of 10:1 [19, 20, 68] is usually maintained in uremia but can be disrupted in some other clinical conditions. This ratio may rise [19, 20, 68] as a result of an increase in BUN in catabolic states, in prerenal azotemia, in uremic patients after a high protein intake, by absorption of blood from the gut after gastrointestinal bleeding, when urinary tract obstruction causes renal reabsorption of urea, or when, as a consequence of the implantation of the ureters into the lumen of the gut, urea is absorbed from the gastrointestinal tract.

The ratio of BUN to plasma creatinine may be lower [20] as BUN decreases as a result of starvation, after a low protein intake, in advanced liver failure, or as a result of an increase in plasma creatinine as seen after muscular breakdown in muscular subjects. Creatinine dialyzes less well than urea [20, 68], and patients in chronic dialysis may have plasma creatinine levels that are proportionately higher than the BUN.

In advanced renal failure [44] at levels of GFR of 20 ml/min and less, as the remaining nephrons undergo an osmotic diuresis, the reabsorption of urea by the renal tubules diminishes and the urea clearance, which is usually lower than the GFR, approximates the clearance of inulin. Similarly, as a tubular maximum secretory rate for creatinine is exceeded at these levels of renal insufficiency [1, 44], creatinine clearance, which at higher levels of GFR overestimates the clearance of inulin, decreases toward the GFR. Therefore, the mean values of urea and creatinine clearance correspond more closely to the clearance of inulin at such low levels of GFR [44], and this measurement has been recommended for the evaluation of the progression of renal failure in patients in terminal uremia.

Summary

As the automated method for creatinine determination is being adopted by most institutions, the measurement of creatinine is gaining in accuracy and reliability, and it is now possible to obtain more uniform information on the use of creatinine as an index of renal function. Although the technical difficulties of creatinine determination have been overcome to a large extent, there are still significant limitations on the validity of creatinine for the evaluation of GFR. These problems are exemplified by the uncertainties that have been introduced by the existence of a secretory mechanism in the renal handling of creatinine; by the effects of various factors, such as diet and exercise, on creatinine metabolism; by the shifting in the ratios of plasma true creatinine-noncreatinine chromogens and of creatinine clearance-inulin clearance in progressive renal failure; and, more significantly, by the induction of an extrarenal mechanism of creatinine metabolism and excretion in uremia.

In spite of all these disadvantages, however, creatinine is the only known substance in endogenous concentration in the body of which the clearance approximates the clearance of inulin, thus making its use for the estimate of GFR both practical and economical. If a lack of availability of a more reliable method makes the use of creatinine necessary for the evaluation of renal function, creatinine clearance is preferred over plasma creatinine concentration because the former correlates better with inulin clearance. Because of the difficulties inherent in prolonged urine collections, the ability of the patient to cooperate is critical in deciding among a 1-hour creatinine clearance, a 24-hour creatinine clearance, and a plasma creatinine determination. A single measurement of creatinine can be misleading in evaluating renal function, but serial determinations are helpful in detecting the direction of changes in renal disease.

References

1. Anderson, C. F., Jaecks, D. M., Ballon, H. S., et al. Renal handling of creatinine in nephrotic and non-nephrotic patients. *Clin. Sci.* 38:555, 1970.
2. Aviram, A., Ben-Ishay, D., Chowers, I., et al. Low plasma creatinine in diabetes mellitus. *J. Lab. Clin. Med.* 67:473, 1966.
3. Baldwin, D. S., Sirota, J. H., and Villarreal, H. Diurnal variations of renal function in congestive heart failure. *Proc. Soc. Exp. Biol. Med.* 74:578, 1950.
4. Berlyne, G. M., Varley, H., Nilwarangkur, S., et al. Endogenous-creatinine clearance and glomerular-filtration rate. *Lancet* 2:874, 1964.
5. Bleiler, R. E., and Schedl, H. P. Creatinine excretion: Variability and relationship to diet and body size. *J. Lab. Clin. Med.* 59:945, 1962.
6. Bloch, K., and Schonheimer, R. The biological precursors of creatinine. *J. Biol. Chem.* 138:167, 1941.
7. Bonsness, R. W., and Taussky, H. H. On the colorimetric determination of creatinine by the Jaffe reaction. *J. Biol. Chem.* 158:581, 1945.
8. Borsook, H., and Dubnoff, J. W. The hydrolysis of phosphocreatine and the origin of urinary creatinine. *J. Biol. Chem.* 163:493, 1947.
9. Camara, A. A., Arn, K. D., Reimer, A., et al. The twenty-four hour hourly endogenous creatinine clearance as a clinical measure of the functional state of the kidneys. *J. Lab. Clin. Med.* 37:743, 1951.
10. Carter, W. J., Faas, F. H., and Wynn, J. O. Role of starvation in production of creatinuria in experimental hyperthyroidism. *Metabolism* 26:1243, 1977.
11. Chasson, A. L., Grady, H. J., and Stanley, M. A. Determination of creatinine by means of automatic chemical analysis. *Am. J. Clin. Pathol.* 35:83, 1961.
12. Chiou, W. L., and Hsu, F. H. Pharmaco-kinetics of creatinine in man and the implications in the monitoring of renal function and in dosage regimen modifications in patients with renal insufficiency. *J. Clin. Pharmacol.* 15:427, 1975.
13. Cockroft, D. W., and Gault, M. H. Prediction of creatinine clearance from serum creatinine. *Nephron* 16:31, 1976.
14. Crawford, B. Depression of the exogenous creatinine/inulin or thiosulfate ratios in man by Diodrast and p-aminohippuric acid. *J. Clin. Invest.* 27:171, 1948.
15. Davison, J. M., Uldahl, P. R., and Walls, J. Renal function studies after nephrectomy in renal donors. *Br. Med. J.* 1:1050, 1976.
16. Dean, R. F. A., and McCance, R. A. Inulin, diodone, creatinine and urea clearances in newborn infants. *J. Physiol.* (Lond.) 106:431, 1947.

17. DeWardener, H. E. *The Kidney: An Outline of Normal and Abnormal Structure and Function* (4th ed.). Edinburgh: Churchill/Livingstone, 1973. Pp. 33–41.
18. Doolan, P. D., Alpen, E. L., and Theil, G. B. A clinical appraisal of the plasma concentration and endogenous clearance of creatinine, *Am. J. Med.* 32:65, 1962.
19. Dossetor, J. B. Creatininemia versus uremia: The relative significance of blood urea nitrogen and serum creatinine concentrations in azotemia. *Ann. Intern. Med.* 65:1287, 1966.
20. Dunea, G., and Freedman, P. Serum creatinine. *J.A.M.A.* 204:163, 1968.
21. Dunea, G., and Freedman, P. Renal clearance studies. *J.A.M.A.* 205:171, 1968.
22. DuVigneaud, V., Cohn, M., Chandler, J. P., et al. The utilization of the methyl group of methionine in the biological synthesis of choline and creatine. *J. Biol. Chem.* 140:625, 1941.
23. Edwards, K. D. G., and Whyte, H. M. Plasma creatinine level and creatinine clearance as tests of renal function. *Australas. Ann. Med.* 8:218, 1959.
24. Effersøe, P. Relationship between endogenous 24-hour creatinine clearance and serum creatinine concentration in patients with chronic renal disease. *Acta Med. Scand.* 156:429, 1957.
25. Enger, E., and Blegen, E. M. The relationship between endogenous creatinine clearance and serum creatinine in renal failure. *Scand. J. Clin. Lab. Invest.* 16:273, 1964.
26. Findley, R., Jr. The excretion of endogenous "creatinine" by the human kidney. *Am. J. Physiol.* 123:260, 1938.
27. Folin, O. Laws governing the chemical composition of urine. *Am. J. Physiol.* 13:66, 1905.
28. Friedman, E. A., and Rubin, J. E. Nephropathy in diabetes mellitus. *Cardiovasc. Med.* 2:239, 1977.
29. Friedman, S. A., Raiszner, A. E., Rosen, H., et al. Functional defects in the aging kidney. *Ann. Intern. Med.* 76:41, 1972.
30. Goldman, R. Creatinine excretion in renal failure. *Proc. Soc. Exp. Biol. Med.* 85:446, 1954.
31. Greenblatt, D. J., Ransil, B. J., Harmatz, J. S., et al. Variability of 24-hour urinary creatinine excretion by normal subjects. *J. Clin. Pharmacol.* 16:321, 1976.
32. Heinemann, H. O. Creatinine Clearance. In F. H. Netter (Ed.), *The Ciba Collections of Medical Illustrations.* Summit, N.J.: Ciba Pharmaceutical Company, 1973. Vol 6, p. 45.
33. Hoberman, H. D., Sims, E. A. H., and Peters, J. H. Creatine and creatinine metabolism in the normal adult studied with the aid of isotope nitrogen. *J. Biol. Chem.* 172:45, 1948.
34. Husdan, H., and Rapoport, A. Estimation of creatinine by the Jaffe reaction: A comparison of three methods. *Clin. Chem.* 14:222, 1968.
35. Jackson, S. Creatinine in urine as an index of urinary excretion rate. *Health Phys.* 12:843, 1966.
36. Jeliffe, R. W. Estimation of creatinine clearance when urine cannot be collected (letter to the editor). *Lancet* 1:975, 1971.
37. Jeliffe, R. W. Creatinine clearance: Bedside estimate (letter to the editor). *Ann. Intern. Med.* 79:604, 1973.
38. Jones, J. D., and Burnett, P. C. Implication of creatinine and gut flora in the uremic syndrome: Induction of "creatininase" in colon contents of the rat by dietary creatinine. *Clin. Chem.* 18:280, 1972.

39. Jones, J. D., and Burnett, P. C. Creatinine metabolism in humans with decreased renal function: Creatinine deficit. *Clin. Chem.* 20:1204, 1974.
40. Jones, J. D., and Burnett, P. C. Creatinine metabolism and toxicity. *Kidney Int.* 7(Suppl. 3):S-294, 1975.
41. Kampman, J., Siersbaeck-Nielsen, K., Kristensen, M., et al. Rapid evaluation of creatinine clearance. *Acta Med. Scand.* 196:517, 1974.
42. Kassirer, J. P. Clinical evaluation of kidney function: Glomerular function. *N. Engl. J. Med.* 285:385, 1971.
43. Kim, K. E., Onesti, G., Ramirez, Q., et al. Creatinine clearance in renal disease: A reappraisal. *Br. Med. J.* 4:11, 1969.
44. Lubowitz, H., Slatopolsky, E., Shankel, S., et al. Glomerular filtration rate: Determination in patients with chronic renal disease. *J.A.M.A.* 199:252, 1967.
45. Mandel, E. E., Jones, F. L., Willis, M. J., et al. Renal excretion of creatinine and inulin in man. *J. Lab. Clin. Med.* 42:621, 1953.
46. Miller, B. F., and Winkler, A. W. The renal excretion of endogenous creatinine in man: Comparison with exogenous creatinine and inulin. *J. Clin. Invest.* 17:31, 1938.
47. Mogensen, C. E. Kidney function and glomerular permeability to macromolecules in juvenile diabetes mellitus with specific reference to early changes. *Dan. Med. Bull.* 19(Suppl. 3):1, 1972.
48. Ogden, D. A. Donor and recipient function 2 to 4 years after renal homotransplantation. *Ann. Intern. Med.* 67:998, 1967.
49. Pasternack, A., and Kuhlbäck, B. Diurnal variations of serum and urine creatine and creatinine. *Scand. J. Clin. Lab. Invest.* 27:1, 1971.
50. Ransil, B. J., Greenblatt, D. J., and Koch-Weser, J. Evidence for systemic temporal variation in 24-hour urinary creatinine excretion. *J. Clin. Pharmacol.* 17:108, 1977.
51. Rapoport, A., and Husdan, H. Endogenous creatinine clearance and serum creatinine in the clinical assessment of kidney function. *Can. Med. Assoc. J.* 99:149, 1968.
52. Refsum, H. E., and Stromme, S. B. Relationship between urine flow, glomerular filtration, and urine solute concentration during prolonged heavy exercise. *Scand. J. Clin. Lab. Invest.* 35:775, 1975.
53. Rehberg, P. B. Studies on kidney function: I. The rate of filtration and reabsorption in the human kidney. *Biochem. J.* 20:447, 1926.
54. Richardson, J. A., and Philbin, P. E. The one-hour creatinine clearance rate in healthy man. *J.A.M.A.* 216:987, 1971.
55. Roche, M., Benedict, J. D., Yü, T. F., et al. Origin of urinary creatine in progressive muscular dystrophy. *Metabolism* 1:1, 1952.
56. Rowe, J. W. The influence of age on renal function. *Res. Phys.* 49, Feb. 1978.
57. Rowe, J. W., Andres, R., Tobin, J. D., et al. Age-adjusted standards for creatinine clearance. *Ann. Intern. Med.* 84:567, 1976.
58. Savory, J., Pu, P. H., and Sunderman, F. W., Jr. A biuret method for determination of protein in normal urine. *Clin. Chem.* 14:1160, 1968.
59. Schloerb, P. R. Total body water distribution of creatinine and urea in nephrectomized dogs. *Am. J. Physiol.* 199:661, 1960.
60. Shaffer, P. The excretion of kreatinin and kreatin in health and disease. *Am. J. Physiol.* 23:1, 1908.
61. Shannon, J. A. The renal excretion of creatinine in man. *J. Clin. Invest.* 14:403, 1935.
62. Simenhoff, M. L., Saukkonen, J. J., Burke, J. F., et al. Amine metabolism and the small bowel in uraemia. *Lancet* 2:818, 1976.

63. Sims, E. A. H., and Krantz, K. E. Serial studies of renal function during pregnancy and the puerperium in normal women. *J. Clin. Invest.* 37:1764, 1958.
64. Sirota, J. H., Baldwin, D. S., and Villarreal, H. Diurnal variations of renal function in men. *J. Clin. Invest.* 29:187, 1950.
65. Smith, H. W. The Reliability of Inulin as a Measure of Glomerular Filtration. In H. W. Smith (Ed.), *The Kidney: Structure and Function in Health and Disease.* New York: Oxford University Press, 1955. Pp. 231–238.
66. Spriggs, E. I. On the excretion of creatinine and uric acid in some diseases involving the muscles. *Q. J. Med.* 1:63, 1907.
67. Srivastava, S. S., Mani, K. V., Soni, C. M., et al. Effect of muscular exercises on urinary excretion of creatine and creatinine. *Indian J. Med. Res.* 55:953, 1967.
68. Tobias, F. J., McLaughlin, R. F., Jr., and Kopper, J., Jr. Endogenous creatinine clearance: A valuable clinical test of glomerular filtration and a prognostic guide in chronic renal disease. *N. Engl. J. Med.* 266:317, 1962.
69. Turner, W. J., and Merlis, S. Vicissitudes in research: The twenty-four hour urine collection. *Clin. Pharmacol. Ther.* 12:163, 1971.
70. Winberg, J. The 24-hour true endogenous creatinine clearance in infants and children without renal disease. *Acta Paediatr.* 48:443, 1959.

2. Glomerular Filtration Rate and Renal Plasma Flow

Cristobal G. Duarte, Lila R. Elveback, and Robert R. Liedtke

The introduction of inulin as a test of renal function was a result of the empirical observation [61] that glucose is not excreted in the urine of the aglomerular fish; it was then theorized that a metabolically inert carbohydrate that, after being filtered, is not handled by the renal tubular cells of species with glomerular nephrons [61] could be used for the measurement of glomerular filtration rate (GFR). In the course of investigating several substances that may have such properties, it was found that the clearance of xylose was lower than the clearance of inulin [55] and that values of xylose clearance could be brought up closer to those of inulin clearance by blocking a reabsorptive process of xylose by the administration of phlorizin. Further evaluation of inulin [61] revealed that this substance, which is a polysaccharide with a molecular weight of approximately 5000, is metabolically inert and nontoxic, is not bound to plasma proteins, and is not excreted in the urine of the aglomerular fish [49]; inulin can be recovered quantitatively from the urine after being administered to species with glomerular nephrons, it has no detectable intrinsic effects on renal function, and its renal clearance is independent of variations in plasma concentration of inulin. These indirect lines of evidence [55, 61] justified the widespread acceptance of inulin as a test for GFR, and the following, more recent findings consolidated even further the role of inulin clearance as the standard test for GFR: (1) the concentration of inulin has been determined in the fluid collected from Bowman's space by micropuncture [31, 32, 37] and was found to be identical to that in plasma, thus demonstrating that inulin is freely filtered at the glomerulus; and (2) there is total recovery of radiolabeled inulin both from the urine [30, 41] after inulin is microinjected into the lumen of a proximal tubule and from a distal tubule [41] after the substance is microperfused through the more proximal portions of the corresponding nephron, and none of the inulin introduced into the lumen of the tubule [30, 41] appears in the peripheral blood or in the urine of the contralateral kidney, thus demonstrating that inulin is not reabsorbed by the renal tubular epithelial cells. These results demonstrate that inulin fulfills all the requirements proposed by Homer Smith [63] for a substance that is handled by the kidneys exclusively by glomerular filtration (see Chap. 1), and thus the clearance of inulin is the standard test for the measurement of GFR.

Because of the way in which inulin is handled by the nephrons [12], the excretory rate of inulin in the urine in a unit time is equal to the filtered load

This work was done while Dr. Duarte was Director of Laboratory Nephrology, Mayo Clinic Foundation, Rochester, Minn.

of inulin at the glomerulus (as calculated by multiplying the plasma concentration of inulin by the GFR) under steady-state conditions and at constant plasma levels of inulin. This relationship can be expressed as follows: Plasma inulin (P_{in})(mg/ml) × GFR(ml/min) = urine inulin (U_{in})(mg/ml) × Urine flow (V)(ml/min). Therefore,

$$\text{GFR(ml/min)} = \frac{U_{in}(\text{mg/ml}) \times \dot{V}(\text{ml/min})}{P_{in}(\text{mg/ml})}$$

Inulin, however, is not in endogenous concentration in the body, and studies of renal clearance must be performed by specialized technical personnel over a period of several hours. There must be constant intravenous infusion of inulin preceded by a priming dose to maintain plasma concentration of inulin constant throughout the study; complete urine collections must be obtained at each clearance period; and blood samples must be drawn at well-timed intervals. Although the procedure for determining inulin clearance has been greatly simplified by (1) the automation of the chemical determination of inulin in the laboratory, and (2) by the administration to the patient of a gamma-emitting radiolabeled compound of sufficient energy to monitor bladder emptying without the need for urethral catheterization (see Chap. 3), there is persistent interest in further simplifying the procedure for determining GFR.

Although creatinine is endogenous in the body and thus does not need to be infused for studies of renal function, it is generally felt that creatinine is not a satisfactory method for the correct estimation of GFR, as discussed in Chapter 1. The search for simple yet reliable methods has continued [25] and has resulted in the introduction of new procedures, some of which are now in use and others of which are still in the process of being evaluated (see Chap. 4). The administration of gamma-emitting radiolabeled compounds for the determination of renal clearance by the standard method (continuous intravenous infusion) simplifies the processing of the samples, which can be measured more easily in the laboratory by gamma scintillation counting, but the usual procedures for a standard clearance study must still be followed. The determination of GFR after subcutaneous injection of a radiolabeled compound obviates the need for a constant intravenous infusion, thus greatly simplifying the procedure. The methods for the measurement of GFR and renal plasma flow with radioisotopes by constant intravenous infusion (standard method) and after subcutaneous administration, as related to the standard inulin clearance, will be studied in this chapter; the noninvasive methods for studying renal function will be discussed in Chapter 4.

Standard and Simplified Methods for the Measurement of GFR with Radioisotopes

Most of the studies for the measurement of GFR with radioisotopes have been performed with the use of [^{125}I] iothalamate sodium. The following experimental data demonstrate similarities between the renal handling of inulin and iodinated iothalamate: the binding of [^{125}I] iothalamate sodium to proteins is negligible [3]; the renal clearance of iothalamate remains constant [56] independent of variations in plasma activity; [^{125}I] iothalamate sodium is not excreted in the urine of the aglomerular fish [28]; iodinated iothalamate that has been microinjected into the lumen of superficial nephrons [39] can be recovered completely from the urine of the ipsilateral kidney, although recovery was not complete [39] when the ureteral pressure was elevated; stop-flow studies in the dog [28] demonstrated that radiolabeled iothalamate was handled by the kidneys by glomerular filtration, with none being reabsorbed or secreted; and in studies performed simultaneously [24, 40] an excellent correlation was demonstrated between the renal clearance of [^{125}I] iothalamate sodium and that of inulin by standard methods (constant intravenous infusion).

A significant simplification in the measurement of GFR was achieved when it was demonstrated that the plasma activity of [^{125}I] iothalamate sodium remained constant [1, 35] after it was administered subcutaneously with the addition of epinephrine to delay absorption from the subcutaneous depot, and that there was a good correlation between the renal clearance of iothalamate by this subcutaneous method and the clearance of inulin performed simultaneously by constant intravenous infusion. Although the plasma activity of radiolabeled iothalamate was less stable in subjects with normal renal function when epinephrine was omitted from the subcutaneous injection of iothalamate [44], a high correlation between the clearance of radioiodinated iothalamate by subcutaneous injection without epinephrine and the simultaneous clearance of inulin by standard methods [44] was demonstrated. Reservations have been expressed [44] concerning the possible effects of epinephrine on renal function when it is given in the course of studies of renal clearance. Furthermore, a good correlation has been demonstrated between the clearance of inulin by constant intravenous infusion [17] and the clearance of [^{131}I] iothalamate sodium at a constantly decreasing activity of this substance in plasma after a single intravenous bolus injection of radioiodinated iothalamate.

We evaluated a correlation between the clearance of inulin by standard methods and the simultaneous clearance of [^{125}I] iothalamate sodium either by a standard method ($n = 98$), after subcutaneous administration without epinephrine ($n = 103$), or by intravenous bolus injection and urine collection ($n = 83$). The methods that were followed for the standard clearance studies of inulin and standard and subcutaneous iothalamate are described in Chapter 3. For the bolus studies, 0.2 μCi/kg of [^{125}I] iothalamate sodium was given intravenously. The results, which are shown in Figures 2–1A, 2–1B, and 2–1C, are given in terms of natural logarithms. There was a linear and significant correlation between the standard clearance of inulin and each of the iothalamate clearances. The following differences were noted, however: the intercept of the regression line is not significantly different from zero in the standard studies (Fig. 2–1A), whereas it is significantly different from zero when the standard

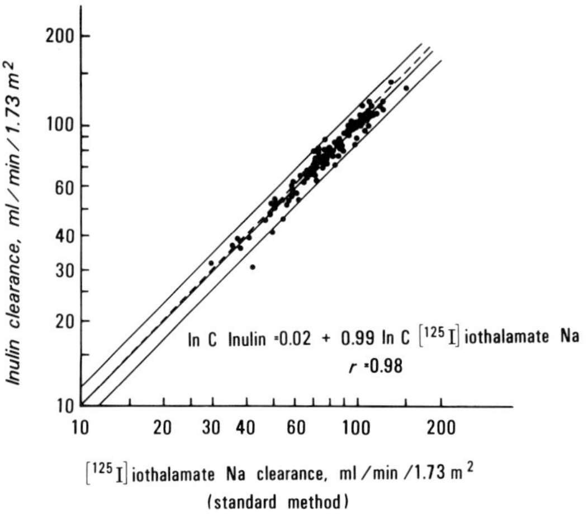
200
100
60
40
30
20
10
Inulin clearance, ml / min / 1.73 m²
ln C Inulin = 0.02 + 0.99 ln C [125I] iothalamate Na
r = 0.98
10
20
30
40
60
100
200
[125I] iothalamate Na clearance, ml / min / 1.73 m²
(standard method)

A

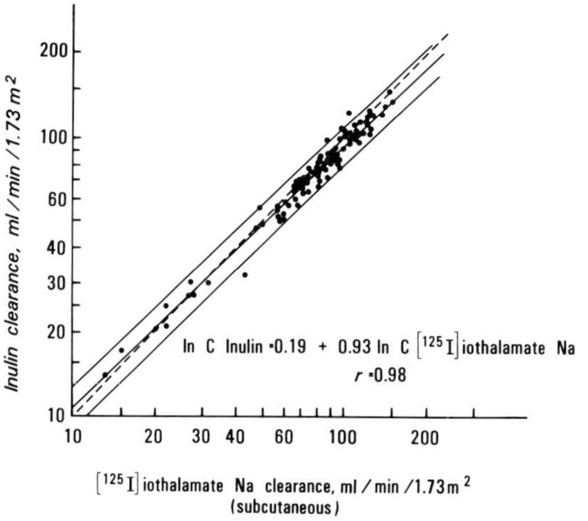
200
100
60
40
30
20
10
Inulin clearance, ml / min / 1.73 m²
ln C Inulin = 0.19 + 0.93 ln C [125I] iothalamate Na
r = 0.98
10
20
30
40
60
100
200
[125I] iothalamate Na clearance, ml / min / 1.73 m²
(subcutaneous)

B

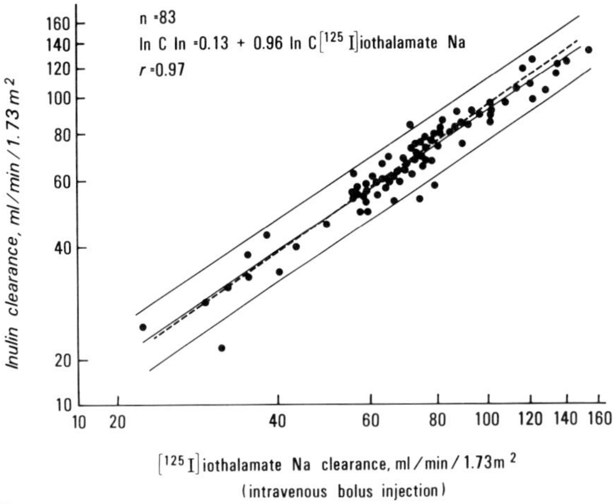

C

Figure 2–1
Correlation between the natural logarithms of standard inulin clearance and the clearance of [^{125}I] iothalamate sodium by standard methods (A), by subcutaneous injection (B), and after intravenous bolus injection (C). The middle solid line represents the regression line, the outer solid lines the confidence intervals ($\hat{y} \pm 1.96$ SE $\hat{Y}$), and the broken line the line of identity.

inulin clearance studies were correlated with both the subcutaneous iothalamate (Fig. 2–1B) and the intravenous bolus clearance studies (Fig. 2–1C); and the regression lines are approximately the same in the three studies (Figs. 2–1A, 2–1B, and 2–1C).

Different values of mean [^{125}I] iothalamate sodium clearance and its corresponding estimated mean inulin clearance for each of the three studies are given in Table 2–1. The mean values of iothalamate clearance were higher than those of the corresponding inulin clearance in the three studies, but a better approximation with the clearance of inulin was obtained when the clearance of iothalamate was determined by the standard method. The residual variation about the regression line ($s_{y \cdot x}$) was narrower when both clearances were determined by the standard method, and the 95-percent confidence limit intervals were considerably higher when inulin clearance was correlated with the intravenous bolus iothalamate study (Fig. 2–1 and Table 2–1).

Since each point plotted in Figures 2–1A, 2–1B, and 2–1C represents the mean value of three consecutive clearance periods in the same patient, it is of interest to determine the degree of variability in the same individual for each clearance period. The result of such study is shown in Figure 2–2, where it can be seen that the variability was approximately the same for the standard clearance of inulin and the clearance of iothalamate by the standard and the sub-

Table 2–1. Relationship between ln Inulin Clearance and ln [125I] Iothalamate Sodium Clearance

Standard Studies [a]			Subcutaneous Iothalamate [b]		Intravenous Bolus Iothalamate [c]	
[125I] Iothalamate Sodium Clearance	Inulin Clearance Estimate		Inulin Clearance Estimate		Inulin Clearance Estimate	
Mean	Mean	Interval	Mean	Interval	Mean	Interval
30	29	26–34	30	26–35	30	25–37
40	39	34–45	39	34–46	40	33–48
50	49	43–56	48	41–56	50	41–60
60	58	51–67	57	49–67	59	49–71
70	68	60–78	66	57–77	69	57–83
80	78	68–89	75	64–87	78	65–94
100	97	85–110	92	79–108	97	80–117
110	106	93–121	101	87–118	106	88–128
120	116	102–132	110	94–128	115	96–139
130	125	110–143	118	102–138	125	103–151
140	135	118–154	127	109–148	134	111–162
150	145	127–165	135	116–158	143	119–173

[a] Standard studies: $\ln Cl_{in} = 0.02 + 0.99 \ln Cl$ [125I] iothalamate sodium; $s_{y \cdot x} = 0.06$.
[b] Subcutaneous iothalamate: $\ln Cl_{in} = 0.19 + 0.94 \ln Cl$ [125I] iothalamate sodium; $s_{y \cdot x} = 0.07$.
[c] Intravenous bolus iothalamate: $\ln Cl_{in} = 0.13 + 0.96 \ln Cl$ [125I] iothalamate sodium; $s_{y \cdot x} = 0.09$.

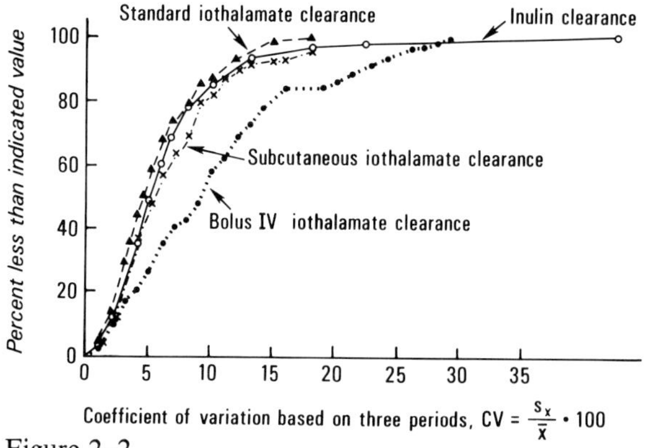

Figure 2–2
Cumulative frequency of distribution of the coefficient of variance of inulin clearance and the clearance of iothalamate in the studies shown in Figure 2–1.

cutaneous methods, but it was much greater for the intravenous bolus iothalamate clearance study. As Figure 2–2 shows, in approximately 90 percent of the clearance studies of standard inulin, standard iothalamate, and subcutaneous iothalamate, the coefficient of variation was 10 percent or less, whereas in only 58 percent of the bolus iothalamate clearance studies was the coefficient of variation 10 percent or less. In conclusion, the clearance of inulin by standard methods correlated better with the clearance of [^{125}I] iothalamate sodium by the standard method. The differences between the standard inulin clearance and the clearance of iothalamate by subcutaneous administration are not clinically significant, and the clearance of subcutaneous iothalamate without epinephrine is a good screening test (better than creatinine; see Chap. 1) for the estimation of GFR. The larger standard deviation and the significant variation between consecutive clearance periods in the same individual makes the clearance of [^{125}I] iothalamate sodium by bolus injection with urine collection a not very reliable method for determining GFR.

Another study was performed by us in order to determine the adequacy of changes between the standard clearance of inulin and each of the three iothalamate studies. Taking 80 ml/min as the lowest normal value for GFR, the points showing a lack of correlation (i.e., normal levels of either inulin or iothalamate clearance corresponding to abnormally low values of the other clearance) were investigated. When the clearance of iothalamate was determined by the standard method, there was lack of agreement with the standard clearance of inulin in 8 percent of the subjects, and the clearance of iothalamate tended to overestimate or underestimate the clearance of inulin in the same proportion. When the clearance of iothalamate was performed by the subcutaneous method, there was a lack of correlation with the standard inulin method in 11 percent of the subjects, and the clearance of iothalamate overestimated inulin clearance in those

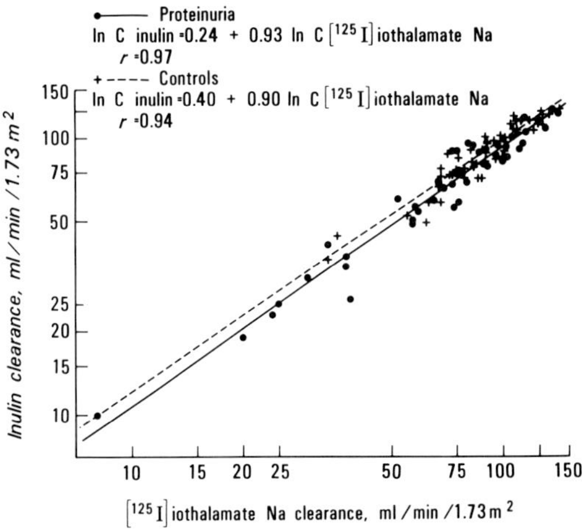

Figure 2–3
Correlation between the clearances of inulin and [^{125}I] iothalamate sodium by standard methods in nonproteinuric controls and in patients with significant proteinuria.

instances. When the clearance of iothalamate was performed by the intravenous bolus injection, there was a lack of correlation with the standard clearance of inulin in 6 percent of the subjects.

Because it has been reported that the clearance of creatinine is disproportionately higher than the clearance of inulin in patients with proteinuria as compared with nonproteinuric controls [8] (see Chap. 1), we studied the correlation between the clearances of inulin and [^{125}I] iothalamate sodium by standard methods in 46 patients with significant proteinuria (24-hour urinary excretion of protein $\geqslant$ 3.5gm) [52] and in 56 nonproteinuric controls (24-hour urinary excretion of protein $\leqslant$ 270 mg). The results of this study are shown in Figure 2–3. There was a linear and significant correlation between both clearances in both clinical conditions, and the regression equations were not significantly different (Fig. 2–3). The cumulative percent difference between both clearances in the two conditions is shown graphically in Figure 2–4. The clearance of [^{125}I] iothalamate sodium was greater than the clearance of inulin in 77 percent of the proteinuric patients and in 65 percent of the nonproteinuric controls, but this difference was not significant. Thus the correlation between the clearances of inulin and iothalamate is essentially the same whether the patient is proteinuric or not.

Other radiolabeled compounds whose clearance has been reported to correlate well with the clearance of inulin when both are determined simultaneously by standard methods include [^{57}Co] cyanocobalamin [3], [^{51}Cr] EDTA [26], [^{99m}Tc] pertechnetate [21], [^{131}I] diatrizoate [67], and [^{169}Yb] DTPA, but

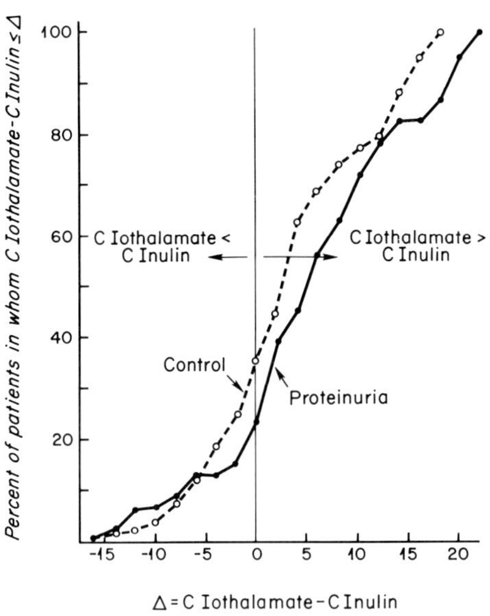

Figure 2–4
Cumulative percent difference between the clearances of inulin and [^{125}I] iothalamate sodium in proteinuric and nonproteinuric controls in the studies shown in Figure 2–3.

the clearance of some of these compounds has been reported to be variably lower than the clearance of inulin [3, 21, 67].

Other methods have been described that simplify the determination of GFR even further by obviating the need for urine collection. The plasma clearance technique assumes that after equilibration has been achieved following an intravenous bolus injection of a marker of GFR, the rate of decline in plasma concentration or activity is related to the rate at which the administered substance is cleared by glomerular filtration [2, 5, 70]. The GFR, therefore, can be determined by this method by serial sampling of blood without urine collection. The constant infusion technique, or pump method [23], assumes that the rate of intravenous infusion needed to maintain the plasma concentration of inulin at constant levels is proportional to the rate of the renal clearance of inulin; however, difficulties have been encountered in obtaining equilibration of the infused substance in blood [7, 18], especially in patients with edema, and results by the constant infusion method may yield significantly higher values than by the standard method [58]. A highly significant correlation was found [14] when the standard clearance of inulin was measured simultaneously with that of iothalamate by external monitoring of the disappearance of [^{125}I] iothalamate sodium, although in patients with edema, the clearance of iothalamate by this method may overestimate the GFR.

Although these simplified methods (plasma clearance, constant intravenous infusion, and external monitoring) have the significant advantage of eliminating one of the big problems in the clearance studies by obviating the need for urine collections, they lack the precision of the standard and the subcutaneous methods [9] for the determination of GFR, and therefore they should be reserved for particular instances in which the measurement of GFR by standard methods is not practical (e.g., in pediatric patients, when patient cooperation is difficult to obtain) or for cases in which urine cannot be collected (e.g., in patients with ureteral reflux, urinary incontinence, or urinary tract obstruction, or when the ureter has been diverted into the bowels). A detailed description of simplified and noninvasive methods for the measurement of GFR and new developments in the field are given in Chapter 4.

Renal Plasma Flow

A substance that is cleared completely in a single passage through the kidneys by a process of glomerular filtration and tubular secretion [62] can be used to measure the renal plasma flow (RPF). Initially, iodopyracet (Diodrast) was used to measure RPF [62], but later it became evident that the clearance of para-aminohippurate (PAH) was equal to the clearance of Diodrast and had the following properties [62]: PAH is nontoxic; it does not penetrate red blood cells in humans; it is less extensively bound to proteins than Diodrast; it is handled by the nephron by a process of glomerular filtration and proximal tubular secretion, and its concentration in plasma and urine can be easily determined by reliable methods. Experimental data from isolated perfused tubules of rabbits [69] revealed that PAH is secreted along the length of the proximal tubule, but that the rate of uptake of PAH at the peritubular membrane and subsequent diffusion from the cell into the tubular lumen was considerably greater in the straight portion. Approximately 8 percent of the PAH perfusing the kidneys bypasses functional renal tissue, and thus the term *effective renal plasma flow* (ERPF) has been considered to be more appropriate [62] when referring to the clearance of PAH, which is calculated by the following formula:

$$\text{Clearance PAH (ml/min)} = \frac{\text{Urine PAH (mg/dl)} \times \text{Urine flow } (V) \text{ (ml/min)}}{\text{Plasma PAH (mg/dl)}}$$

Like inulin, PAH is not in endogenous concentration in the body, and studies of RPF by standard methods with PAH require the specialized procedures that have been mentioned in this chapter for the determination of GFR with inulin. Therefore, attempts have been made to simplify the measurement of RPF by the introduction of radiolabeled compounds. The radionuclide used most frequently for the determination of RPF is [^{131}I] iodohippurate sodium, and an excellent correlation has been found between its clearance and PAH clearance in studies performed simultaneously by standard methods [13, 53, 54], al-

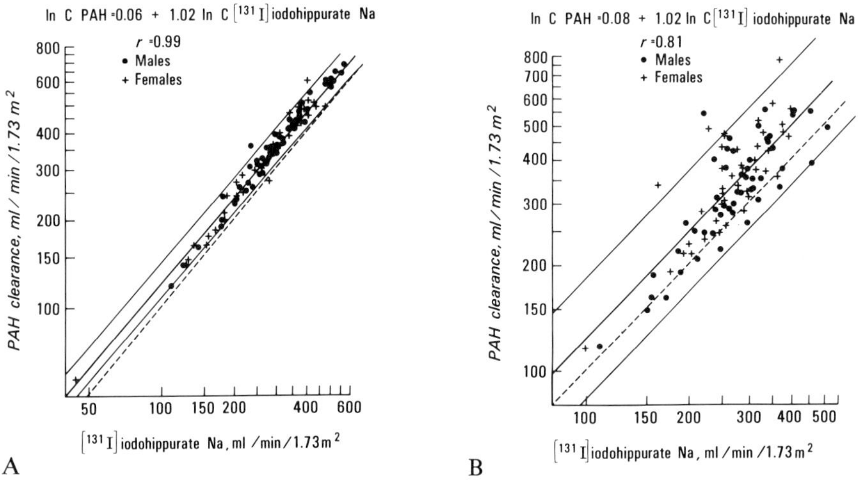

Figure 2–5
Correlation between the standard clearance of PAH and the clearance of [^{131}I] iodohippurate sodium by the standard method (A) and after subcutaneous injection (B). The lines are as in Figure 2–1.

though the clearance of radioiodinated hippurate has been reported to be consistently lower by 83 to 87 percent [13, 53, 54]. The reason for this discrepancy has not been established but has been related to the amount of free iodine present in the radiolabeled hippurate preparation [13], to the delay in excretion of [^{131}I] iodohippurate [54] due to protein binding, and/or to a possible interference in the tubular transport of [^{131}I] iodohippurate sodium [64] when studies are performed simultaneously with PAH clearance.

We studied a correlation between the clearance of PAH and that of [^{131}I] iodohippurate sodium by the simultaneous standard method (constant intranenous infusion; n = 101), and between the standard clearance of PAH and simultaneous clearance of [^{131}I] iodohippurate sodium after a single subcutaneous injection of 5 μCi of this substance (n = 98). The methods that were followed for the standard clearance studies of PAH and [^{131}I] iodohippurate sodium are described in Chapter 3. As demonstrated in Figure 2–5A, there was a significant linear correlation with a positive slope when both clearances were performed by the standard method; although there was also a linear correlation with a positive slope when the standard clearance of PAH was correlated with the subcutaneous clearance of [^{131}I] iodohippurate sodium (Fig. 2–5B), the scatter was greatly increased and the correlation was appreciably lower. Different mean values of [^{131}I] iodohippurate sodium clearance and its corresponding estimated PAH clearance, as well as the deviation around the regression line, are shown in Table 2–2. For any given value of the clearance of [^{131}I]

Table 2–2. Relationship Between ln PAH Clearance and ln [131I] Iodohippurate Sodium Clearance

	Standard Studies [a]		Subcutaneous Iodohippurate [b]	
[131I] Iodohippurate Sodium Clearance	PAH Clearance Estimate		PAH Clearance Estimate	
Mean	Mean	Interval	Mean	Interval
150	176	154–202	185	122–279
200	236	206–271	248	164–374
250	296	259–340	312	206–471
275	327	285–374	344	228–519
300	357	312–409	376	249–568
325	387	338–444	408	270–616
350	418	365–479	440	291–665
375	448	391–514	472	313–713
400	479	418–549	505	334–762
420	503	439–577	531	351–801
450	540	471–619	570	377–860
470	564	493–647	596	394–899
500	601	525–689	635	420–958

[a] Standard studies: ln ClPAH = 0.06 + 1.02 ln Cl[131I] iodohippurate sodium; $s_{y \cdot x} = 0.068$.
[b] Subcutaneous iodohippurate: ln ClPAH = 0.08 + 1.02 ln Cl[131I] iodohippurate sodium; $s_{y \cdot x} = 0.21$.

iodohippurate sodium, the corresponding estimated PAH clearance is higher in both studies, and the intervals are significantly greater for the subcutaneous studies (Fig. 2–5 and Table 2–2). Therefore, although the clearance of [131I] iodohippurate sodium is consistently lower than the clearance of PAH, there is an excellent correlation between the two when studies are performed by the standard method; unfortunately, however, the clearance of radiolabeled hippurate is not a good test for RPF after its subcutaneous administration.

Methods have been described in which the measurement of RPF has been simplified by subcutaneous administration [25], by the constant infusion technique without urine collection (pump method) [23], or by a single intravenous injection and determination of the plasma clearance of a marker of RPF [10, 68]; however, these simplified methods have not been accepted for general use. A detailed description of simplified and noninvasive methods for studies of RPF is given in Chapter 4.

Normal Values

Values of renal function are lower in young infants than in adults [6, 22, 71]. In infants 2 to 8 days of age of both sexes [22], GFR ranges from 16.3 to 44.6 ml/min/1.73 m², and RPF from 23.5 to 125 ml/min/1.74 m². GFR and RPF increase with growth; a mean value of 124 ml/min/1.73 m² is reached at 12 to

20 weeks of age for GFR, and a mean value of 646 ml/min/1.73 m^2 has been reported for RPF at 30 weeks of age [71]. GFR and RPF then remain constant at these levels until they start to decline in the second [59], third [20], or after the fourth decade [10] of life. After age 45 to 50, GFR has been found to decline at a rate of 13 ml per decade, and RPF at a rate of 70 ml per decade [70]. With advancing age [65, 66], there is a decrease in renal mass affecting mainly the cortex [33]; the renal perfusion decreases as a result of a fall in cardiac output and a reduction in the renal vascular bed; and there is a process of glomerular hyalinization [38, 65], with a reduction in the nephron population [47] but without functional compensation of the remaining units. After uninephrectomy, however [45, 59], hypertrophy and hyperplasia of the remaining kidney occur, with a partial return of GFR and RPF to prenephrectomy levels.

The filtration fraction (FF) is the fraction of plasma in the glomerulus that is transferred to Bowman's space as a filtrate [70]; it is calculated by the formula GFR/RPF $\times$ 100 and normally varies between 18 and 22 percent. The FF remains constant until age 60 [20] and then increases.

In studies performed throughout the day [58], the RPF was found to remain constant, but a fall in the GFR was detected between 12:00 P.M. and 4:00 A.M. In subjects with congestive heart failure and edema [4], this pattern is reversed and the GFR increases during sleep. In studies performed to determine the variability in methodology and in renal function in the same individual [19], it was found that the day-to-day variability was greater than the fluctuations in sequential clearance studies, but daily variations were less pronounced in older persons. The GFR increases by 50 percent in pregnancy [57] and returns to control levels in the puerperium. The RPF increases by 25 percent during the early and middle stages of pregnancy [57], returns to control values during the last trimester of pregnancy, and then falls below control levels in the puerperium. The changes in renal function during pregnancy [57] have been related to an increased activity of hormones from the adrenal and thyroid glands. The FF increases during pregnancy [57]. During exercise, the GFR and RPF decline [15], probably as a result of diversion of blood flow from the kidneys and other organs to the working muscles, and the FF decreases. A high protein intake [46] has been reported to increase GFR and RPF.

In patients with acromegaly and gigantism [27, 34], the kidneys, the glomeruli, and the proximal convoluted tubules increase in size and there is an elevation in GFR and RPF, but the FF does not change. The initial changes in GFR in diabetics [43] may be the result of increased growth hormone activity. There is significant elevation in GFR in newly diagnosed, untreated, young diabetics [43], and since the RPF remains normal, the FF increases. With greater duration of the disease and initiation of insulin therapy [43], diabetic patients experience a fall in GFR. With increased duration of the diabetes and onset of proteinuria [43], there is a significant fall in GFR and RPF in patients with diabetic nephropathy.

Indications and Contraindications for the Determinations of GFR and RPF

The measurements of GFR and RPF are an essential part of the functional evaluation of prospective kidney donors, and these determinations must be repeated periodically in the donor and recipient after transplantation. The measurements of GFR and RPF are also indicated in those clinical conditions in which there is evidence of renal dysfunction and the necessity to document the severity of the renal impairment. However, the values of renal function may be abnormally low in the absence of intrinsic renal disease [47], in conditions such as dehydration and in states of fear or anxiety. On the other hand, GFR and RPF may not decline for a while in the presence of renal disease [47] until there is a substantial reduction in renal functional mass.

In renal disease, the rate of progression or regression of the process and the resolution of the impairment can be monitored by serial measurements of GFR and RPF. These determinations may also be helpful in relating the degree of dysfunction to the onset of some of the complications of uremia. Thus with mild reductions in renal function (at a GFR of 60 to 70 ml/min) it may be possible to detect significant elevations in the plasma activity of parathyroid hormone, and the administration of phosphate binders for the prevention of the osteodystrophy of uremia is indicated at this time. In untreated patients, hyperparathyroidism may become clinically symptomatic at a GFR of 20 to 30 ml/min [47]. It has been recommended that the intake of proteins be restricted at a GFR of 30 to 40 ml/min [47]; depending on the rate of progression of the disease, fistula formation in preparation for dialysis should be instituted early to allow for maturation, and hemodialysis should be initiated at a GFR of approximately 10 ml/min [47].

The effectiveness of drugs that act by blocking the renal tubular transport of electrolytes, such as diuretics and uricosuric agents [47], diminishes as the delivery of fluid to their sites of action within the nephron decreases with the fall in GFR. Thus thiazide diuretics may become ineffective at a GFR of $\leqslant 30$ ml/min, and loop diuretics [47] may fail to elicit a diuretic response at a GFR of $\leqslant 10$ ml/min. In order to avoid retention in the body and toxicity, the dosage of drugs that are metabolized and excreted by the kidneys [47] must be adjusted to the degree of renal impairment. The measurement of GFR [42] has been used to quantitate the residual function in dialysis patients, and in some centers the frequency and duration of dialysis are determined by the residual renal function (see Chap. 5).

The FF may be a helpful indicator in clarifying the mechanism of changes in renal function in some clinical conditions. In primary glomerular disease and in pyrogenic reactions [47], the FF is reduced as a result of a primary fall in GFR. In congestive heart failure [70] there is a greater reduction in RPF than in GFR, and the FF increases. In essential hypertension [48] there may be vasoconstriction of the afferent arteriolar capillary, and since there may also be an increased postglomerular resistance, the RPF falls in greater proportion than the GFR and the FF increases. In studies performed in patients with essential hypertension over a period of time [48], there was a progressive decrease in RPF and an elevation in FF that was more pronounced in malignant hypertension. In renovascular hypertension of unilateral renal artery stenosis [11], although the function of each kidney may be quite different, the ratio of FF of normal versus constricted kidney has been reported to be one. Others, however, have found a lower FF in the constricted side (see Chap. 6).

Protein binding is not a problem with the radioisotopes that are more commonly used for studies of renal function, namely, [^{125}I] iothalamate sodium and [^{131}I] iodohippurate sodium [16]. Since the total content of free iodine in these substances is negligible, their administration is not contraindicated in patients with iodine hypersensitivity. In such patients, in order to block a possible uptake of radioiodine by the thyroid gland, sodium perchlorate should be given to the patient instead of the usual dose of a saturated solution of potassium iodine (see Chap. 3). The radiation exposure with the two radioisotopes [16] is much lower than for most routine radiographic studies. However, the administration of radioisotopes is contraindicated in pregnant women, because of the danger of causing genetic defects in the fetus, in lactating mothers, and in growing children. In such instances, measurement of inulin and PAH clearance can be carried out instead. Radiation exposure is greater when clearance studies with radioisotopes are performed frequently in the same person by the standard technique, and in patients with renal failure, total body radiation must be maintained at the normal level by adjusting the dosage of radioisotopes to be administered to the degree of renal impairment (see Chap. 3). A procedure has been described that makes it possible to measure GFR by the fluorescent excitation of nonradioactive iothalamate [29], thus saving the patient from exposure to radiation.

Since the prior administration of some radioisotopes for other studies may interfere with the counting of [^{125}I] and [^{131}I] in blood and urine, a renogram should not be performed on the same day before studies of renal function with these two radioisotopes; however, the renogram can be performed after the clearance studies. Determinations of GFR and RPF should not be performed in the presence of factors that may alter renal function, such as when the kidneys are undergoing an osmotic diuresis that has been induced by the administration of dyes given for an excretory urogram or after arteriography; when the body is dehydrated as a consequence of the effects of diuretics, enemas, or laxatives; during overhydration; or during therapeutic action of antihypertensive agents.

Conclusions

Of all the methods that have been studied for the evaluation of GFR in the present and the preceding chapter, the clearance of radiolabeled iothalamate by constant intravenous infusion (standard method) gives the best correlation with the clearance of inulin. Other tests to estimate GFR, in descending order of accuracy, are the clearance of [^{125}I] iothalamate sodium by subcutaneous injection, the clearance of endogenous creatinine, and the plasma concentration of creatinine.

The clearance of [^{131}I] iodohippurate sodium by the standard method, although consistently lower, shows an excellent correlation with the clearance of PAH and can be used to estimate RPF. The clearance of radiolabeled iodohippurate after subcutaneous injection is not a good substitute for the standard method, and in those instances in which the FF or the RPF needs to be determined, standard studies must be performed.

References

1. Adefuin, P. Y., Gur, A., Siegel, N. J., et al. Single subcutaneous injection of iothalamate sodium I^{125} to measure glomerular filtration rate. *J.A.M.A.* 235:1456, 1976.
2. Alving, A. S., and Miller, B. F. A practical method for the measurement of glomerular filtration rate (inulin clearance): With an evaluation of the clinical significance of this determination. *Arch. Intern. Med.* 66:306, 1940.
3. Anderson, C. F., Sawyer, T. K., and Cutler, R. E. Iothalamate sodium I^{125} vs. cyanocobalamin Co^{57} as a measure of glomerular filtration rate in man. *J.A.M.A.* 204:653, 1968.
4. Baldwin, D. S., Sirota, J. H., and Villarreal, H. Diurnal variations of renal function in congestive heart failure. *Proc. Soc. Exp. Biol. Med.* 74:578, 1950.
5. Barnett, H. L. Renal physiology in infants and children: I. Method for estimation of glomerular filtration rate. *Proc. Soc. Exp. Biol. Med.* 44:654, 1940.
6. Barnett, H. L., Hare, K., McNamara, H., et al. Measurement of glomerular filtration rate in premature infants. *J. Clin. Invest.* 27:691, 1948.
7. Berger, E. Y., Farber, S. J., and Earle, D. P., Jr. Comparision of the constant infusion and urine collection techniques for the measurement of renal function. *J. Clin. Invest.* 27:710, 1948.
8. Berlyne, G. M., Varley, H., Nilwarangkur, S., et al. Endogenous-creatinine clearance and glomerular-filtration rate. *Lancet* 2:874, 1964.
9. Blaufox, M. D. Measurement of Renal Function with Radioactive Materials. In M. D. Blaufox (Ed.), *Progress in Nuclear Medicine: Evaluation of Renal Function and Disease with Radionuclides.* Baltimore: University Park Press, 1972. Chap. 2, pp. 9–20.
10. Blaufox, M. D., and Merrill, J. P. Simplified Hippuran clearance: Measurement of renal function in man with simplified Hippuran clearances. *Nephron* 3:274, 1966.
11. Britton, K. E., and Brown, N. J. G. Physiological Problems. In K. E. Britton, N. J. G. Brown (Eds.), *Clinical Renography.* Chicago: Year Book, 1972. Chap. 4, pp. 60–86.
12. Britton, K. E., and Brown, N. J. G. How Does the Kidney Work? In K. E. Britton, N. J. G. Brown (Eds.), *Clinical Renography.* Chicago: Year Book, 1972. App. 2, pp. 243–263.
13. Burbank, J. K., Tauxe, W. M., Maher, F. T., et al. Evaluation of radioiodinated Hippuran for estimation of renal plasma flow. *Proc. Staff Meet. Mayo Clin.* 36:372, 1961.

14. Cangiano, J. L., Genuth, S. M., Renerts, L., et al. Simplified measurement of glomerular filtration rate. *Invest. Urol.* 9:34, 1971.
15. Chapman, C. B., Henschel, A., Minckler, J., et al. The effect of exercise on renal plasma flow in normal male subjects. *J. Clin. Invest.* 27:639, 1948.
16. Cohen, M. L. Radionuclide clearance techniques. *Semin. Nucl. Med.* 4:23, 1974.
17. Cohen, M. L., Smith, F. G., Jr., Midell, R. S., et al. A simple, reliable method of measuring glomerular filtration rate using single, low dose sodium iothalamate I^{131}. *Pediatrics* 43:407, 1969.
18. Cole, B. R., Ciangiacomo, J., Ingelfinger, J. R., et al. Measurement of renal function without urine collection: A critical evaluation of the constant-infusion technic for determination of inulin and para-aminohippurate. *N. Engl. J. Med.* 287:1109, 1972.
19. Davies, D. F., and Shock, N. W. The variability of measurement of inulin and Diodrast tests of kidney function. *J. Clin. Invest.* 29:491, 1950.
20. Davies, D. F., and Shock, N. W. Age changes in glomerular filtration rate, effective renal plasma flow, and tubular excretory capacity in adult males. *J. Clin. Invest.* 29:496, 1950.
21. Dayton, D. A., Maher, F. T., and Elveback, L. R. Renal clearance of technetium (^{99m}Tc) as pertechnetate. *Mayo Clin. Proc.* 44:549, 1969.
22. Dean, R. F. A., and McCance, R. A. Inulin, diodone, creatinine and urea clearances in newborn infants. *J. Physiol.* 106:431, 1947.
23. Earle, D. P., Jr., and Berliner, R. W. A simplified clinical procedure for measurement of glomerular filtration rate and renal plasma flow. *Proc. Soc. Exp. Biol. Med.* 62:262, 1946.
24. Elwood, C. M., Sigman, E. M., and Treger, C. The measurement of glomerular filtration rate with ^{125}I-sodium iothalamate (Conray). *Br. J. Radiol.* 40:581, 1967.
25. Findley, T., and White, H. L. Measurement of Diodrast and inulin clearances in man after subcutaneous administration. *Proc. Soc. Exp. Biol. Med.* 45:623, 1940.
26. Garnett, E. S., Parsons, V., and Veall, N. Measurement of glomerular-filtration rate in man using a ^{51}Cr/edetic acid complex. *Lancet* 1:818, 1967.
27. Gershberg, H., Heinemann, H. O., and Stumpf, H. H. Renal function studies and autopsy report in patients with gigantism and acromegaly. *J. Clin. Endocrinol. Metab.* 17:337, 1957.
28. Griep, R. J., and Nelp, W. B. Mechanism of excretion of radioiodinated sodium iothalamate. *Radiology* 93:807, 1969.
29. Guesry, P., Kaufman, L., Orloff, S., et al. Measurement of glomerular filtration rate by fluorescent excitation of non-radioactive meglumine iothalamate. *Clin. Nephrol.* 3:134, 1975.
30. Gutman, Y., Gottschalk, C. W., and Lassiter, W. E. Micropuncture study of inulin absorption in the rat kidney. *Science* 147:753, 1965.
31. Harris, C. A., Baer, P. G., Chirito, E., et al. Composition of mammalian glomerular filtrate. *Am. J. Physiol.* 227:972, 1974.
32. Hendrix, J. P., Westfall, B. B., and Richards, A. N. Quantitative studies of the composition of glomerular urine: XIV. The glomerular excretion of inulin in frogs and necturus. *J. Biol. Chem.* 116:735, 1937.
33. Hollenberg, N. K., Adams, D. F., Solomon, H. S., et al. Senescence and the renal vasculature in normal man. *Circ. Res.* 34:309, 1974.
34. Ikkos, D., Ljunggren, H., and Luft, R. Glomerular filtration rate and renal plasma flow in acromegaly. *Acta Endocrinol. (Kbh.)* 21:226, 1956.
35. Israelit, A. H., Long, D. L., White, M. G., et al. Measurement of glomerular

filtration rate utilizing a single subcutaneous injection of ^{125}I-iothalamate. *Kidney Int.* 4:346, 1973.
36. James, A. E., Jr., Hosain, F., DeLand, F. H., et al. ^{169}Ytterbium diethylenetriaminepentaacetic acid (^{169}YB DTPA): A versatile radiopharmaceutical. *J. Can. Assoc. Radiol.* 22:136, 1971.
37. Le Grimellec, C., Poujeol, P., and de Rouffignac, C. ^{3}H-inulin and electrolyte concentration in Bowman's capsule in rat kidney: Comparison with artificial ultrafiltration. *Pfluegers Arch.* 354:117, 1975.
38. Ljungqvist, A., and Lagergren, C. Normal intrarenal arterial pattern in adult and aging human kidney: A microangiographical and histological study. *J. Anat.* 96:285, 1962.
39. Lorentz, W. V., Jr., Lassiter, W. E., and Gottschalk, C. W. Renal tubular permeability during increased intrarenal pressure. *J. Clin. Invest.* 51:484, 1972.
40. Maher, F. T., Nolan, N. G., and Elveback, L. R. Comparison of simultaneous clearances of ^{125}I-labeled sodium iothalamate (Glofil) and of inulin. *Mayo Clin. Proc.* 46:690, 1971.
41. Marsh, D., and Frasier, C. Reliability of inulin for determining volume flow in rat renal cortical tubules. *Am. J. Physiol.* 209:283, 1965.
42. Milutinovic, J., Cutler, R. E., Hoover, P., et al. Measurement of residual glomerular filtration rate in the patient receiving repetitive hemodialysis. *Kidney Int.* 8:185, 1975.
43. Mogensen, C. E. Kidney function and glomerular permeability of macromolecules in juvenile diabetes mellitus with specific reference to early changes. *Dan. Med. Bull.* 19:1, 1972.
44. Ott, N. T., and Wilson, D. M. A simple technique for estimating glomerular filtration rate with subcutaneous injection of ^{125}I iothalamate. *Mayo Clin. Proc.* 50:664, 1975.
45. Pabico, R. C., McKenna, B. V., and Freeman, R. B. Renal function before and after unilateral nephrectomy in renal donors. *Kidney Int.* 8:166, 1975.
46. Pullman, J. N., Alving, A. S., Dern, R. J., et al. The influence of dietary protein intake on specific renal functions in normal man. *J. Lab. Clin. Med.* 44:320, 1954.
47. Renkin, E. M., and Robinson, R. R. Glomerular filtration. *N. Engl. J. Med.* 290:785, 1974.
48. Reubi, F. C., Weidmann, P., Hodler, J., et al. Changes in renal function in essential hypertension. *Am. J. Med.* 64:556, 1978.
49. Richards, A. M., Westfall, B. B., and Bott, P. A. Renal excretion of inulin, creatinine and xylose in normal dogs. *Proc. Soc. Exp. Biol. Med.* 32:73, 1934.
50. Rosenbaum, J. L., Kramer, M. S., Raja, R. M., et al. Determination of inulin and *p*-aminohippurate clearances without urine collection. *Nephron* 10:347, 1973.
51. Rowe, J. W. The influence of age on renal function. *Res. Staff Phys.* 49, Feb. 1978.
52. Savory, J., Pu, P. H., and Sunderman, F. W., Jr. A biuret method for determination of protein in normal urine. *Clin. Chem.* 14:1160, 1968.
53. Schwartz, F. D., and Madeloff, M. S. Simultaneous renal clearances of radiohippuran and PAH in man. *Clin. Res.* 9:208, 1961.
54. Schwartz, F. D., and Madeloff, M. S. Use of radiohippuran in diagnosis of unilateral renal disease. *J. Urol.* 87:244, 1961.
55. Shannon, J. A., and Smith, H. W. The excretion of inulin, xylose and urea by normal and phlorizinized man. *J. Clin. Invest.* 14:393, 1935.
56. Sigman, E. M., Elwood, C., Reagan, M. E., et al. The renal clearance of I^{131}-labeled sodium iothalamate in man. *Invest. Urol.* 2:432, 1965.

57. Sims, E. A. H., and Krantz, K. E. Serial studies of renal function during pregnancy and the puerperium in normal women. *J. Clin. Invest.* 37:1764, 1958.
58. Sirota, J. H., Baldwin, D. S., and Villarreal, H. Diurnal variations of renal function in men. *J. Clin. Invest.* 29:187, 1950.
59. Skov, P. E., and Hansen, H. E. Glomerular filtration rate, renal plasma flow and filtration fraction in living donors before and after nephrectomy. *Acta Med. Scand.* 195:97, 1974.
60. Slack, T. K., and Wilson, D. M. Normal renal function. C_{In} and C_{PAH} in healthy donors before and after nephrectomy. *Mayo Clin. Proc.* 51:296, 1976.
61. Smith, H. W. Measurement of the Filtration Rate. In H. W. Smith (Ed.), *The Kidney: Structure and Function in Health and Disease.* New York: Oxford University Press, 1955. Chap. 3, pp. 39–62.
62. Smith, H. W. Clearances Involving Tubular Excretion. In H. W. Smith (Ed.), *The Kidney: Structure and Function in Health and Disease.* New York: Oxford University Press, 1955. Chap. 6, pp. 143–202.
63. Smith, H. W. The Reliability of Inulin as a Measure of Glomerular Filtration. In H. W. Smith (Ed.), *The Kidney: Structure and Function in Health and Disease.* New York: Oxford University Press, 1955. Chap. 9, pp. 231–238.
64. Smith, H. W., Finkelstein, H., Aliminosa, L., et al. The renal clearance of substituted hippuric acid derivatives and other aromatic acids in dog and man. *J. Clin. Invest.* 24:388, 1945.
65. Takazakura, E., Wasabu, N., Handa, A., et al. Intrarenal vascular changes with age and disease. *Kidney Int.* 2:224, 1972.
66. Tauchi, H., Tsuboi, K., and Okutomi, J. Age changes in the human kidney of the different races. *Gerontology* 17:87, 1971.
67. Tauxe, W. M., Burbank, J. K., Maher, F. T., et al. Renal clearance of radioactive ortho-iodohippurate and diatrizoate. *Mayo Clin. Proc.* 39:761, 1964.
68. Tauxe, W. M., Maher, F. T., and Taylor, W. F. Effective renal plasma flow: Estimation from theoretical volumes of distribution of intravenously injected ^{131}I orthohippurate. *Mayo Clin. Proc.* 46:524, 1971.
69. Tune, B. M., Burg, M. B., and Patlack, C. S. Characteristics of *p*-aminohippurate transport in proximal renal tubules. *Am. J. Physiol.* 217:1057, 1969.
70. Wesson, L. G. Renal Hemodynamics in Physiologic States. In L. G. Wesson (Ed.), *Physiology of the Human Kidney.* New York: Grune & Stratton, 1969. Chap. 6, pp. 96–108.
71. West, J. R., Smith, H. W., and Chasis, H. Glomerular filtration rate, effective renal blood flow, and maximal tubular excretory capacity in infancy. *J. Pediatr.* 32:10, 1948.

3. Laboratory Protocols and Methods for the Measurement of Glomerular Filtration Rate and Renal Plasma Flow

Robert R. Liedtke and Cristobal G. Duarte

Determinations of Glomerular Filtration Rate and Renal Plasma Flow by Standard Methods

At the time when the patient makes an appointment for tests to determine the glomerular filtration rate (GFR) and renal plasma flow (RPF), any special requests and problems are discussed with the clinical service and the age, sex, height, and weight of the patient are recorded. Because it is important to know the level of renal function in order to be able to prepare the solutions to be infused for these studies, as will be discussed later, the results of previous determinations of GFR and RPF are also recorded; if no such results are available, a rough estimation of renal function is obtained by a recent plasma creatinine determination. It is also important to screen for other tests which, if performed on the same day prior to these studies, may interfere with the determinations of GFR and RPF; such tests include an excretory urogram, which by causing an osmotic diuresis may induce changes in renal function, and the previous administration of radioisotopes for a renogram, renal scan or other studies, which may interfere with the counting of activity in plasma and urine if radioisotopes are also used for the determination of GFR and RPF. A renogram and a renal scan can be performed the same day after studies of renal function with radioisotopes.

Because genetic defects can be induced by radiation exposure when studies of renal function are performed with radioisotopes, women of childbearing age are screened for pregnancy, and a pregnancy test is performed if there is any doubt. If a female patient has delivered recently and is nursing her child, radioisotopes should not be administered. Studies of renal function with inulin and sodium para-aminohippurate (PAH) can be performed in pregnant women and in lactating mothers. Medications that may cause changes in renal function, such as diuretics and antihypertensive agents, should be discontinued for 48 hours before studies of renal function except when they are considered essential by the treating physician. Sulfa drugs and procaine give falsely elevated readings for PAH.

The patient is given an appointment to report to the renal function laboratory and is advised that the test will last approximately 3 hours. He is instructed not

This work was done while Dr. Duarte was Director of Laboratory Nephrology, Mayo Clinic Foundation, Rochester, Minn.

to eat solid foods for 4 hours before the test and to drink four glasses of water within the hour preceding the test. A cup of coffee or tea can be substituted for one of the glasses of water if so desired by the patient. The patient is also told to empty his bladder 1 hour before reporting for the study and not to void again until instructed to do so by the nurse.

After the patient arrives at the laboratory, his name, hospital or clinic number, and other personal data are corroborated and he is asked to empty his bladder. A 15-ml aliquot of this urine is saved to be used as a blank and is labeled U_{0}°. The patient is asked to disrobe, to put on a hospital gown, and to get into bed; blankets are supplied as needed for comfort. The nature, course, and expected duration of the test are explained to the patient. Any unexpected problems are noted, and the patient's blood pressure is measured and recorded. Optimal physical and mental comfort is an important factor in obtaining satisfactory clearance results. The clinical history of the patient should be available to be reviewed by the physician in charge of the renal function laboratory.

The Clearance of Inulin and PAH

LABORATORY PROTOCOL. Before the patient arrives at the laboratory, the priming and sustaining infusions of inulin and PAH are prepared according to the desired plasma levels that must be reached and maintained constant throughout the study. Ampules of inulin can be obtained that contain 50 ml of a 10% solution (Arnar-Stone Laboratories, Mount Prospect, Ill.). This is a supersaturated solution in which excess solid inulin is present; solution is effected by heating inulin in boiled water, after which the solution remains clear for several days. Ampules of PAH can be obtained in 10-ml vials of a 20% solution (Merck, Sharp, and Dohme, West Point, Pa.). Inulin and PAH can be obtained in powder form from the same sources for the preparation of the standard solutions.

The priming solutions of inulin and PAH can be estimated according to the following calculations:

$$\frac{\text{Milliliters of stock}}{\text{Kilograms of body weight}} = \frac{\text{Space of distribution} \times \text{Desired plasma level}}{\text{Concentration of the stock solution}}$$

Considering that the space of distribution of inulin is 20 percent, that the desired plasma level is 250 mg per kilogram, and that the concentration of inulin in the stock solution is 10 percent, the volume of inulin to be used as the priming dose will be

$$\frac{0.20 \times 1 \text{ kg} \times 250 \text{ mg/kg}}{100 \text{ mg/ml}} = \frac{0.5 \text{ ml of stock solution of inulin}}{\text{Kilograms of body weight}}$$

For PAH the space of distribution is 40 percent of body weight, the ideal plasma level is 25 mg per kilogram, and the concentration of the stock solution is 20 percent. Therefore, the priming dose of PAH will be as follows:

$$\frac{0.40 \times 1 \text{ kg} \times 25 \text{ mg/kg}}{200 \text{ mg/dl}} = \frac{0.05 \text{ ml of stock solution of PAH}}{\text{Kilograms of body weight}}$$

The priming solution of inulin and PAH is prepared by diluting the correct volume of the stock solution of inulin (0.5 ml/kg body weight) and PAH (0.05 ml/kg body weight) to 50 ml with normal saline in a 60-ml syringe, and 10 μCi of [^{131}I] hippurate sodium is added for the monitoring of bladder emptying, as will be discussed later.

The concentrations of inulin and PAH in plasma are maintained constant throughout the study by the continuous infusion of a sustaining solution of inulin and PAH. The sustaining doses of inulin and PAH are estimated according to the following calculations:

$$\frac{\text{Normal clearance} \times \text{Desired plasma concentration} \times \text{Duration of the test (min)}}{\text{Concentration of the stock solution}}$$
$$= \text{Volume of the stock solution}$$

For inulin the normal clearance is 125 ml/min, the desired plasma concentration is 25 mg/dl, the duration of the test is 200 minutes, and the concentration of the stock solution is 10 percent, and therefore, substituting, we obtain:

$$\frac{125 \text{ ml/min} \times 25 \text{ mg/dl} \times 200 \text{ min}}{100 \text{ mg/ml}} = 62.5 \text{ ml of stock solution of inulin}$$

For PAH the normal clearance is 600 ml/min, the desired plasma level is 2.5 mg/dl, the duration of the test is 200 minutes, and the concentration of the stock solution is 20 percent, and therefore, substituting, we obtain:

$$\frac{600 \text{ ml/min} \times 2.5 \text{ mg/dl} \times 200}{200 \text{ mg/ml}} = 15 \text{ ml of the stock solution of PAH}$$

These figures have been calculated for a person with a normal renal function and therefore must be corrected for the estimated values of renal function for a particular individual. The renal function can be roughly estimated by dividing 100 by the plasma concentration of creatinine in males and 80 by the plasma creatinine in females. Therefore, a male patient with a plasma concentration of creatinine of 2 mg/dl will have an estimated function of 50 percent of normal (100/2), and the sustaining doses of inulin and PAH should be reduced by 50 percent.

The sustaining infusion is prepared by diluting the appropriate amounts of inulin and PAH to 200 ml with normal saline in a glass bottle, and 10 μCi of [^{131}I] hippurate sodium is added for monitoring bladder emptying. Sterility must be maintained at all times.

A needle is placed in a superficial vein of the forearm, and 10 ml of heparinized blood is drawn, the blood is spun, and the plasma is separated to be used as a blank and is labeled P_0. U_0 and P_0 must be collected before the administration of the test substances. Then the priming infusion of inulin and PAH is injected through this needle over a 2-minute period, and the needle is connected to the sustaining infusion of inulin and PAH, which is delivered at the rate of 1 ml/min as controlled by a constant infusion pump. A needle is inserted in the vein of the other forearm for the collection of the remaining blood samples.

A period of 45 minutes is allowed to elapse after the administration of the priming infusion and the initiation of the sustaining infusion of inulin and PAH for equilibration; the activity of the radioactive Hippuran in the full bladder is then determined by applying the probe of a gamma spectrometer (portable Geiger counter) over the suprapubic area. The patient is then instructed to empty his bladder, and after the patient is placed back in bed, the counting over the empty bladder with the Geiger counter is repeated and compared with the background, which is the probe applied over the precordium. If the same reading is obtained over the bladder and the background, a complete urine collection has been obtained and the bladder is therefore empty. Readings over the bladder that are significantly higher than the background indicate that a significant volume of residual urine has been retained in the bladder; in these instances the patient is encouraged to try to empty his bladder again. If these efforts are fruitless because of lower urinary tract obstruction, an indwelling catheter is placed in the patient's bladder for the rest of the study after approval has been obtained from the treating physician. A urine culture is obtained at the time the catheter is inserted, and the patient is treated prophylactically with a sulfa drug. Two days later another urine culture is obtained. Methods have been described for estimating residual bladder urine without urethral catheterization [6, 8].

Once a complete emptying of the bladder has been achieved, another 10-ml sample of blood is drawn (P1) and a 30-minute urine collection is started from the time the bladder was empty (first clearance period). At the end of this 30-minute period a complete urine collection is obtained, the urinary volume is determined to the nearest milliliter, a 15-ml urine sample is saved (U1), and another 10-ml blood sample is drawn (P2). The collection of blood and urine is timed accurately. Two additional 30-minute clearance periods are collected, the succeeding blood samples being labeled P3 and P4 and the urine collections U2 and U3. Depending on the urinary flow, the patient may have to be hydrated by oral administration of water. Clearance periods with urinary flows that are lower than 3ml/min or higher than 10 ml/min are discarded because of the possible effects of dehydration or overhydration on renal function; in such instances additional clearance periods are collected until the ideal urinary flows are achieved. A complete record is carefully maintained throughout the study, and the data sheet is sent to the laboratory together with the 15-ml aliquots of urine and plasma samples for chemical analysis.

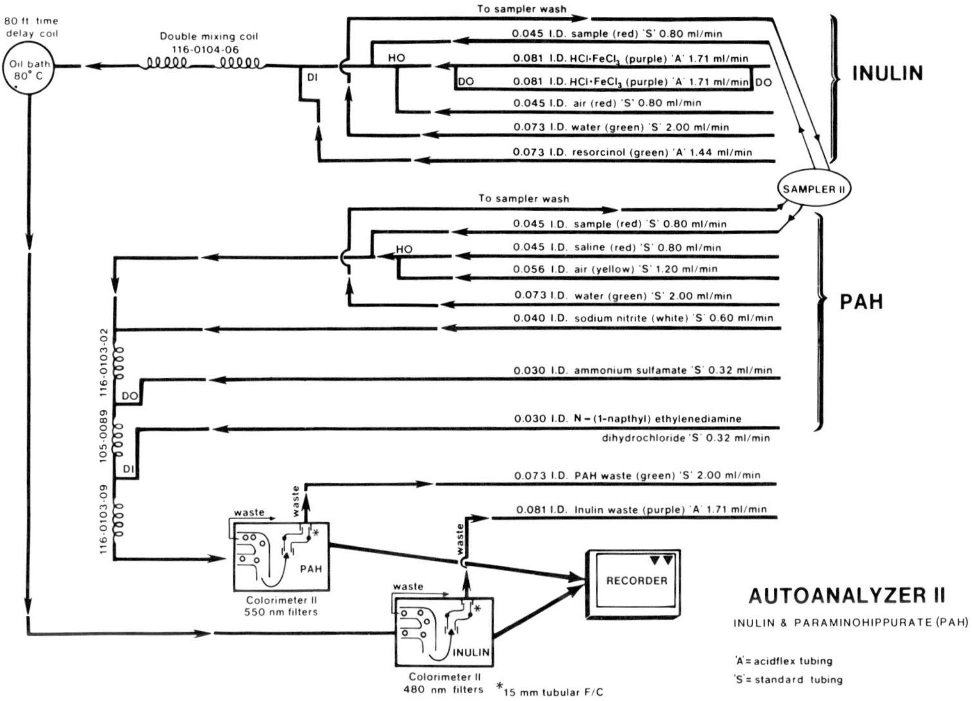

Figure 3–1
AutoAnalyzer flow diagram for the simultaneous determination of inulin and PAH.

CHEMICAL DETERMINATIONS OF INULIN AND PAH. Inulin and PAH are analyzed simultaneously in a Technicon AutoAnalyzer. Inulin is determined by a modification of the method of Fjeldbo and Stamey [3] in which inulin is hydrolyzed to fructose with concentrated HCl and $FeCl_3$ and then reacts with resorcinol, producing a red condensation product that is measured spectrophotometrically at 480 nm. PAH is determined by a modification of the procedure described by Harvey and Brothers [4] in which PAH is diazotized by sodium nitrate; the excess sodium nitrate is neutralized by ammonium sulfamate, and the diazotized PAH combines with *N*-1-naphthyl ethylene dihydrochloride to form a red-purple complex that is read at 550 nm.

The AutoAnalyzer consists of a Sampler II with a 60-sample per hour CAM with a 2:1 pick up-to-rinse ratio, a Proportioning Pump II, an 80°C heating bath containing an 80-foot coil, two flow-through colorimeters with 15-mm cell paths, and a two-channel recorder. The flow diagram, which is illustrated graphically in Figure 3–1, describes the various kinds of tubing, connectors, mixing coils, time delay coils, filters, and so forth and the sequence in which they are connected. The apparatus for inulin and PAH is joined as one system, utilizing the same sampler, proportioning pump, and recorder.

The reagents for the determination of inulin are as follows:

1. Resorcinol (0.15% in 95% ethanol). Dissolve 1.5 gm of resorcinol in approximately 500 ml of 95% ethanol in a 1-liter volumetric flask. Dilute to the 1-L mark with 95% ethanol and mix well. Prepare fresh daily.
2. Acid ferric chloride
   a. Stock solution. Dissolve 89.0 mg of $FeCl_3 \cdot 6\ H_2O$ in approximately 500 ml of concentrated HCl in a 1-L volumetric flask. Add concentrated HCl to the 1-L mark. The solution may be stored at room temperature for up to 2 months.
   b. Working solution. Dilute the stock solution 1 : 10 with concentrated HCl. The solution may be stored at room temperature for up to 1 week.
3. Precipitating reagents for the preparation of protein-free plasma filtrates [7].
   a. Cadmium sulfate. Dissolve 8.0 gm of $CdSO_4 \cdot 8\ H_2O$ in 39.4 ml of 1 N H_2SO_4 in a 1-L volumetric flask. Dilute to the 1-L mark with distilled water. May be stored at room temperature for 6 months.
   b. Sodium hydroxide (1.0 N). Dissolve 40 gm of NaOH in approximately 500 ml of distilled water in a 1-L volumetric flask (cool while dissolving). Dilute to the 1-L mark with distilled water and mix well. May be stored at room temperature for up to 6 months.

The reagents used to determine PAH are as follows:

1. Sodium nitrite. Dissolve 0.125 gm $NaNO_2$ in 50 ml of concentrated HCl in a 500-ml volumetric flask. Dilute to the 500-ml mark with distilled water and mix well. Store at 4°C; prepare fresh every 2 days.
2. Ammonium sulfamate. Dissolve 1.625 gm of $NH_4SO_3NH_2$ in approximately 200 ml of distilled water in a 500-ml volumetric flask. Dilute to the 500-ml mark with distilled water and mix well. Store at 4°C; prepare fresh weekly.
3. *N*-(1-naphthyl) ethylenediamine dihydrochloride (NEDD). Dissolve 1.05 gm of NEDD in 200 ml of absolute ethanol in a 1-L volumetric flask. Dilute to the 1-L mark with distilled water.
4. Physiological saline. Dissolve 9.0 gm of NaCl in approximately 500 ml of distilled water in a 1-L volumetric flask. Dilute to the 1-L mark with distilled water. Mix well. Add 2 ml of Brig-35 wetting agent and mix well. May be stored at room temperature for 6 months.
5. Precipitating reagents. Same as for inulin.

The standard solutions contain both inulin and PAH and are prepared as follows:

Stock Standards

1. Dry the inulin and PAH at 80°C for 2 hours. Store in a desiccator.
2. Place 1.0 gm of inulin in a 250-ml beaker. Add 50 ml of distilled water and a 1-inch magnetic stir bar. Place the beaker on a stirring hot plate. Stir on medium heat for 30 minutes or until the inulin dissolves. Use caution to avoid splashing.
3. Cool to room temperature and add 0.10 gm of PAH. Stir without heating until the PAH dissolves.
4. Transfer the contents of the beaker except the stir bar to a 200-ml volumetric flask. With repeated rinses using distilled water, quantitatively transfer the residual solution to the volumetric flask. Use caution to avoid overfilling the flask. Dilute to the 200 ml mark with distilled water. Prepare a fresh solution every time new standards are made. The stock standard solution has a concentration of 0.5% inulin and 0.05% PAH.

Working standard solutions. Dilute the stock standard as follows:

Working Standard Concentration		Milliliters of Stock Diluted to 500 ml with Distilled Water
Inulin (mg/dl)	PAH (mg/dl)	
0.1	0.01	0.1
0.5	0.05	0.5
1.0	0.10	1.0
2.0	0.20	2.0
3.0	0.30	3.0
4.0	0.40	4.0
5.0	0.50	5.0
6.0	0.60	6.0
7.0	0.70	7.0
8.0	0.80	8.0
9.0	0.90	9.0
10.0	1.00	10.0

Prepare fresh solution every 2 weeks. Store at 4° C.

After the instrument has been set up according to the flow diagram, the following steps are taken before each day's analysis:

1. Rinse the system for 20 minutes by pumping water through the reagent and sample lines. Check the analyzer visually for malfunctions (e.g., lines not drawing, leaks, bad bubble pattern).

2. Transfer the reagent lines to the proper reagent reservoirs and pump another 20 minutes.
3. After pumping reagents for 20 minutes, set the baseline to 98%T.
4. Set the 0%T using a zero aperture, then recheck the 98% baseline.
5. Place several high-range standards through the analyzer and make sure that the baseline returns to 98%T.

When the instrument has been checked out, analyze the standard curve by placing the standards into the sample tray in order, in duplicate, starting with the lowest concentration. Following the curve, analyze urine and plasma control samples. Make sure that the instrument is in control before proceeding with sample analysis. The samples are prepared for analysis in the following ways:

Plasma. Precipitation of plasma proteins [7].

1. Add 6.5 ml of cadmium sulfate to 0.5 ml of plasma in a 13 × 100 ml glass tube and mix.
2. Add 0.5 ml of 1 N NaOH to the tube and mix.
3. Centrifuge at 2000 rpm for 10 minutes. The supernatant is used for analysis.

Urine

1. Dilute the urine samples with distilled water, using volumetric flasks and pipettes. Use the estimated function as a guide to the proper dilution. Usually a 1 : 200 or 1 : 400 dilution is needed, but this may vary from 1 : 100 to 1 : 1000 in order to reach the analytical range, which ideally is 25 to 90%T. The samples are then analyzed in the following sequence in *duplicate* for each patient in a group:
   a. A plasma and urine control.
   b. All the patient's urine (diluted) in order, starting with U_0.
   c. All the patient's plasma supernatants in order, starting with P_0.
   d. A midrange standard.
2. Read the second peak in each set of duplicates.
3. Plot the standard curve on semilogarithmic paper with %T on the *y* axes and concentration (mg/dl) on the *x* axes. Using the %T for the unknown plasmas and urines, look up the concentration in milligrams per deciliter. Make sure that the standard and controls are in range before accepting the data.

The formula $\dfrac{UV}{P}$

where U = urine concentration (mg/dl),
V = urine volume (ml/min), and
P = plasma concentration (mg/dl)

is used to calculate the GFR (inulin clearance) and ERPF (PAH clearance) for each period. This clearance is corrected for the standard surface area of 1.73 m^2 by the following formula [2]:

$$\text{Uncorrected clearance} \times \frac{1.73 \text{ m}^2}{\text{Patient's surface area}} = \text{Corrected clearance}$$

The valid periods, those with flows between 3 and 10 ml/min where there has been complete bladder emptying, are averaged to obtain the GFR and ERPF for the patient. The formula

$$\text{FF} = \frac{\text{GFR}}{\text{ERPF}} \times 100$$

is used to calculate the filtration fraction (FF).

The Clearance of [^{125}I] *Iothalamate Sodium and of* [^{131}I] *Hippurate Sodium*

LABORATORY PROTOCOL. The clearance of iothalamate sodium labeled with ^{125}I (Glofil, Abbott Laboratories, North Chicago, Ill.) approximates the clearance of inulin, and the clearance of *o*-iodohippurate sodium (Hipputope, Squibb and Sons, Princeton, N.J. or Hippuran, Abbott Laboratories, North Chicago, Ill.) approximates the clearance of PAH. Doses of these agents are determined to provide approximately 1000 counts per minute of each agent per milliliter of plasma and to sustain these levels during the test.

Priming Solutions

1. The priming solution of [^{125}I] iothalamate sodium is prepared according to the following calculations:

$$0.214\ \mu\text{Ci [}^{125}\text{I] iothalamate sodium} \times \text{kilograms of body weight} = [^{125}\text{I] iothalamate sodium required}$$

$$\frac{\mu\text{Ci [}^{125}\text{I] iothalamate sodium required}}{\mu\text{Ci/ml [}^{125}\text{I] iothalamate sodium in stock solution}} = \text{Milliliters to be withdrawn from stock solution, to be used as priming dose}$$

2. The priming solution of [^{131}I] hippurate sodium is prepared as follows:

$$0.119\ \mu\text{Ci [}^{131}\text{I] hippurate sodium} \times \text{kilograms of body weight} = \text{Microcuries of hippurate required}$$

$$\frac{\mu\text{Ci [}^{131}\text{I] hippurate sodium required}}{\mu\text{Ci/ml [}^{131}\text{I] hippurate sodium in stock solution}} = \text{Milliliters to be withdrawn from stock solution, to be used as priming dose}$$

Sustaining Solutions

1. For [^{125}I] iothalamate sodium:

20 μCi [^{125}I] iothalamate sodium $\times$ estimated function in percent (up to 100%)
= μCi [^{125}I] iothalamate sodium required

$$\frac{\mu\text{Ci } [^{125}\text{I}] \text{ iothalamate sodium required}}{\mu\text{Ci/ml } [^{125}\text{I}] \text{ iothalamate sodium in stock solution}}$$
= Milliliters to be withdrawn from stock solution for sustaining infusion

2. For [^{131}I] hippurate sodium:

67 μCi [^{131}I] hippurate sodium $\times$ estimated function in percent (up to 100%)
= μCi [^{131}I] hippurate sodium required

$$\frac{\mu\text{Ci } [^{131}\text{I}] \text{ hippurate sodium required}}{\mu\text{Ci/ml } [^{131}\text{I}] \text{ hippurate sodium in stock solution}}$$
= Milliliters to be withdrawn from stock solution for sustaining infusion

[^{125}I] iothalamate sodium and [^{131}I] hippurate sodium are placed in a 250-ml bottle and brought to a total volume of 200 ml by the addition of normal saline. Sterility must be maintained at all times. The function is estimated from plasma concentration of creatinine as follows:

Males: $$\frac{1.00 \times 100}{\text{Serum creatinine}} = \text{Percent estimated function}$$

Females: $$\frac{0.80 \times 100}{\text{Serum creatinine}} = \text{Percent estimated function}$$

Before the study is started, a heparinized blood sample and a urine sample are collected and the patient is given three to five drops of a saturated solution of potassium iodide in 20 ml of water to be taken orally in order to block the possible uptake by the thyroid glands of the iodine-labeled radioisotopes. If the patient is allergic to iodine, 5 ml of sodium perchlorate is given instead. The priming solutions of [^{125}I] iothalamate sodium and [^{131}I] hippurate sodium are administered intravenously over a 2-minute period, and then the sustaining infusions are started and delivered at a rate of 1 ml/min. A urinary flow between 3 and 10 ml/min is maintained throughout the test by oral hydration with water.

After the priming infusions have been given and the sustaining solutions are started, a period of 45 minutes is allowed to elapse for equilibration. The patient is then instructed to void three times at 30-minute intervals, and a blood sample is drawn at the end of each urine collection. The completeness of bladder emptying is determined by applying the probe of a gamma counter over the region of the urinary bladder and comparing the counts of [^{131}I] hippurate sodium with those obtained over the heart. When the bladder is empty, the counts over the empty bladder should be equal to those read over the precordial area. A significant difference suggests incomplete emptying; if this is the case, the length of urine collection is prolonged because in some instances the patient is able to achieve a more complete emptying when the bladder is fuller. If catheterization is indicated because of urinary retention, approval is first obtained from the treating physician, a urine culture is obtained at the time the catheter is placed, and the patient is given prophylactic medication for urinary infection. Another urine culture is obtained two days later.

COUNTING THE SAMPLES. A gamma counter (Searle 1185) is used for counting the samples. The instrument is calibrated with ^{129}Iodine as a standard, and spillover of [^{131}I] counts into the [^{125}I] channel as well as background are determined in each of the three channels. Then 2 ml of plasma or urine is placed in a 16 × 125 mm screw-cap polyethylene tube and counted for 5 minutes. Counts are corrected automatically for spillover (for [^{125}I] iothalamate sodium) and for background (for [^{125}I] iothalamate sodium and [^{131}I] hippurate sodium).

The clearance of either [^{125}I] iothalamate sodium or [^{131}I] hippurate sodium is calculated according to the formula:

$$\frac{\text{Urine} \times V}{\dfrac{P_1 \times P_2}{2}} = \text{Uncorrected clearance}$$

Determinations of GFR and RPF by Simplified Methods with Urine Collection

The Clearance of Creatinine

LABORATORY PROTOCOL. The clearance of creatinine can be used as a screening test for GFR, especially in those instances in which more reliable tests with radioisotopes, such as the clearance of iothalamate by subcutaneous injection, cannot be performed because the administration of radioisotopes is contraindicated. In addition to the shortcomings already discussed of creatinine as a test of renal function (see Chap. 1), the clearance of creatinine has the disadvantage that with this procedure completeness of bladder emptying is not monitored.

The clearance of creatinine is usually determined with a 1-hour or a 24-hour urine collection. For the 24-hour creatinine clearance, the patient is instructed to empty his bladder at 7:00 A.M. on the first day of the test; this urine is then discarded and a blood sample is drawn. All the urine passed over the following 24 hours is collected, including the specimen obtained when the patient voids the next morning at 7:00 A.M., following which another blood sample is drawn. To avoid any losses of urine, the patient is instructed to try to pass his urine prior to having a bowel movement.

For the 1-hour creatinine clearance, the patient is encouraged to drink three to four glasses of water within the hour preceding the test and not to eat for 4 hours before reporting for the study. He should empty his bladder 1 hour before the test and should not void again until so instructed by the nurse. When the patient reports for the study, he is then asked to empty his bladder; this urine is discarded; 7 ml of blood is drawn into a heparinized syringe; the patient is asked to wait in the lobby for 1 hour or until he has the sensation of a full bladder; and he is asked to drink a glass of water every 20 minutes. After 1 hour the patient reports to the desk attendant in the lobby and is directed to the clearance room, where the operations of having the patient empty his bladder and collecting another blood sample are repeated. In all these studies a protocol is carefully maintained; the times of urine and blood collections are accurately reported; the volume of urine is measured; and the protocol, an aliquot of urine, and the plasma samples are sent to the chemistry laboratory after the patient has been discharged.

CHEMICAL DETERMINATION OF CREATININE. A method described by Chasson, Grady, and Stanley [1] has been adapted for the determination of creatinine with an AutoAnalyzer [9]. The components of the AutoAnalyzer include a Sampler II with a 60 samples per hour cam with a 2 : 1 sample to rinse ratio, a Proportioning Pump II, a dialyzer bath utilizing a type "C" membrane, a 20-foot time delay coil immersed in a room-temperature water bath, a flow-through colorimeter with a 15-mm tubular flow cell set at 505 nm, and a single pen recorder. The flow diagram listed in the Technicon methodology [9] describes the various kinds of tubing, connectors, mixing coils, time delay coils, filters, and so on, as well as the sequence of flow through the system.

The reagents for the determination of creatinine are as follows:

1. *Saline* (0.9%). Place 9.0 gm of reagent-grade NaCl in a 1-liter volumetric flask. Add approximately 500 ml of distilled water and dissolve the sodium chloride. Dilute to the 1-liter mark with distilled water and shake well to mix.
2. *Sodium hydroxide* (0.5N). Place 40 gm of reagent-grade NaOH pellets in a 2-liter volumetric flask; add approximately 1 liter of distilled water and swirl to dissolve the pellets (cool in an ice bath while dissolving). Dilute to the 2-liter mark with distilled water and mix well.
3. *Saturated picric acid.* Place 13 gm of reagent-grade picric acid in 1 liter of distilled water and shake well. Allow the solution to stand at room temperature for 48 hours, mixing occasionally. Filter out the excess crystals and store the clear solution in a polyethylene bottle.
4. *Stock standard* (1 mg creatinine per milliliter). Add 1.0 gm creatinine to a 1-L volumetric flask, add approximately 500 ml 0.1 N HCl, and mix until dissolved. Dissolve to the 1-L mark with 0.1 N HCl and mix well.
5. *Working standards.* Dilute the stock standard in the following proportions with 0.02 N HCl.

Standard Concentration	Milliliters of Stock	Diluted to
1 mg/100 ml	1	100 ml
3 mg/100 ml	3	100 ml
5 mg/100 ml	5	100 ml
7 mg/100 ml	7	100 ml

The following procedure is used for daily operation:

1. Before each day's run:
   a. Rinse the system for 30 minutes with the reagent lines in distilled water. Check visually all tubing and coils for crimping or breaks.
   b. Transfer the reagent lines to the proper reagent bottles and pump for another 30 minutes.
   c. After the equilibration period, turn on the recorder and check 0%T by placing a zero aperture in the colorimeter. If necessary, set 0 with the 0 control knob. Remove the 0 aperture and set the baseline to 98% with the gain control knob. Allow the baseline to run for at least 15 minutes to determine that it is stable. Readjust if necessary.
   d. Analyze a standard curve and urine and plasma controls. Determine that the instrument is "in control."
2. Patient samples are analyzed and grouped together for each individual in the following sequence:
   a. A standard curve.
   b. All the urine samples diluted according to concentration.
   c. All plasmas undiluted.
   d. A control plasma and urine sample.
3. The %T values for the standard curve for all patient samples and controls are recorded. A graph is prepared by plotting standard concentration against %T on semilogarithmic paper. The concentration of the controls is determined and checked to ensure that they are "in control." The concentration of the patient's samples is then determined from the standard curve graph.
4. The clearance of creatinine is calculated in the same manner as for inulin or PAH, except that the concentration of creatinine in the urine and plasma samples is substituted.

The Clearance of [^{125}I] *Iothalamate Sodium by Subcutaneous Injection and Urine Collection* [5]

The advantages of this test over the standard methods for the determination of GFR are as follows: it can be performed over a shorter period of time in a greater number of patients, and it does not require the number of specialized personnel and the continuous use of laboratory space that are needed for the standard studies, thus providing the advantages of efficiency and economy. The emptying of the bladder is monitored in this test, and therefore complete urine collections can be obtained. The clearance of subcutaneous iothalamate is a more reliable screening test for GFR than is the clearance of creatinine.

The contraindications for this test are the same as those indicated for the standard methods for the measurement of GFR with radioisotopes. One additional disadvantage is that the subcutaneous administration of radiolabeled hippurate does not correlate well with the clearance of PAH, and thus the RPF cannot be determined simultaneously with the clearance of subcutaneous iothalamate (see Chap. 2). Therefore, when the RPF and the filtration fraction need to be determined, as in patients with congestive heart failure, standard renal clearance studies must be performed.

LABORATORY PROTOCOL. The patient is told that the test will last approximately 2 hours. He is instructed to drink three to four glasses of water within the hour before the test (a cup of black coffee may be substituted for one of these glasses) and not to drink or eat anything else for 4 hours before reporting for the study. He should empty his bladder 1 hour before the test and should not void again until instructed to do so by the nurse.

The patient is given three to five drops of a saturated solution of potassium iodide in 20 ml of water orally. If he has a previous history of iodine hypersensitivity, he is given 5 ml of sodium perchlorate instead. The test starts with the subcutaneous injection of 0.2 μCi/kg of body weight of [^{125}I] iothalamate sodium in the upper arm. Depending on the decay of the radioisotope and the size of the patient, the volume of solution injected varies from a minimum volume of 0.07 ml (for a small person injected with a fresh solution) to 0.35 ml (for the largest person 10 days after the radioisotope was received). A total of 5 μCi of [^{131}I] hippurate sodium is added to the iothalamate solution for the purpose of monitoring the emptying of the bladder. After the injection, the patient is asked to wait in the lobby for half an hour and to drink a glass of water to maintain hydration. The patient is then recalled to the clearance room, and the counting obtained by applying a gamma counter over the area of the bladder is recorded. This operation is repeated after the patient is asked to empty the bladder completely, and this counting is compared with that obtained over the precordium as a background. The counting over the empty bladder and the heart should be approximately the same, and if this is the case, the urine is discarded and the test is started. If the counting over the bladder is higher than that over the heart, the patient is asked to try again to empty his bladder completely. After a complete bladder emptying has been obtained, 7 ml of heparinized blood is drawn, and the exact time of the voiding and blood collection is recorded. The patient is then asked to wait in the lobby for 1 hour or until he has the sensation of a full bladder and to drink a glass of water approximately every 20 minutes. When he is able to void again the patient reports to a desk attendant who directs him to the clearance room, where the same operations are repeated (i.e., obtaining a complete bladder collection and a blood sample and accurate reporting of the time of these collections). This urine sample is saved and is sent to the laboratory together with the blood samples. The patient is then discharged.

COUNTING OF THE SAMPLES. The counting of the samples is as described for the standard methods for iothalamate clearance. The calculations are as follows:

$$\frac{U\ [^{125}I]\ \text{iothalamate sodium} \times V}{\dfrac{P_1\ [^{125}I]\ \text{iothalamate sodium} + P_2\ [^{125}I]\ \text{iothalamate sodium}}{2}} = \text{Uncorrected clearance}$$

$$\text{Corrected clearance} = \text{Uncorrected clearance} \times \frac{1.73\ m^2}{\text{Patient surface area } m^2}$$

where U [^{125}I] iothalamate sodium = counts in 2 ml of urine for 5 minutes,

P_1 [^{125}I] iothalamate sodium = counts in 2 ml of initial plasma sample for 5 minutes,

P_2 [^{125}I] iothalamate sodium = counts in 2 ml of final plasma sample for 5 minutes, and

V = urine flow in milliliters per minute.

References

1. Chasson, A. L., Grady, H. J., and Stanley, M. A. Determination of creatinine by means of automatic chemical analysis. *Am. J. Clin. Pathol.* 35:83, 1961.
2. Du Bois, E. F. The Estimation of the Surface Area of the Body. In *Basal Metabolism in Health and Disease.* Philadelphia: Lea & Febiger, 1924. Chap. 7, pp. 136–147.
3. Fjeldbo, W., and Stamey, T. A. Adapted method for determination of inulin in serum and urine with an AutoAnalyzer. *J. Lab. Clin. Med.* 107:353, 1968.
4. Harvey, R. B., and Brothers, A. J. Renal extraction of p-aminohippurate and creatinine measured by continuous in vivo sampling of arterial and renal vein blood, *N. Y. Acad. Sci.* 102:46, 1962.
5. Ott, N. T., and Wilson, D. M. A simple technique for estimating glomerular filtration rate with subcutaneous injection of (^{125}-I) iothalamate. *Mayo Clin. Proc.* 50:664–668, 1975.
6. Shand, B. S., MacKenzie, J. C., Cattell, W. R., et al. Estimation of residual urine volume with ^{131}I Hippuran. *Br. J. Urol.* 40:196, 1968.
7. Smith, H. W., Finkelstein, N., Aliminosa, L., et al. Renal clearance of substituted hippuric acid and derivatives and other aromatic acids in dog and man. *J. Clin. Invest.* 24:388, 1945.
8. Strauss, B. S., and Blaufox, M. D. Estimation of residual urine and urine flow rates without urethral catheterization. *J. Nucl. Med.* 11:81, 1970.
9. Technicon AutoAnalyzer methodology, File N-11b. Chauncey, N.Y.: Technicon Instrument Corporation.

4. Noninvasive Methods for the Measurement of Renal Function

Claudio Bianchi

The measurement of renal function is required to investigate suspected renal disease, to follow the course of the disease, and to assess therapy. A correct evaluation of this function requires the determination of the glomerular filtration rate (GFR) and, in some cases, the effective renal plasma flow (ERPF). The determination of these parameters on a large scale in renal patients is limited, however, by notable difficulties in technique. In fact, the conventional method for their measurement requires the continuous intravenous administration of adequate substances (inulin or analogues for GFR, para-aminohippurate for ERPF) as well as vesical catheterization for total urine collection. Such procedures, in addition to involving possible errors, present potential risks to the patients examined. The errors consist of the possibilities of an unstable blood concentration of tracer during clearance due to an incorrect infusion rate and an incomplete collection of urine through the catheter. The main risk is infection resulting from bladder catheterization.

Although the clearance of endogenous creatinine is not subject to these practical limitations, it overestimates the GFR and is subject to large errors due to the variability in tubular excretion of creatinine and the difficulty of obtaining complete urine collections [1, 11, 22, 30, 34, 36, 37, 42, 53]. Furthermore, the possible effect of drug treatment on creatinine clearance has been indicated [25]. Therefore there is a need to use noninvasive methods, with simple and accurate procedures, for determining GFR and ERPF.

Isotopic techniques have allowed considerable progress in this direction. They have been employed both in the determination of total renal function (i.e., the sum of function of both kidneys) and in the measurement of unilateral renal clearance.

Measurement of Total Renal Function

Two noninvasive methods are available to measure total renal function. Both methods are designed to determine GFR as well as ERPF without bladder catheterization and consist of the administration of tracers by a single intravenous injection. One of these methods involves the indirect measurement of total renal function based on an analysis of the plasma disappearance curve of tracers, and thus it provides the plasma clearance. The other method provides direct measurement of renal clearance. It is based on the measurement by external counting of the accumulation of tracers in the bladder (the bladder cumulative method).

Plasma Clearance Method

RATIONALE. Plasma clearance is the volume per minute of plasma cleared of the studied substance without considering the organs involved in the elimination of the substance. If the substance employed is eliminated only through the kidneys, the plasma clearance corresponds to the renal clearance.

The plasma clearance of a tracer is determined from an analysis of its plasma disappearance curve. In the plasma curve of glomerular tracers and iodohippurate sodium (Hippuran, the only tracer available for the determination of ERPF), it is possible to distinguish two parts. In the first part the plasma concentration of the tracer falls rapidly but at a progressively diminishing rate (70 to 90 minutes in the case of the glomerular tracers and 35 to 50 minutes in the case of Hippuran). After these intervals, the plasma concentration decreases at an exponential rate in the second part of the curve.

The first part of the curve denotes the diffusion of the tracer in its distribution volume and its excretion. It must be noted that the distribution volume of renal tracers approximates the extracellular space. The second part of the curve refers only to the excretion of the tracer. If only the kidneys are involved in the elimination of the tracer, this part of the curve denotes the level of kidney function.

The beginning of the second part of the curve indicates that the tracer has reached a dynamic equilibrium; from this point, the tracer concentration decreases at the same exponential rate in all compartments in which it is distributed. This process takes place within 90 minutes after the injection for the glomerular tracers and within 50 minutes for Hippuran.

The mathematical model for this approach is an open two-compartment system in which the tracer is injected into the first compartment, equilibrates with a second compartment, and is excreted from the first one via the kidneys and other organs involved in its excretion.

The graphic analysis shows that the plasma disappearance curve of the renal tracers is the sum of two exponential terms (Fig. 4–1), the faster one due mainly to diffusion and the slower one to excretion.

MATERIALS. To measure GFR and ERPF by the plasma clearance method, inulin and para-aminohippurate have been employed in the past [27, 46]. However, practical difficulties have limited the use of these nonradioactive tracers (see under Discussion). Presently, radioactive tracers are preferred. The tracers available for the measurement of GFR are diatrizoate and iothalamate, both labeled with [^{125}I] or [^{131}I]; ethylenediamine tetra-acetic acid (EDTA) labeled with [^{51}Cr]; and diethylenetriamine penta-acetic acid (DTPA) labeled with [^{99m}Tc] [2, 3, 16, 28, 29, 31, 38, 47]. For the measurement of ERPF, only Hippuran labeled with [^{125}I] or [^{131}I] is currently available [14, 16, 19, 29, 31, 39, 52].

For the simultaneous measurement of GFR and ERPF (and, therefore, from their ratio, or the filtration fraction) it is necessary to use tracers whose physi-

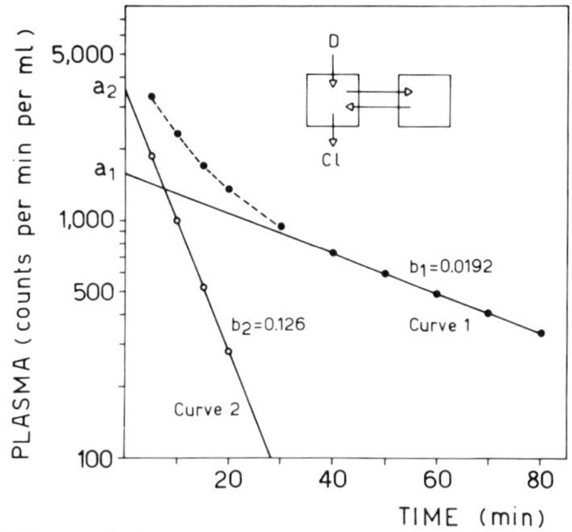

Figure 4–1
A typical plasma disappearance curve of [^{131}I] Hippuran. By means of graphic analysis two exponential terms, slow and fast, are identified (curve 1 and curve 2). The appropriate model is an open two-compartment system in which the tracer (*D*) is introduced into the first compartment, equilibrates with a second compartment, and is cleared from the first one.

cal properties enable accurate counting in mixtures. For this purpose it is possible to utilize diatrizoate (or iothalamate) and Hippuran, one labeled with [^{125}I], the other with [^{131}I], or [^{99m}Tc] DTPA together with [^{131}I] Hippuran.

PROCEDURE. To measure either GFR or ERPF, we employ doses of about 50 μCi of [^{131}I] diatrizoate or [^{131}I] Hippuran. For the simultaneous determination of these parameters, [^{131}I] diatrizoate and [^{125}I] Hippuran in the respective doses of 50 μCi and 100 μCi are used. The tracers are rapidly injected into an antecubital vein. Following this procedure we obtain, using an indwelling needle in the contralateral arm to prevent radioactive contamination of the blood drawn, a series of blood samples of 3 ml each by means of heparinized syringes.

To obtain a well-defined plasma disappearance curve (and therefore a correct calculation of plasma clearance), numerous blood samples are required. To measure the GFR, blood samples are withdrawn at 5, 10, 20, 40, 60, 80, 100, 120, 140, and 160 minute intervals after tracer injection. Dynamic equilibrium is achieved in all patients (regardless of body size or edema) within 90 minutes. To determine ERPF, blood samples are drawn at 5, 10, 15, 20, 30, 40, 50, 60, 70, and 80 minute intervals after tracer injection; equilibrium is attained within 50 minutes. When GFR and ERPF are measured simultaneously, in order to define with sufficient accuracy the equilibrium time and the exponential slope of diatrizoate and Hippuran curves we draw samples at 5, 10, 15, 20, 40, 50, 60, 70, 80, 100, 120, 140, and 160 minute intervals after tracer injection. The radioactivity of 1 ml of plasma of each blood sample is measured in a well-type counter.

CALCULATION. Plasma clearance is calculated by means of graphic analysis of the plasma disappearance curve (Fig. 4–1). The values of radioactivity of each sample of plasma, expressed as counts per minute (cpm) per milliliter of plasma, are plotted on semilogarithmic paper in ordinate against time in abscissa. The linear terminal portion of the curve, which is obtained by visual fit, is extrapolated back to time zero (curve 1). The values at various times of the extrapolated portion of curve 1 are subtracted from the corresponding observed readings. The resulting differences are replotted to yield curve 2, which is a straight line.

Plasma clearance is obtained by the following equation, which has been derived previously by Sapirstein and colleagues in their studies of creatinine and PAH clearances [40, 48]:

$$\mathrm{Cl} = \frac{Db_1b_2}{a_1b_2 + a_2b_1} \qquad (1)$$

where D is the dose of injected tracer, b_1 and b_2 are the slopes of the two exponential terms of the plasma disappearance curve (slow and fast, respectively), and a_1 and a_2 represent their intersections with the ordinate.

To calculate the injected dose, the syringe containing the tracer to be injected (syringe 1) and another syringe (syringe 2) containing an aliquot of this dose (generally one-half) are weighed on a precision balance. The contents of syringe 1 are injected into the patient, and the contents of syringe 2 are emptied into a 1-liter flask fllled with water. Both syringes are weighed once again, and 1 ml of the diluted aliquot is counted. The injected dose, D, expressed in counts per minute, is calculated as:

$$D = \frac{\text{Weight of dose}}{\text{Weight of aliquot}} \times \frac{\text{Counts per minute}}{\text{Milliliter of diluted aliquot}} \times 1000.$$

The following example refers to the calculation of plasma clearance of [^{131}I] Hippuran for ERPF determination (see Fig. 4–1).

The radioactivities of plasma samples are as follows:

Time (Minutes after Tracer Injection)	Plasma Radioactivity (cpm/ml)
5	3,300
10	2,300
15	1,700
20	1,350

Time (Minutes after Tracer Injection)	Plasma Radioactivity (cpm/ml)
30	950
40	730
50	600
60	490
70	420
80	340

These values are plotted on semilogarithmic paper against time. The disappearance curve is then resolved into the sum of two exponential functions in the manner described above.

The data required for the calculation of the plasma clearance are as follows:

D (dose administered) = 46,800,000 cpm
a_1 (intercept of the slow component of the plasma curve): 1570 cpm/ml
Half time ($T\frac{1}{2}$) of the slow component of the plasma curve: 36 min
b_1 (slope ($0.693/T\frac{1}{2}$) of the slow component of the plasma curve): 0.0192/min
a_2 (intercept of the fast component of the plasma curve): 3550 cpm/ml
Half time of the fast component of the plasma curve: 5.5 min
b_2 (slope of the fast component of the plasma curve): 0.126/min

According to Equation 1, the plasma clearance of [^{131}I] Hippuran is then

$$\frac{46{,}800{,}000 \times 0.0192 \times 0.126}{(1{,}570 \times 0.126) + (3{,}550 \times 0.0192)} = 426 \text{ ml/min.}$$

SIMPLIFIED PLASMA CLEARANCE. The determination of the total clearance by the method described above involves some practical limitations. In fact, to describe fully the entire curve in this way is both time-consuming to the investigator and inconvenient to the patient, since it requires that many blood samples be withdrawn. These limitations explain why numerous simplified techniques have been proposed over the years. All these simplified techniques tend to reduce the number of blood samples needed. Their mathematical model is a single-compartment system rather than a two-compartment system as described above. They are based on the assumption that the tracer is distributed in only one compartment and is eliminated by the kidneys.

In practice, two to three blood samples are drawn and the values of the plasma radioactivity are plotted on semilogarithmic paper in ordinate against time in abscissa. The experimental points are connected by a straight line, and this is extrapolated back to zero time.

The clearance is calculated as:

$$\text{Cl} = \frac{Db}{a} \qquad (2)$$

where D = the dose of injected tracer,
b = the slope of the single exponential term, and
a = its intersection with the ordinate.

The time intervals at which blood samples are drawn differ widely according to different authors; they vary from 60 to 300 minutes after tracer injection for GFR [24, 32, 46] and from 7 to 60 minutes for ERPF determination [20, 35, 46]. Estimation of GFR based on a single blood sample withdrawn 3 hours after the tracer injection has also been described [33].

Other simplified yet more sophisticated techniques have been proposed; they are based on the determination by means of external counting of the disappearance curve of radioactivity recorded over a highly vascularized area. It is assumed that such a curve is similar to the plasma disappearance curve. The detector is positioned over the patient's head [14, 16, 21] or over the precordium [29, 43, 45, 47, 51]. One to two blood samples are generally drawn to calibrate the values of the curve obtained by external counting.

In the segment preceding the exponential slope, the plasma curve and the curve obtained by external counting seem quite different. In fact, the latter is considerably slower than the former. This phenomenon is attributed to the extravascular diffusion of the tracers (both glomerular tracers and Hippuran) whereby the external counter records simultaneously the decrease of activity in the plasma and an increase in the interstitial space [14, 16].

The slopes of the slower exponential term obtained by the plasma curve and by external counting are similar for glomerular tracers [16, 47], whereas conflicting results are reported for Hippuran [16, 21, 29].

Neither of these simplified techniques based on external counting has achieved wide acceptance.

DISCUSSION. The plasma clearance method of measuring total renal function is important because it avoids the two principal disadvantages of the conventional technique (i.e., continuous intravenous infusion of tracers and vesical catheterization). Nevertheless, this method is valid only if the tracers employed are eliminated exclusively through the kidneys so that plasma clearance is equal to renal clearance. Unfortunately, this condition is not satisfied due to the fact that many of the tracers used for the determination of renal function are also eliminated to varying degrees by extrarenal pathways (generally in the bile) [16, 17, 19, 23, 26, 41, 49, 50]. Such extrarenal elimination is minimal in normal subjects but becomes important in patients with severely damaged renal function, in whom the plasma clearance often exceeds the renal clearance to a significant degree.

In addition to the possible cause of errors just mentioned, some practical difficulties inherent to the execution of plasma clearance should be noted. This method has little application with nonradioactive tracers because of the necessity of rapid injection of a large volume of liquid and, above all, because the rapid decrease in plasma concentration makes it difficult to define the plasma disappearance curve with accuracy. The use of radioactive tracers overcomes these difficulties because of the low volume of doses to be injected and the lower incidence of error obtained in the measurement of plasma concentration of the radioactive tracers. Nevertheless, it is still necessary to obtain numerous blood samples to define the plasma curve correctly and to identify its two exponential terms according to the two-compartment analysis, and this involves considerable difficulty.

The simplified techniques are based on a single-compartment analysis and therefore require the identification of only one exponential term. They are more suitable for routine clinical use because fewer blood samples are required. However, the accuracy of these techniques is unsatisfactory. In general, the more simplified the techniques, the greater the inaccuracies appear to be. Furthermore, it should be noted that the analysis of only one exponential term of the plasma curve results in an overestimation of the plasma clearance.

The techniques based on external counting provide many points to plot, thus reducing the chances of error. Nevertheless, the differences in their shape in the segment preceding the exponential slope, in comparison with the plasma curve, discourage their use. This also applies when Hippuran is used, where the slopes of the exponential terms determined by external counting and by the plasma curve are different.

In conclusion, the conventional plasma clearance method may be utilized in renal investigation as long as the limitations described above are considered. The simplified techniques, however, which are often based on confused and unwarranted assumptions, will provide only a rough estimation of renal function and thus should be discarded in all precise clinical investigation.

In general, the direct measurement of renal clearance is preferable to its indirect determination obtained by means of plasma clearance or its simplifications.

Bladder Cumulative Method for the Measurement of Renal Clearance

Renal clearance is the volume per minute of plasma cleared of the studied substance by the kidneys. The conventional method for its determination (described in Chapters 1, 2, and 3 of this book) requires, in addition to intravenous infusion of the tracer at a constant rate, the complete collection of urine by means of vesical catheterization. Since the bladder cumulative method (described in this section) has been available for the past few years, the use of vesical catheterization for this purpose seems to be an unnecessary hazard. The bladder cumulative method furnishes the direct measurement of renal clearance by means of a single injection of the tracer and external counting over the bladder, thereby avoiding bladder catheterization and continuous intravenous infusion of the tracer [3].

RATIONALE. At a constant plasma concentration, the renal clearance of a substance is as follows:

$$\mathrm{Cl} = \frac{U \times V}{P} \tag{1}$$

where U and P represent the urinary and plasma concentrations of the substance, respectively, and V represents the urine output in milliliters per minute. Equation 1 is used during steady state for the calculation of renal clearances of endogenous substances (i.e., creatinine) and exogenous substances (i.e., different tracers employed for the study of renal function). In the latter case, constant plasma concentration is obtained by means of an intravenous infusion at a constant rate.

To measure the renal clearance of an exogenous substance after a single intravenous injection, the total amount of substance eliminated with the urine must be divided by the integral of its plasma concentration. Equation 1 then becomes

$$\mathrm{Cl} = \frac{\Delta U}{\int_{t_1}^{t_2} P(t)\, dt} \tag{2}$$

where ΔU is the amount of substance eliminated with the urine during the period of clearance, P is its plasma concentration, and t_1 and t_2 are the time limits, beginning and end, of the clearance.

When radioactive gamma-emitting tracers of sufficient energy are employed, ΔU, the numerator of Equation 2, can be determined simply by external counting, thus measuring the increase in radioactivity over the bladder in the interval between t_1 and t_2.

The integral of plasma concentration in the period of clearance (the denominator of Equation 2) is easily measured when dynamic equilibrium is attained, that is, when the plasma curve is exponential. At this point a minimum of two blood samples are required to define the slope, which is a straight line on semilogarithmic paper. The integral is then

$$\int_{t_1}^{t_2} P(t)\, dt = \frac{a}{b}\,(e^{-bt_1} - e^{-bt_2}) \tag{3}$$

where a and b represent respectively the intersection with the ordinate and the slope of the exponential term. In practice, to calculate the integral it is sufficient to draw only one blood sample at the midpoint of clearance. The radioactivity of this sample is considered to be a mean of the plasma radioactivity during the period of clearance. In this way, it is assumed that the decrease in plasma radioactivity is linear instead of exponential. The differences between the results obtained with this simplification and by Equation 3 are minimal. The slower the exponential slope (i.e., the greater the reduction of renal function) the smaller these differences are. The integral denominator of Equation 2 can be then easily calculated as the product of the plasma concentration at the midpoint of clearance times the duration of the clearance:

$$\int_{t_1}^{t_2} P(t)\,dt = P(T\tfrac{1}{2}) \times (t_2 - t_1) \tag{4}$$

It should be noted that the numerator and the denominator of Equation 2 are measured by different techniques (external counting for bladder radioactivity, well-type counting for plasma radioactivity), and thus they have to be brought back to the same units. To accomplish this, ΔU is corrected by means of a calibration factor, k, which permits one to convert the external counting values to the same units with which the plasma activity has been measured. For calculation of the k value, at the end of the clearance period a urine sample is collected by free micturition and an aliquot is counted in the same well-counter with which the plasma activity has been determined. The calibration factor is then obtained as the ratio between total radioactivity of the collected urines, ΔE, and decrease of the external counting rate over the bladder consequent to the vesical emptying (ΔB):

$$k = \frac{\Delta E}{\Delta B} \tag{5}$$

In conclusion, the renal clearance is obtained by external counting over the bladder as

$$\mathrm{Cl} = \frac{\Delta U \times k}{P(T\tfrac{1}{2}) \times (t_2 - t_1)}. \tag{6}$$

MATERIAL. The bladder cumulative method requires gamma-emitting tracers of sufficient energy for external detection. For the measurement of GFR we use [^{131}I] diatrizoate or [^{99m}Tc] DTPA. Other widely available tracers, such as [^{131}I] iothalamate or [^{51}Cr] EDTA, are also suitable. Tracers labeled with [^{125}I], however, are not usable because the emission energy of this isotope is not sufficient for external counting over the bladder. To measure ERPF, [^{131}I] Hippuran is employed.

External counting over the bladder requires a scintillation counter provided with a suitable collimator to minimize the effect of difference in volume of the bladder. The volume of the bladder is, in fact, widely variable, and these geometric variations produce differences in the values obtained by external counting. The type of detector we use allows one to measure vesical radioactivity in a wide range of bladder volumes (up to 400 ml); it consists of a 3- × 2-inch NaI(Tl) scintillation counter placed into a truncated cone collimator. At its widest point (surface closest to patient) it measures 12.5 cm in internal diameter and 14 cm in external diameter, with a total length of 29 cm. Details regarding this apparatus have already been published [3].

It is useful to remember that in order to establish the reliability of a scintillation counter for external counting over the bladder, it is necessary to verify that the results obtained are independent of bladder volume. The simplest method to prove this point consists of introducing into the bladder (in patients already catheterized) a low radioactive dose (2 to 3 μCi) of the isotope to be employed, for instance [^{131}I], and then measuring the relative bladder activity by external counting. The volume of the bladder is then progressively increased by the introduction of normal saline solution through the catheter (50 ml each time, up to a minimum of 300 ml). After each volume increment the radioactivity of the bladder is counted. If the apparatus used is reliable, the results will not vary.

PROCEDURE. At present, the bladder cumulative method is employed mainly for the determination of GFR, using [^{131}I] diatrizoate as a tracer. The procedure described here refers to one such measure. To obtain full cooperation of the patient, it is advisable to inform him prior to the test about the more important aspects of the procedure.

Time (min)	
0	Approximately 0.6 μCi of [^{131}I] diatrizoate per kilogram of body weight is rapidly injected intravenously. Dynamic equilibrium, that is, exponential decrease of the plasma disappearance curve, is also attained in edematous patients within 90 minutes. The clearance period begins after this time has elapsed, but it is advisable not to wait much longer, thus avoiding too low values of plasma radioactivity.
0–80	To obtain an adequate urine output during the clearance period, the patient is hydrated by oral administration of approximately 1 liter of tap water.
80–85	To avoid excessive bladder filling, the patient is asked to urinate before the beginning of the clearance. The urine is discarded.
85–90	The patient lies down on the couch and the counter is placed over the bladder, with the pubic symphysis used as a reference point.
90	The clearance period is initiated and lasts for 30 minutes, during which time the bladder radioactivity is repeatedly measured at 1-minute counting intervals (Fig. 4–2).
105	At the midpoint of the clearance, a venous blood sample is drawn

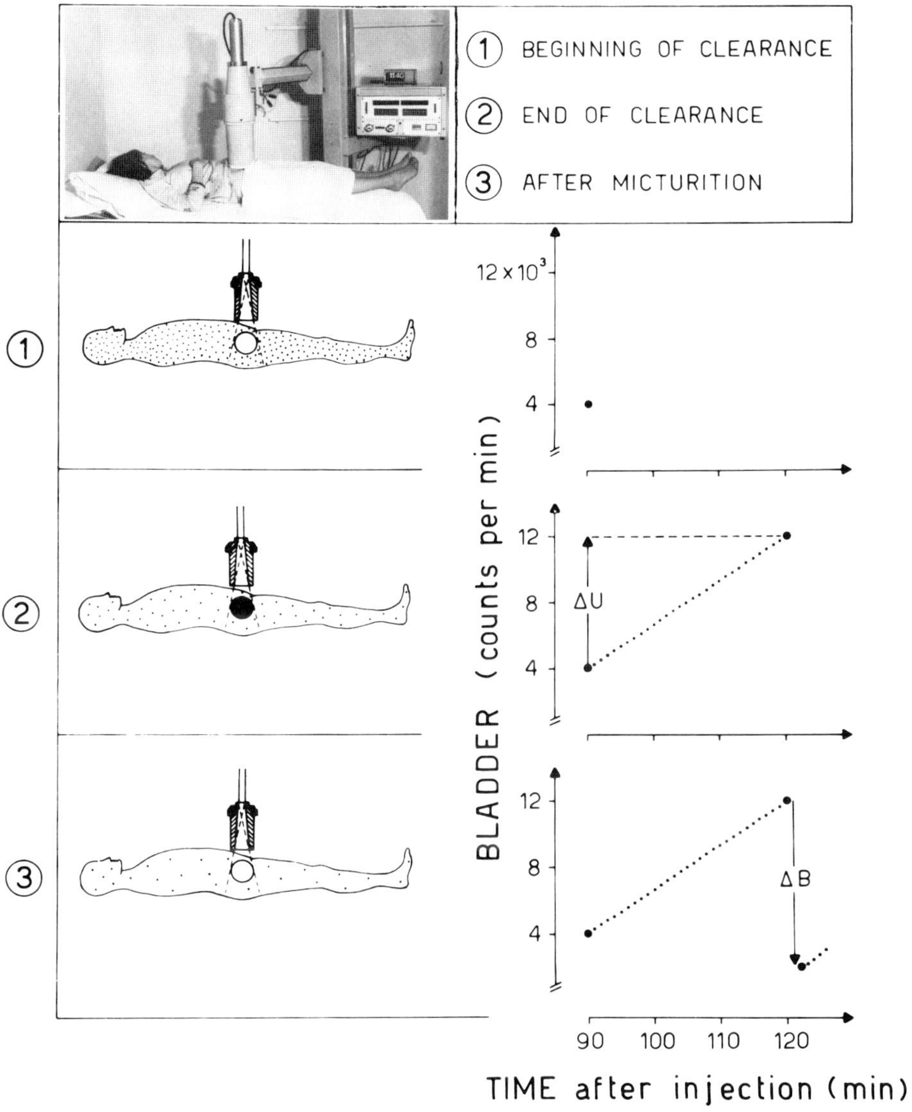

Figure 4–2
The bladder cumulative method for the measurement of total renal clearance (right plus left kidney). *Step 1: Beginning of clearance.* The diffusion of the tracer in the body is completed and dynamic equilibrium is attained. The result of the first measurement by external counting of bladder radioactivity is shown. *Step 2: End of clearance.* The body radioactivity has decreased, and a significant aliquot of radioactivity has accumulated in the bladder. The entire bladder accumulation curve has been recorded. ΔU indicates the amount of radioactivity accumulated in the bladder during the clearance. *Step 3: After micturition.* The bladder is empty. ΔB indicates the decrease of the external counting rate over the bladder due to vesical emptying.

from a vein of the contralateral arm in a heparinized syringe (to avoid radioactive contamination of the sample).

120 The clearance period ends.

120–122 For measurement of the calibration factor, the patient is asked to urinate and the urine is collected. After micturition the patient lies down again and the counter is repositioned. If the subject has been instructed properly, the whole operation (micturition and reposition of the counter) is completed within 2 minutes.

122–127 The radioactivity of the bladder is again measured at 1-minute counting intervals for 5 more minutes. The urine volume is then measured, the blood is centrifuged, and an aliquot of both urine and plasma is counted in duplicate in the same well-type counter.

At the end of the examination the patient is asked to drink freely during the subsequent 6 hours and to urinate frequently in order to reduce the radiation-absorbed dose.

The method described above for measuring GFR does not vary when different tracers are used, except insofar as the injected dose is concerned. In those instances in which a tracer with a shorter half-life is employed (e.g., [^{99m}Tc] DTPA), the dose must be greater. When [^{131}I] Hippuran is used for the measurement of ERPF, a slight modification of the method is employed. In fact, Hippuran attains equilibrium more rapidly and the rate of its plasma disappearance curve is faster in comparison with the glomerular tracers. For these reasons, it is recommended that higher doses of Hippuran be used (about 1.2 μCi/kg body weight) than of [^{131}I] diatrizoate. It is also advisable to begin the clearance after the fiftieth minute following the injection (instead of the ninetieth minute as in GFR).

CALCULATION. The data required for the calculation of GFR by the bladder cumulative method are as follows (derived from the schema in Figure 4–2):

1. Bladder radioactivity at the beginning of the clearance period: 4000 cpm
2. Bladder radioactivity at the end of the clearance period: 12,000 cpm
3. Bladder radioactivity after micturition: 2000 cpm
4. Urine radioactivity: 20,000 cpm/ml
5. Volume of urine: 300 ml
6. Plasma radioactivity: 2000 cpm/ml
7. Duration of the clearance period: 30 min

The increment in bladder radioactivity during the clearance period, ΔU, is given in this example:

$$12{,}000 - 4000 = 8000$$

If the increment of bladder radioactivity is regular (as observed in a great majority of the patients examined), ΔU can be simply calculated as the difference between the actual counting values. However, when the passage of urine into the bladder is less regular, it may be necessary to interpolate the bladder counting curve and to calculate ΔU as the difference between the interpolated values. For this reason, in every patient the time course of bladder radioactivity is measured during the entire clearance period and not only at the beginning and at the end.

The calibration factor, *k,* is given by the ratio of the urine radioactivity times the urine volume (ΔE) over the difference between the bladder count rate at the end of the clearance period and that after micturition (ΔB). It is therefore

$$\frac{20{,}000 \times 300}{12{,}000 - 2000} = 600$$

If the time required for micturition is short enough (2 to 3 minutes), it is sufficient to calculate the decrement of bladder radioactivity following micturition as the difference between the actual counting rate values (as in the preceding example). However, if the required time is longer, it is necessary to extrapolate the bladder radioactivity curve during the clearance period up to the point at which counting over the bladder is started again after micturition and to take the extrapolated value as the value of bladder radioactivity at the end of the clearance period. Similarly, if the bladder curve after micturition has a regular course, the initial counting value may be taken as the measurement of the residual bladder radioactivity. If the course is irregular, this value has to be obtained by interpolation.

The product $\Delta U \times k$, the numerator of Equation 6 (see under Rationale), is therefore

$$8000 \times 600 = 4{,}800{,}000$$

The integral of plasma concentration in the denominator of Equation 6 is given, as discussed above, by the product of plasma radioactivity at the middle of the clearance period $[P(T\frac{1}{2})]$ times the duration of the clearance itself. In this example it is

$$2000 \times 30 = 60{,}000$$

GFR, the ratio between total radioactivity eliminated through the kidneys during the clearance period (corrected by the calibration factor) and plasma radioactivity at the middle of the clearance period times duration of the clearance (see Equation 6) is then

$$\frac{4{,}800{,}000}{60{,}000} = 80 \text{ ml/min.}$$

DISCUSSION. Before its routine use in diagnostics, the bladder cumulative method was compared in a large number of cases to the conventional method; the results of the two techniques are in agreement [5, 7, 15, 16, 18]. Later the method was employed for the measurement of GFR in hospitalized and ambulatory patients of different ages and body sizes and with different degrees of renal function. Up to the present at our Kidney Service, more than 18,000 GFR measurements have been carried out using this method without any significant inconveniences being encountered.

Like the plasma clearance method, the bladder cumulative method is important because it allows one to measure renal function with a single intravenous injection of tracer and without vesical catheterization. Since its execution is rather simple, it can be carried out by nurses or technicians.

In contrast to the plasma clearance method, the bladder cumulative method does not require an exact determination of the administered dose of tracer. It does involve the need for obtaining, at the end of the clearance period, a certain amount of urine by free micturition. However, it is not necessary for the patient to empty the bladder completely; it is necessary to collect only that quantity of urine needed to determine a significant decrease of activity by external bladder counting. Consequently, this method can also be used in patients with incomplete voiding.

The calculation of results is definitely less time-consuming with the bladder cumulative method than with the plasma clearance method.

An important advantage of our technique is that it gives a direct measurement of renal clearance, unlike the methods based on the plasma disappearance curve. In fact, plasma clearance is equal to renal clearance if the kidneys represent the only way of eliminating the tracer. Thus the bladder cumulative method lends itself well to the use of the different radioactive tracers available, even when these tracers are eliminated to a significant extent by extrarenal pathways (as in patients with low renal function).

In some instances the bladder cumulative method can give false results, for example, in patients with urinary incontinence, vesical malformations, and vesicoureteric reflux. In the last two conditions, part of the radioactive urine can be situated outside the field of the bladder counter. False results can also occur in obstructive uropathy (where the passage of urine from pelvis to bladder is irregular) and rarely in patients with pelvic kidney, where the ectopic kidney can be partially situated in the field of the vesical detector. A notably irregular bladder accumulation curve leads one to suspect the existence of abnormalities that can easily be demonstrated by radiological methods (e.g., intravenous pyelography, voiding cystourethrography).

For both the bladder cumulative and the plasma clearance methods, the radiation dose to the patient is within a range that is quite acceptable for use in adults and children.

In our experience with both tests, the bladder cumulative method is better understood and accepted by the patient. Consequently, it lends itself well to repetitive tests, particularly on an outpatient basis. Therefore, in our opinion the bladder cumulative method is preferable to the plasma clearance method (and to the various modifications of the latter) for two reasons: it gives a direct measurement of renal function, and it has a better clinical applicability. We are now in the process of standardizing this method in order to obtain the simultaneous measurement of GFR and ERPF (and the resulting filtration fraction) because of the keen clinical interest in this determination.

Measurement of Differential Renal Function

The measurement of divided renal function is indicated in the evaluation of hypertensive patients with unilateral renal disease, such as renovascular hypertension (RVH) or unilateral pyelonephritis (PN). This measurement is currently carried out by determining the clearance of each kidney by means of bilateral ureteral catheterization. With this technique it is possible to ascertain, along with the functional capacity of each kidney, the type of unilateral renal disease. This possibility is based on the glomerulotubular imbalance of the ischemic kidney, which determines an increased tubular reabsorption of water and consequently a urinary hyperconcentration of nonreabsorbable substances. However, the method of bilateral ureteral catheterization can be used in only a limited number of patients due to the inconveniences of catheterization. In fact, leakage of urine into the bladder caused unreliable results in some of the cases observed. Furthermore, ureteral catheterization exposes the patient to notable risks such as pain, hematuria, and infection. All these factors justify research into new, noninvasive methods for the measurement of unilateral renal function.

A rather simple method that gives a clinically useful estimate of renal function is that proposed by Raynaud [44], which is based on the measurement of the mercury renal uptake level using $^{197}HgCl_2$. This technique provides figures that can be used to judge the impairment of individual kidneys without reference to the usual parameters of renal function (GFR and ERPF).

By means of another noninvasive technique, the stop-flow method, it seems possible to measure the function of each kidney and simultaneously to ascertain the type of renal disease. Since the instrumentation and the procedure for the stop-flow method have recently been described in detail [4], only a brief outline is given here. The procedure is based on the measurement by external counting of the increase in radioactivity recorded over each kidney during a venous infusion of a gamma-emitting tracer eliminated through the kidney, when urine flow to the bladder is stopped. The situation under which such a measurement can be performed is represented schematically in Figure 4–3. An infusion of suitable tracers (generally [^{131}I] diatrizoate or [^{99m}Tc] DTPA for GFR, [^{131}I] Hippuran for ERPF) is performed intravenously. Simultaneously, a counter over each kidney detects renal activity and a third counter records the activity accumulated in the bladder.

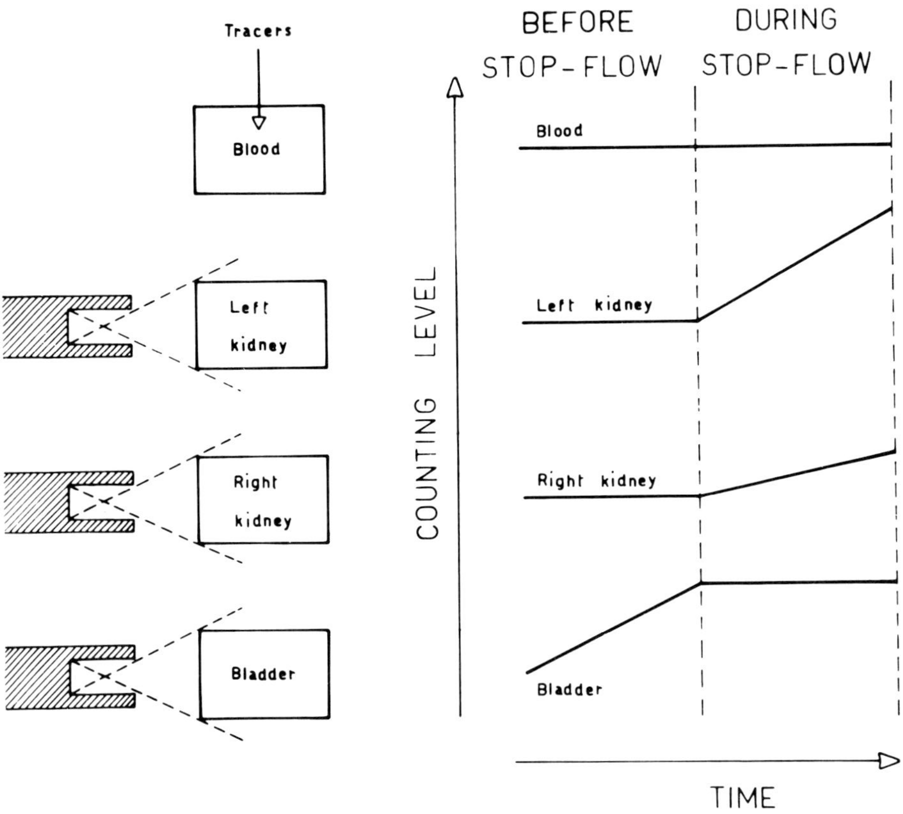

Figure 4–3
The stop-flow method for the measurement of divided renal clearance. A difference in function between the two kidneys (i.e., a reduced function of the right kidney) can be noted.

During the period of free-flow, after constant levels of activity in the blood are attained, the activity over both kidneys remains constant, whereas bladder activity increases progressively with time. During the period of stop-flow (indicated as broken lines in Fig. 4–3), as the urinary flow to the bladder is blocked, blood activity remains unaltered and the counting over each kidney increases progressively at a rate that is proportional to the functional activity of each organ. Thus, a difference in function will be manifested by an unequal activity between both kidneys (as shown in Fig. 4–3), and the difference will be proportional to the renal clearance, i.e.,

$$\Delta L : \Delta R = Cl_L : Cl_R \qquad (1)$$

where ΔL and ΔR are the increase of radioactivity over the left and right kidneys, respectively, and Cl_L and Cl_R are the left and right clearances.

The unilateral clearance (for example, of the left kidney) may be obtained from Equation 1, as follows:

$$Cl_L = \frac{\Delta L}{\Delta L + \Delta R} \times \text{Total clearance} \qquad (2)$$

The total clearance is generally measured before the stop-flow by the bladder cumulative method described above or by the conventional method.

Considerable experience with this technique has proved its reliability for the measurement of unilateral renal function [4, 6, 10, 12, 13]. Recently we considered the possibility of also employing the method to ascertain the type of unilateral renal disease. This recent research is based on the observation that in RVH the filtration fraction of the ischemic kidney is significantly lower than that of the contralateral one, whereas in PN there is no difference between the two sides [4, 8, 9].

We are now investigating the possibility of employing the stop-flow method for the simultaneous measurement of GFR (by [^{99m}Tc] DTPA) and ERPF (with [^{131}I] Hippuran), and then of the filtration fraction; the preliminary results seem promising [4].

In contrast to any other noninvasive method proposed up to now, the stop-flow method seems to be suitable both for measuring the functional capacity of each kidney and for defining the type of unilateral renal disease.

Acknowledgment

Dr. Michael A. De Luca (Chief, Pharmacy Service, U.S. Army Hospital, Leghorn, Italy) is gratefully thanked for his valuable help and criticism in the preparation of this chapter.

References

1. Berlyne, G. M., Varley, H., Nilwarangkur, S., et al. Endogenous-creatinine clearance and glomerular-filtration rate. *Lancet* 2:874, 1964.
2. Bianchi, C. Valore comparativo nell'indagine nefrografica del diodrast, dell'hypaque e del PAI marcati con ^{131}I. *Minerva Nucl.* 5:157, 1961.
3. Bianchi, C. Measurement of the Glomerular Filtration Rate. In M. D. Blaufox (Ed.), *Evaluation of Renal Function and Disease with Radionuclides.* Basel: Karger, 1972. Pp. 21–53.
4. Bianchi, C., Bonadio, M., Donadio, C., et al. Filtration fraction in unilateral hypertensive renal disease and a new noninvasive method for its measurement. *Contrib. Nephrol.* 11:29, 1978.
5. Bianchi, C., Coli, A., Gallucci, L., et al. The measurement of glomerular filtration rate in children by ^{131}I-hypaque and external counting. *J. Nucl. Biol. Med.* 11:144, 1967.
6. Bianchi, C., Coli, A., Giannotti, P., et al. A new approach to the measurement

of divided renal plasma flow by I^{131}-Hippuran and external counting in humans. *Radioaktive Isotope in Klinik und Forschung,* Vol. 7, pp. 136–144 (München/Berlin: Urban and Schwarzenberg, 1966).
7. Bianchi, C., Coli, A., Meozzi, A., et al. The glomerular filtration rate in clinical practice: The reliability of the hypaque-I^{131} and external counting method. Proc. Int. Congr. *Radioisotopes in the diagnosis of diseases of the kidneys and urinary tract,* Liège, 1967, pp. 161–164; ICS 178 (Amsterdam: Excerpta Medica, 1967).
8. Bianchi, C., Coli, A., Palla, R., et al. Alterazioni emodinamiche renali nelle nefropatie monolaterali con ipertensione arteriosa. *Boll. Soc. Ital. Cardiol.* 20:1169, 1975.
9. Bianchi, C., Coli, A., Palla, R., et al. Renal hemodynamic changes in unilateral hypertensive kidney diseases. *Kidney Int.* 10:185, 1976.
10. Bianchi, C., Coli, A., Palla, R., et al. Unilateral Renal Clearances by External Counting in the Study of Hypertension. In W. Horst (Ed.), *Frontiers of Nuclear Medicine.* Berlin: Springer, 1971. Pp. 272–289.
11. Bianchi, C., Coli, A., Palla, R., et al. The reliability of ^{140}La-DTPA for the determination of glomerular filtration rate in man. *J. Nucl. Biol. Med.* 17:158, 1973.
12. Bianchi, C., Coli, A., Palla, R., et al. Divided renal plasma flow measurement: The improvement of a new technique. Proc. Int. Congr. *Radioisotopes in the diagnosis of diseases of the kidneys and urinary tract,* Liège, 1967, pp. 273–277; ICS 178 (Amsterdam: Excerpta Medica, 1967).
13. Bianchi, C., Giannotti, P., and Coli, A. Studio preliminare sulla determinazione mediante radio-hippuran-^{131}I della portata plasmatica di ciascun rene nell'uomo. *Minerva Med.* 56:4224, 1965.
14. Bianchi, C., and Toni, P. Possibilità di impiego dello *o*-iodo-ippurato di sodio (hippuran), marcato con ^{131}I, per la valutazione della portata renale plasmatica. *Minerva Nucl.* 6:34, 1962.
15. Bianchi, C., and Toni, P. Mesure du taux de filtration glomérulaire chez l'homme par comptage externe, avec un indicateur émetteur de rayons gamma (Hypaque-I^{131}). *Proc. 2nd Int. Congr. Nephrol.,* Prague, 1963, pp. 517–523; ICS 78 (Amsterdam: Excerpta Medica, 1963).
16. Bianchi, C., and Toni, P. L'usage des indicateurs radioactifs et de la gammagraphie dans la mesure du débit plasmatique rénal et du taux de filtration glomérulaire. *Radioaktive Isotope in Klinik und Forschung,* Vol. 5, pp. 301–316 (München/Berlin: Urban and Schwarzenberg, 1963).
17. Bianchi, C., and Toni, P. La determinazione delle clearances renali mediante traccianti radioattivi. *Minerva Nefrol.* 10:116, 1963.
18. Bianchi, C., and Toni, P. The measurement of the renal clearance of γ-emitting tracers by the use of external counting. *Experientia* 20:148, 1964.
19. Blaufox, M. D. Compartment Analysis of the Radiorenogram and Kinetics of ^{131}I Hippuran. In M. D. Blaufox (Ed.), *Evaluation of Renal Function and Disease with Radionuclides.* Basel: Karger, 1972. Pp. 107–124.
20. Blaufox, M. D., and Merrill, J. P. Simplified Hippuran clearance: Measurement of renal function in man with simplified Hippuran clearances. Nephron 3:274, 1966.
21. Blaufox, M. D., Potchen, E. J., and Merrill, J. P. Measurement of effective renal plasma flow in man by external counting methods. *J. Nucl. Med.* 8:77, 1967.
22. Bröchner-Mortensen, J., and Rödbro, P. Selection of routine method for determination of glomerular filtration rate in adult patients. *Scand. J. Clin. Lab. Invest.* 36:35, 1976.

23. Bröchner-Mortensen, J., and Rödbro, P. Comparison between total and renal plasma clearance of [^{51}Cr] EDTA. *Scand. J. Clin. Lab. Invest.* 36:247, 1976.
24. Bröchner-Mortensen, J., and Rödbro, P. Optimum time of blood sampling for determination of glomerular filtration rate by single injection [^{51}Cr] EDTA plasma clearance. *Scand. J. Clin. Lab. Invest.* 36:795, 1976.
25. Burry, H. C., and Dieppe, P. A. Apparent reduction of endogenous creatinine clearance by salicylate treatment. *Br. Med. J.* 2:16, 1976.
26. Chamberlain, M. J., and Sherwood, T. The extrarenal excretion of diatrizoate in renal failure. *Br. J. Radiol.* 39:765, 1966.
27. Chanard, J., and Masson, M. Nouvelle méthode de mesure de la clearance rénale de l'acide para-amino-hippurique: Technique simplifiée sans recueil d'urine. *Nouv. Presse Med.* 1:1905, 1972.
28. Chantler, C., Garnett, E. S., Parsons, V., et al. Glomerular filtration rate measurement in man by the single injection method using ^{51}Cr-EDTA. *Clin. Sci.* 37:169, 1969.
29. Cohen, M. L., Patel, J. K., and Baxter, D. L. External monitoring and plasma disappearance for the determination of renal function: Comparison of effective renal plasma flow and glomerular filtration rate. *Pediatrics* 48:377, 1971.
30. Dodge, W. F., Travis, L. B., and Daeschner, C. W. Comparison of endogenous creatinine clearance with inulin clearance. *Am. J. Dis. Child.* 113:683, 1967.
31. Favre, H. Déterminations des fonctions rénales par la technique de l'injection unique: Analyse statistique du modèle bicompartimental proposé par Sapirstein. *J. Urol. Néphrol.* 79:1007, 1973.
32. Favre, H., Falbriard, A., Busset, R., et al. Estimation de la filtration glomérulaire par décroissance plasmatique de l'EDTA ^{51}Cr au moyen de deux prélèvements sanguins tardifs. *J. Urol. Néphrol.* 75:929, 1969.
33. Fisher, M., and Veall, N. Glomerular filtration rate estimation based on a single blood sample. *Br. Med. J.* 2:542, 1975.
34. Hagstam, K. E., Nordenfelt, I., Svensson, L., et al. Comparison of different methods for determination of glomerular filtration rate in renal disease. *Scand. J. Clin. Lab. Invest.* 34:31, 1974.
35. Heierli, C., Sauer, R., Fridrich, R., et al. The value of a simplified slope clearance of Hippuran for the estimation of the renal plasma flow. *Helv. Med. Acta* 36:51, 1971.
36. Hood, B., Attman, P., Ahlmén, J., et al. Renal hemodynamics and limitations of creatinine clearance in determining filtration rate in glomerular disease. *Scand. J. Urol. Nephrol.* 5:154, 1971.
37. Kim, K. E., Onesti, G., Ramirez, O., et al. Creatinine clearance in renal disease: A reappraisal. *Br. Med. J.* 4:11, 1969.
38. Klopper, J. F., Hauser, W., Atkins, H. L., et al. Evaluation of ^{99m}Tc-DTPA for the measurement of glomerular filtration rate. *J. Nucl. Med.* 13:107, 1972.
39. Mailloux, L., and Gagnon, J. A. Measurement of Effective Renal Plasma Flow. In M. D. Blaufox (Ed.), *Evaluation of Renal Function and Disease with Radionuclides.* Basel: Karger, 1972. Pp. 54–70.
40. Mandel, M. J., Vidt, D. G., and Sapirstein, L. A. Disappearance of para-amino-hippuric acid from the plasma of the dog after single intravenous injection. *Am. J. Physiol.* 182:428, 1955.
41. Nelson, C. M. K., Brown, R. C., and Culp, D. A. The extrarenal excretion of urographic contrast material. *J. Urol.* 110:109, 1973.
42. Price, M. Comparison of creatinine clearance to inulin clearance in the determination of glomerular filtration rate. *J. Urol.* 107:339, 1972.
43. Ram, M. D., Holroyd, M., and Chisholm, G. D. Measurement of glomerular filtration-rate using ^{131}I-diatrizoate. *Lancet* 1:397, 1969.

44. Raynaud, C. A technique for the quantitative measurement of the function of each kidney. *Semin. Nucl. Med.* 4:51, 1974.
45. Razzak, M. A., Botti, R. E., MacIntyre, W. J., et al. Determination of renal blood flow by external monitoring of radiohippuran disappearance. *J. Urol.* 100:209, 1968.
46. Rosenbaum, J. L., Kramer, M. S., Raja, R. M., et al. Determination of inulin and p-aminohippurate clearances without urine collection. *Nephron* 10:347, 1973.
47. Sakai, T., Leumann, E. P., and Holliday, M. A. Single injection clearance in children. *Pediatrics* 44:905, 1969.
48. Sapirstein, L. A., Vidt, D. G., Mandel, M. J., et al. Volumes of distribution and clearances of intravenously injected creatinine in the dog. *Am. J. Physiol.* 181:330, 1955.
49. Schoutens, A., and Destailleur, G. Essai de mesure simultanée de la filtration glomérulaire et du débit plasmatique rénal par injection unique d'hypaque et d'hippuran radioactifs. *Acta Clin. Belg.* 23:23, 1968.
50. Segall, H. D. Gallbladder visualization following the injection of diatrizoate. *Am. J. Roentgenol.* 107:21, 1969.
51. Silk, M., and Wagner, H. N., Jr. Measurement of glomerular filtration rate in man by external monitoring of the clearance of radioactive vitamin B_{12}. *Invest. Urol.* 3:609, 1966.
52. Wagoner, R. D., Tauxe, W. N., Maher, F. T., et al. Measurement of effective renal plasma flow with sodium iodohippurate I^{131}. *J.A.M.A.* 187:811, 1964.
53. Winterborn, M. H., Beetham, R., and White, R. H. R. Comparison of plasma disappearance and standard clearance techniques for measuring glomerular filtration rate in children with and without vesico-ureteric reflux. *Clin. Nephrol.* 7:262, 1977.

5. Evaluation of Renal Function in Far Advanced Renal Failure and in Intermittent Dialysis

William J. Johnson

Current clinical practice requires that the physician understand and evaluate renal function. In the past, small differences in renal function during the terminal stages of renal disease evoked little interest because the methods of treatment were largely ineffective in relieving symptoms of uremia or in prolonging the life of the patient. During the past two decades, however, a marked improvement has occurred in dietary, diuretic, and antihypertensive treatment of the patient with advanced renal failure. Dialysis is now well established as an effective method for providing symptomatic relief and extending the life of patients with advanced renal failure. New antibiotics have been introduced that are more effective in controlling infection but are potentially ototoxic and nephrotoxic for this group of patients. These advances require more precise estimates of renal function in order to enable the physician to prescribe the optimal dietary, chemotherapeutic, and dialysis program; to determine more precisely when dialysis should be initiated; and to design the most desirable regimen of dialysis treatment.

During the early phases of chronic renal disease, the manifestations of renal impairment vary greatly. For example, in pyelonephritis the course may be punctuated by evidence of infection, early loss of concentrating power, mild proteinuria, and mild salt wasting, whereas in chronic membranous glomerulonephritis, severe proteinuria, sodium retention, edema formation, and hypertension may dominate the clinical pattern. Eventually, during the late stages of renal failure, the various diseases that lead to progressive renal destruction merge into a common pattern of deranged excretory and regulatory function; this pattern reflects similarities in the altered structure and function of the atrophic kidneys regardless of the specific cause. The reason for this similarity is that all chronic renal diseases result in a reduction in the number of nephrons. In addition, there is disruption of the normal architecture of the kidney involving the long nephrons that penetrate the renal papillae, their accompanying vasa vasorum, and their surrounding medullary interstitium, with a consequent loss of the usual countercurrent concentration mechanism. The remaining functioning nephrons enlarge, but their function is altered because of the excessive solute load excreted by each nephron. As a result of these changes, the excretory function of the kidney is well preserved even in advanced renal failure, but the capacity of the kidney to regulate the volume and composition of body fluids under various stresses is severely limited [38]. In addition, relatively small reductions in extracellular volume (equivalent to 1 to 3 liters of saline) may result in significant reductions in the glomerular filtration rate (GFR) [22, 28]. Therefore, measurements of GFR must be performed under conditions of optimal hydration and sodium balance without inducing water intoxication, acute pulmonary edema, or hypertensive crises.

In patients with normal renal function, the volume of urine excreted each day represents a small fraction of the volume formed by the glomerular filtrate (for example, a volume of 1 to 2 liters of urine is excreted for each 180 liters filtered), whereas in renal failure, it may represent a large proportion of the filtered load (for example, in a patient with a GFR of 1 ml/min, a urine volume of 1.4 L/day approaches the entire glomerular filtrate formed by the kidneys). Serial measurements of the urine volume in such a patient provide an extremely sensitive indicator of renal function and, if combined with an accurate daily weight and blood pressure determined in an upright position, a useful estimate of the state of hydration and sodium balance.

Tests of Urinary Concentration and Dilution

Impairment of the concentrating ability of the kidney under conditions of water deprivation occurs early in renal disease—long before azotemia develops. Pyelonephritis, polycystic renal disease, medullary cystic disease, analgesic nephropathy, and sickle cell disease are only a few of the disorders that characteristically show an early concentrating defect [5]. The mechanism for the concentrating abnormality varies, depending on the type of renal disease and the stage of renal insufficiency. In chronic renal failure, a relative solute diuresis among surviving nephrons may be the basis for the defect [5], whereas in interstitial nephropathy and sickle cell disease, perturbation of the medullary interstitial concentration gradient occurs [31]. Measurement of the maximal concentrating ability is hazardous in chronic renal failure (GFR less than 20 ml/min). Although polyuria is rarely extreme, such patients have an increased obligatory water loss and readily develop extracellular volume depletion, with a large reduction in GFR when fluids are restricted overnight or for longer intervals.

The ability of the kidney to dilute the urine is present until late in the course of renal failure. Although the administration of a water load increases urine volume, the response is sluggish; several days instead of several hours may be required to restore water balance, and water intoxication may result. An increase in body weight and a decrease in serum sodium concentration are reliable signs of water excess, if the patient does not also have hyperglycemia or hyperlipidemia or if he has not been given mannitol intravenously. Testing for maximal diluting capacity is hazardous in the patient with advanced renal failure. Moreover, it does not provide useful information because solute excretion is not significantly enhanced by water loading [34].

Tests of Acid-Base Regulation and Renal Tubular Insufficiency

Most patients with chronic renal failure excrete a urine with a pH of 6.0 or lower. Failure to lower the pH may be due to bacterial infection with urea-splitting organisms, delayed testing of a contaminated urine specimen, or renal tubular disease with bicarbonate wasting. In chronic renal failure, the ability to excrete nonvolatile acid in the form of phosphate buffers (titratable acidity) is well preserved, but the ability to generate ammonia and to excrete acid as ammonium ions is severely limited [11]. Generally, these changes can be explained by a decrease in the number of functioning nephrons, although occasionally they are best explained by an inherited or acquired tubular defect. In the latter explanation, the systemic acidosis is out of proportion to the reduction in GFR, and examination of the urine may show evidence of bicarbonate wasting. As a result of these changes, the pH of arterial blood is usually normal or slightly below normal in the chronically uremic patient, but the buffer capacity, as indicated by a plasma bicarbonate of 15 to 20 mEq/L, is reduced. For this reason, acid loads should not be administered to such patients in an effort to differentiate renal tubular acidosis from acidosis due to reduced numbers of functioning nephrons.

Patients with chronic renal failure often have an increase in the amounts of glucose, amino acids, and oxalate in the urine, rendering these tests of little value in identifying specific tubular defects. Measurement of the tubular reabsorption of phosphate as an index of parathyroid hormone activity has been largely replaced by the more direct radioimmunoassay of the parathyroid hormone itself.

Other Tests of Renal Function

The excretion of phenolsulfonphthalein (PSP) depends on renal plasma flow and proximal tubular function, thus providing a method of measuring their function. When azotemia supervenes, PSP excretion decreases to such an extent that at a GFR of less than 20 ml/min, PSP excretion is minimal, and further changes are too small to be measured accurately [23]. In situations in which renal plasma flow measurements are important, the para-aminohippurate clearance may be performed, or if separate indexes of renal function are needed, the radioisotope renogram may be helpful in showing which kidney has the predominant functional capacity.

Measurement of the solute content of the urine is of little value in estimating renal function. During the polyuric phases, the amounts of nitrogen, creatinine, sodium, and potassium in the urine approach normal [32]. After the onset of oliguria, usually after dialysis has been initiated, the amounts of these solutes excreted are negligible, and the residual renal function that remains is more accurately reflected by the GFR or the volume of urine excreted per day than in its solute content.

For all these reasons, the technique of serial measurements of the GFR is the only suitable method for monitoring changes in renal function in the patient with advanced renal failure. Unfortunately, there is no direct method for measuring GFR. Available techniques depend on measurements of the rate at which a substance excreted solely by glomerular filtration is cleared from the plasma.

Techniques for Measuring GFR

Preparation for Measurement of GFR

Special problems exist in accurately measuring the GFR in patients with advanced renal failure. There is a complex relationship in such patients among the sodium intake, blood pressure, and renal function. The GFR should be measured when the patient is in a state of sodium balance and when his blood pressure is adequately controlled.

As demonstrated by the experiments of Nickel and colleagues [28] and Levin and Cade [22], the response of the patient with advanced renal failure to sodium depletion is in sharp contrast to the normal response. Sodium deprivation in a normal subject, even of as much as 500 mEq, does not lead to significant reduction of the GFR. Adaptive responses lead to a virtual disappearance of sodium from the urine as a result of tubular reabsorption of 99 percent of the filtered load of sodium. In contrast, most patients with chronic renal failure show a 30- to 60-percent reduction of GFR when given a 50-mEq intake of sodium per day. In one study, body weight decreased 1.7 kg, consistent with a decrease of 11 percent in the extracellular fluid volume [22]; none of the patients increased tubular reabsorption beyond 90 to 97 percent.

In chronic renal disease, a close relationship also exists between the extracellular volume and the blood pressure [9]: The blood pressure increases above normal when the extracellular volume or total body sodium exceeds normal or when the vascular compartment is reduced by the increased secretion of renin angiotensin or by other vasoconstrictor influences [4, 6, 9, 12].

Although almost all patients with chronic renal disease excrete more sodium than normal under conditions of salt deprivation, most patients will adapt to moderate restriction in sodium (90 mEq/day) and, on such a program, will stabilize their total body sodium and blood pressure at reasonably normal levels. An increase in sodium intake to more than 100 mEq/day results in sodium retention, hypertension, and an increase in sodium excretion.

About 20 percent of patients with chronic renal disease are normotensive and excrete 200 mEq or more of sodium each day [9, 10, 40]. Generally, these are patients with tubular-interstitial types of renal disease such as medullary cystic disease, interstitial nephritis, bilateral vesicoureteral reflux, hydronephrosis, and postobstructive nephropathy [38].

A small proportion of patients, perhaps 5 to 10 percent, experience severe hypertension and sodium retention, excreting less than 20 mEq of sodium per day. For the most part, these are patients with malignant nephrosclerosis, rapidly progressive or necrotizing glomerulonephritis, or renal artery occlusive disease [10]. Such patients show evidence of severe vasoconstriction and excessively high renin activity, together with severe hypertension without clinical evidence of sodium excess. Although reduction in blood pressure by means of furosemide, sodium restriction, and antihypertensive drugs undoubtedly reduces renal perfusion and GFR temporarily, it is more important to control the hypertension to prevent further vascular damage than it is to increase the GFR by salt loading in such patients.

The following approach is helpful in determining a reasonably safe balance among sodium intake, hypertension, and optimal glomerular filtration rates. If the patient obviously has a history of excessive external gastrointestinal losses or physical findings and blood chemical values that are consistent with fluid and electrolyte depletion, these deficits should be replaced. However, if there is obvious evidence of extracellular fluid excess, this condition should be corrected by restriction of sodium and administration of furosemide. Usually, neither of these extremes is apparent, and the patient should be given 90 mEq of sodium. If body weight, blood pressure in the standing position, and serial plasma creatinine levels remain stable while the patient is on this regimen, nothing further need be done. However, if there is any evidence of sodium depletion, poorly controlled acidosis (plasma bicarbonate less than 18 mEq/L), orthostatic hypotension, or an increasing plasma creatinine level, additional sodium may be given either as sodium bicarbonate (1 to 3 gm) or as a combination of sodium bicarbonate (1 gm) and sodium chloride (2 gm), depending on the severity of acidosis. Even in the patients with a salt-losing tendency, dietary sodium can be reduced gradually over a period of 1 to 3 months without compromising renal function [8].

During the administration of the test, the patient should drink several glasses of water to promote a high urinary output. The time interval during which the urine is collected should be long enough to permit the patient to accumulate sufficient urine to distend the bladder, prompting complete emptying without catheterization.

Use of Plasma Urea and Creatinine as Indexes of GFR

Plasma urea and creatinine levels are commonly used as indexes of GFR. For this purpose, it is assumed that the plasma concentration of either of these products of nitrogen metabolism is inversely related to its excretion. Inasmuch as the clearance equals excretion divided by plasma concentration, this assumption is valid only if the production of the substance is constant (leading to a stable plasma concentration during collection of the urine), the excretion is constant, and the substance is excreted only by the kidney, being freely filterable by the glomerulus and neither secreted nor reabsorbed by the renal tubule.

The main problem with the measurement of urea is the extreme variability in its production. Because urea is the chief end product of nitrogen metabolism, its plasma concentration depends on the dietary intake of protein and the caloric balance; on the endogenous catabolism of protein as a result of stress, trauma, infection, or adrenocortical activity; on the absorption of products of intestinal bleeding; on the ability of the liver to synthesize urea; and on the effects of drugs such as tetracycline, steroids, and thyroxine, as well as on the GFR [16]. As a result of all these factors, the levels of plasma urea can fluctuate markedly without changes in the GFR. The measurement of urea is useful only as an indicator of dietary compliance and the catabolic state of the patient and as an estimate of the severity of nitrogen retention.

The plasma creatinine level more closely fulfills the role of a practical clinical index of GFR. In a given patient, the rate of production is reasonably constant, varying only 10 to 15 percent from the mean value from day to day [35]. Nearly all the creatinine excreted in the urine is derived from the creatinine of muscle, and the rate of production appears to be a function of the muscle mass [39]. Even with extreme variation in meat consumption, creatinine excretion varies only 10 percent [3]. In a given patient, some decrease in creatinine excretion occurs with extreme muscle wasting or advanced old age [3, 33]. As the plasma creatinine level increases, tubular secretion relative to glomerular filtration increases, and entry of creatinine into the intestine and its degradation to sarcosine and other products may prevent plasma creatinine levels from increasing in proportion to a decrease in the GFR [19]. Under these conditions, the values for plasma creatinine may overestimate the GFR by as much as a factor of 4 [20, 36] in a large proportion of patients.

Methods for Determining the GFR

The substances chosen for measuring the GFR must be freely filterable by the glomerulus and neither secreted nor reabsorbed by the renal tubule. An impressive body of evidence indicates that inulin, a fructose polymer, meets these criteria and is the most accurate index of glomerular filtration in man. Unfortunately, the use of inulin is too demanding for routine clinical purposes. Complicated analytical methods are required for its measurement, and a constant intravenous infusion is required in order to maintain stable plasma concentrations.

Numerous other methods have been employed for the measurement of glomerular filtration in man; they include the clearances of mannitol and other hexitols, allantoin clearance, thiosulfate clearance, and the clearances of [^{14}C] inulin, ferrocyanide, cyanocobalamin, [^{51}Cr] EDTA, [^{169}Yb] diethylenetriaminepenta-acetic acid (DTPA), [^{125}I] iothalamate, urea, and endogenous creatinine. Only the last four substances obviate the need for continuous infusion or special procedures in preparing the material or the patient. [^{125}I] iothalamate is easily and accurately measured by radioisotope techniques and can be detected in the bladder urine by these techniques, ensuring complete emptying of the bladder at the end of the collection period.

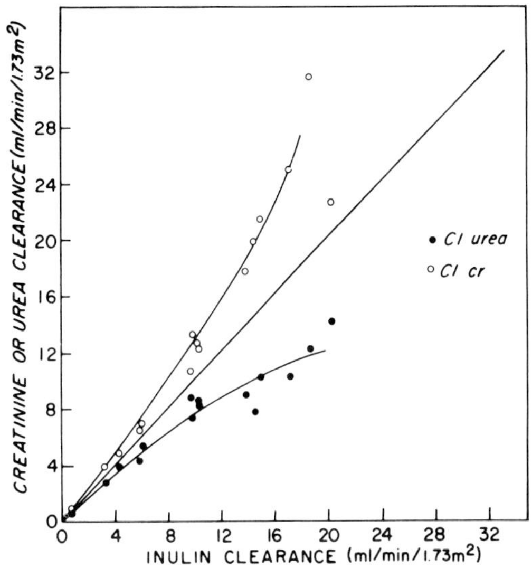

Figure 5–1
Urea or creatinine clearance compared with simultaneous inulin clearance. Points on straight line indicate 1:1 correspondence. (Reprinted, by permission, from H. Lubowitz, E. Slatopolsky, S. Shankel, R. E. Rieselbach, and N. S. Bricker, Glomerular filtration rate determination in patients with chronic renal disease. *J.A.M.A.* 199:252, 1967. Copyright 1967, American Medical Association.)

Urea clearance has been used in the assessment of renal function for many years. However, at higher levels of renal function it grossly underestimates the GFR [24] (Fig. 5–1). This occurs because urea diffuses passively out of the proximal convoluted tubule due to a concentration gradient created by the reabsorption of sodium and water. In chronic renal disease, the fractional reabsorption of salt and water diminishes as the number of nephrons decreases; less urea is reabsorbed; and the urea clearance more closely approximates the inulin clearance, though even at extremely low levels of renal function, urea clearance usually remains lower than inulin clearance.

The creatinine clearance, however, exceeds the inulin clearance because creatinine is eliminated by tubular secretion as well as by glomerular filtration [20, 24, 36]. Almost all the current automated methods for measuring creatinine eliminate noncreatinine chromogens as a factor in the accuracy of the measurement. As more nephrons are destroyed, however, the ability of the kidney to maximally secrete creatinine diminishes and the creatinine clearance more closely approximates the inulin clearance (Fig. 5–1). As the plasma creatinine level increases, more creatinine enters the gastrointestinal tract and is degraded to sarcosine and other products by bacterial activity. Jones and Burnett [19] have shown that 16 to 66 percent of the creatinine formed may be eliminated by

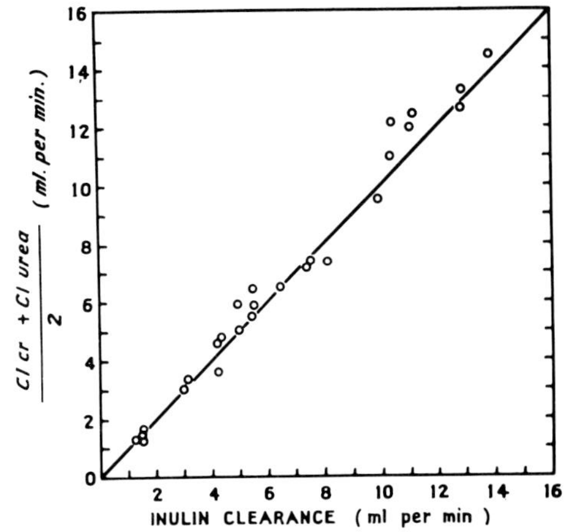

Figure 5–2
Mean urea and creatinine clearances compared with inulin clearance in patients who have inulin clearances of less than 13 ml/min (open circles). Ratio (SE) of $(C_{creat} + C_{urea})/2$ to inulin clearance = 1.009 ± 0.0045. The correlation coefficient is +0.993. (Reprinted, by permission, from S. Lavender, P. J. Hilton, and N. F. Jones, The measurement of glomerular filtration rate in renal disease. *Lancet* 2:1216, 1969.)

the gastrointestinal route. Therefore, the creatinine clearance may overestimate the GFR by as much as 10 to 40 percent [20, 24, 36, 39].

The simultaneous measurement of creatinine and urea clearances and the use of the mean value of the clearance of urea plus creatinine provide a value that corresponds reasonably well to the inulin clearance in patients with a GFR of less than 20 ml/min. Lubowitz and co-workers [24] performed the clearances using short collection periods and an indwelling catheter, but similar results are obtainable using longer collecting periods and spontaneous voiding, which is preferable for routine clinical purposes [21] (Fig. 5–2).

Another approach to measuring the GFR accurately and quickly in ambulatory patients has been the use of [^{125}I] iothalamate [1, 18, 29]. This agent may be administered subcutaneously in a single injection, can be measured accurately by scintillation counting techniques without chemical analysis using very small samples of blood and urine, requires a relatively short period of urine collection, and confirms complete emptying of the bladder by scintillation counting over the bladder, thus obviating the need for catheterization [1, 18, 29]. In addition, the test is relatively inexpensive compared with conventional creatinine and urea clearances, inulin clearance, or other radioisotope techniques (Fig. 5–3).

Many studies have demonstrated that iothalamate is handled by the kidney in a fashion similar to inulin and that the clearance of isotopically labeled

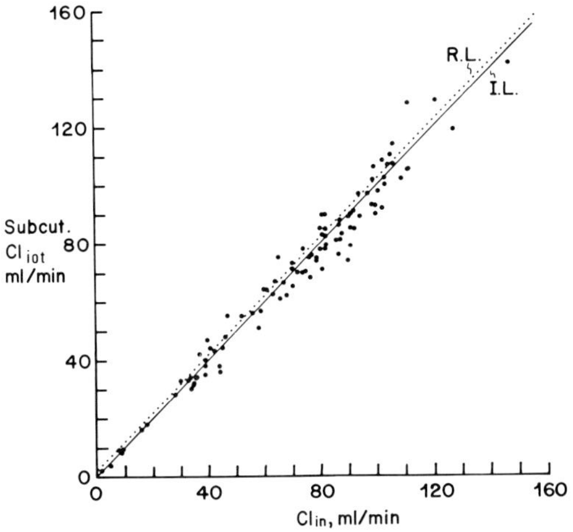

Figure 5–3
Relationship between subcutaneous clearance of [^{125}I] iothalamate (IOT) and intravenous clearance of inulin. $C_{iot} = 1.02\ C_{inulin} - 0.61$; residual standard deviation around regression = 6.37 ml/min; r = 0.982; R. L. = the regression line of the data; I. L. = the identity line. (Reprinted, by permission, from N. T. Ott, and D. M. Wilson, A simple technique for estimating glomerular filtration rate with subcutaneous injection of [^{125}I] iothalamate. *Mayo Clin. Proc.* 50:664, 1975.)

iothalamate administered by constant intravenous infusion or by single subcutaneous injection is nearly identical to the simultaneous inulin clearance [18, 29].

The many other radioisotopic techniques that have been advanced as substitutes for the clearance of inulin have not gained wide acceptance. The use of [^{57}Co] cyanocobalamin to measure GFR was introduced in 1964 and was widely employed for a while because its clearance is virtually identical to the clearance of inulin at all levels of renal function [1, 27]. Unfortunately, this agent requires constant intravenous infusion, and the materials used in the test raise the cost appreciably. Even with massive vitamin B_{12} preloading, significant binding of radioactive cyanocobalamin to plasma protein occurs. In addition, the fraction of bound cyanocobalamin varies considerably from patient to patient and increases during infusion, necessitating correction for binding in each patient and the checking of several samples of blood for binding if the collection period is prolonged [1].

The clearance of [^{51}Cr] EDTA approximates the inulin clearance, but data suggest that tubular reabsorption occurs [7, 13, 15, 41]. A number of investigators have studied the simultaneous clearances of [^{169}Yb] DTPA, [^{113m}In] DTPA, and [^{14}C] inulin, adopting a single injection technique [17, 25, 37]. The plasma clearances of [^{14}C] inulin and the chelate [^{113m}In] DTPA were virtually identical [17, 37]. A high correlation existed in clearance by [^{169}Yb]

DTPA and [^{113m}In] DTPA and with [^{113m}In] DTPA and [^{14}C] inulin, but not between the clearances of [^{169}Yb] DTPA and endogenous creatinine. The mean (SD) ratio of [^{169}Yb] DTPA to creatinine clearance was 1.221 ± 0.748 [37]. In patients with far advanced renal failure, Milutinovic and colleagues [25] found a poor correlation between [^{169}Yb] DTPA and inulin clearances, although only a limited number of measurements were made.

Many practicing clinicians question the need or usefulness of measuring the GFR in patients with advanced renal failure [14]. Although numerous clearance studies are impractical, sometimes a large discrepancy in the patient's symptoms or the untimely appearance of complications of uremia (e.g., uremic pericarditis) might be better understood by performing an iothalamate clearance rather than a creatinine clearance or a single measurement of the plasma creatinine concentration. For example, reference to Skov's publication [36] indicates a plasma creatinine level of 5.3 mg/dl in a patient with the following average plasma clearances: inulin 4.2 ml/min, creatinine 7.6 ml/min, and iothalamate 4.06 ml/min. Obviously, for such a patient dialysis is imminent or overdue when the plasma creatinine level would indicate many months or possibly years of conservative treatment and when the creatinine clearance level overestimates the GFR by a factor of 1.84.

Measurement of GFR in Patients Maintained by Intermittent Dialysis

After the induction of dialysis, residual renal function decreases. Immediately after dialysis is started and during the 24 hours after dialysis, urine flow rates usually decrease; they then increase to optimal levels on the day before the next dialysis (Fig. 5–4). The decrease in urine volume immediately after dialysis is not prevented by maintaining the osmotic load through the addition of urea to the dialysate. When urea is added, however, the interdialytic volume is somewhat higher on the second and third days after dialysis. Similarly, postdialysis oliguria is not prevented by maintenance of total body sodium, weight, and blood pressure by the administration of normal saline intravenously during dialysis, as demonstrated by Falls and colleagues [12]. These workers attributed the decreases in creatinine clearance (30%), urine sodium excretion (40%), and urine volume (12%) to reduction of the extracellular fluid volume (11%) induced by a shift of fluid into the intracellular space as plasma osmolality was reduced (6%), along with removal of urea. Some have attributed this phenomenon to removal of a natriuretic hormone during dialysis [30]. Regardless of the mechanism, there is little value in measuring the GFR during the 24 hours immediately after dialysis when it is at its lowest point.

In addition to the transient decrease in renal function that occurs immediately after dialysis treatment, there is a more gradual loss of residual renal function. Patients with the more rapidly progressive forms of renal disease and accelerated hypertension may become totally anuric within a relatively short span of weeks or months (Fig. 5–5). Total anuria also is not prevented by the maintenance of an osmotic load through the addition of urea to the dialysate nor, in

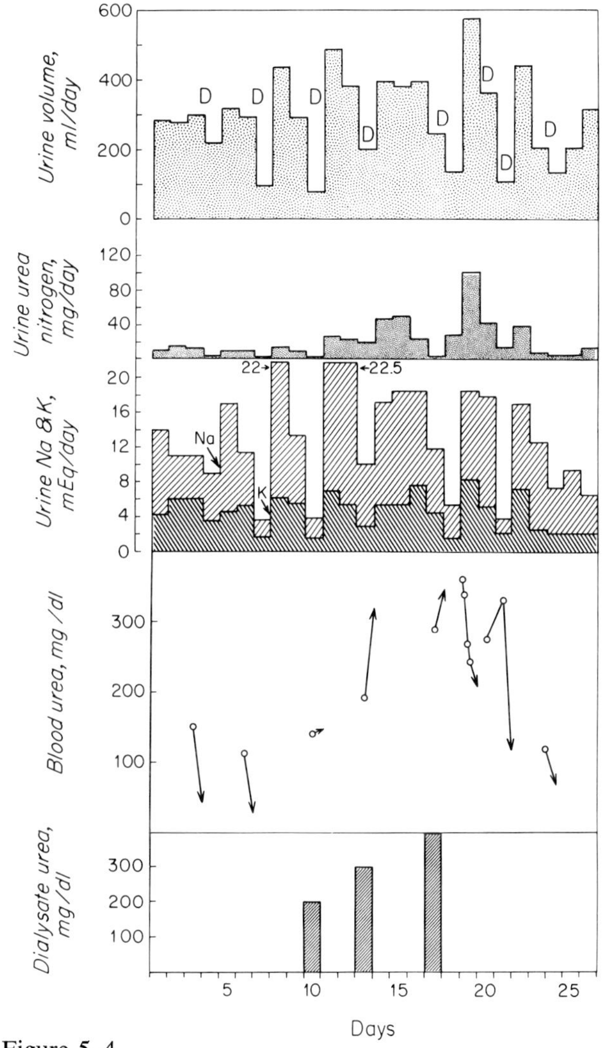

Figure 5–4
Daily urine volume, urea nitrogen, sodium, and potassium excretions in a patient maintained by intermittent hemodialysis. Note the decrease in urine volume and solute excretion after each dialysis. The addition of urea to the dialysate in an amount sufficient to increase blood urea concentration resulted in a slight increase in urine volume the day before dialysis but did not prevent postdialysis oliguria.

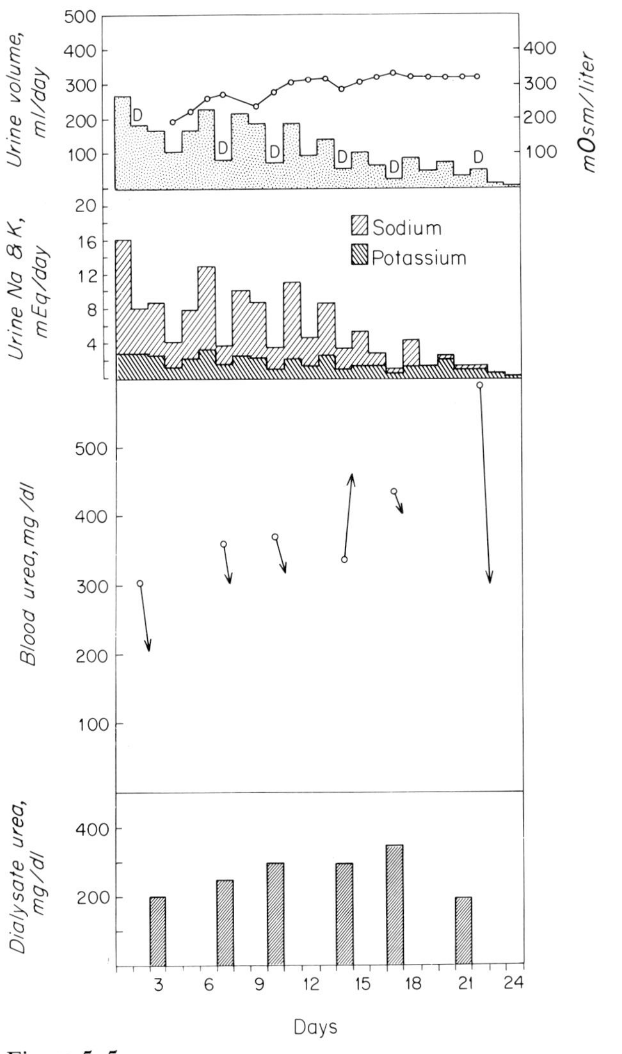

Figure 5–5
Gradual decline in urine volume and sodium and potassium excretion in a patient started on dialysis in spite of the maintenance of blood urea concentration by the addition of urea to the dialysate.

most instances, by the control of hypertension. In other patients, such as those with interstitial forms of nephritis and polycystic kidney disease, renal function may stabilize for many months and sometimes for years. Therefore, the GFR should be measured after the patient has become stabilized on dialysis and at regular intervals until the onset of anuria.

After establishment of the dialysis regimen, the plasma urea and creatinine levels increase to a peak value before dialysis, decrease in an exponential curve during the dialysis procedure, show a slight rebound during the 3 hours after the procedure due to the reestablishment of equilibrium among the various body fluid compartments, and then increase steadily during the remaining inter-dialytic period [2].

Milutinovic and co-workers [25] have shown that in the group of patients with glomerular filtration rates between 1.0 and 5.0 ml/min, the iothalamate clearance by the single injection technique correlates best with the inulin clearance. In patients with glomerular filtration values of less than 1 ml/min, the correlation of the clearances of [^{125}I] iothalamate, creatinine, urea and (urea + creatinine)/2 with the clearance of inulin was satisfactory for clinical purposes. A simple procedure is described for accurately measuring the residual glomerular filtration in patients undergoing repetitive hemodialysis.

By measuring the GFR at the onset of treatment and at regular intervals, it is possible to prescribe more precisely the frequency and duration of dialysis and the type of dialyzer to be employed. Milutinovic and co-workers [26] and Babb and colleagues [2] have advanced the idea that the amount of residual GFR in patients undergoing dialysis is a crucial variable that can effect impressive amounts of solute removal of substances in the molecular weight range of 500 to 5000. Regardless of whether or not this idea is supported by further research, it is possible in patients with appreciable renal function to reduce the duration and frequency of dialysis and therefore to reduce the cost and inconvenience of the treatment. In some patients, reduction of the frequency and length of dialysis actually leads to an improved sense of well-being. At the other extreme, accurate estimates of residual renal function in patients who have a very low GFR despite an appreciable output of urine may avoid inadequate dialysis leading to serious complications such as pericarditis and uremic neuropathy.

References

1. Anderson, C. F., Sawyer, T. K., and Cutler, R. E. Iothalamate sodium I 125 vs. cyanocobalamin Co 57 as a measure of glomerular filtration rate in man. *J.A.M.A.* 204:653, 1968.
2. Babb, A. L., Strand, M. J., Uvelli, D. A., et al. Quantitative description of dialysis treatment: A dialysis index. *Kidney Int.* 7(Suppl. 2):23, 1975.
3. Barrett, E., and Addis, T. The serum creatinine concentration of normal individuals. *J. Clin. Invest.* 26:875, 1947.

4. Blumberg, A., Nelp, W. B., Hegstrom, R. M., et al. Extracellular volume in patients with chronic renal disease treated for hypertension by sodium restriction. *Lancet* 2:69, 1967.
5. Bricker, N. S., Morrin, P. A. F., and Kime, S. W., Jr. The pathologic physiology of chronic Bright's disease: An exposition of the "intact nephron hypothesis." *Am. J. Med.* 28:77, 1960.
6. Cangiano, J. L., Ramirez-Muxó, O., Ramirez-Gonzalez, R., et al. Normal renin uremic hypertension: Study of cardiac hemodynamics, plasma volume, extracellular fluid volume, and the renin angiotensin volume. *Arch. Intern. Med.* 136:17, 1976.
7. Chantler, C., Garnett, E. S., Parsons, V., et al. Glomerular filtration rate measurement in man by the single injection method using ^{51}Cr-EDTA. *Clin. Sci.* 37:169, 1969.
8. Danovitch, G. M., Bourgoignie, J., and Bricker, N. S. Reversibility of the "salt-losing" tendency of chronic renal failure. *N. Engl. J. Med.* 296:14, 1977.
9. Davidson, R. C., and Scribner, B. H. Basal sodium excretion in treatment of hypertension in chronic renal disease. *Cardiovasc. Med.* 1:259, 1976.
10. Davies, D. L., Schalekamp, M. A., Beevers, D. G., et al. Abnormal relation between exchangeable sodium and the renin-angiotensin system in malignant hypertension and in hypertension with chronic renal failure. *Lancet* 1:683, 1973.
11. Elkinton, J. R. Hydrogen ion turnover in health and in renal disease. *Ann. Intern. Med.* 57:660, 1962.
12. Falls, W. F., Jr., Stacy, W. K., Bear, E. S., et al. Dialysis-induced change of extracellular fluid volume in man. *Proc. Clin. Dial. Transplant Forum* 2:155, 1972.
13. Favre, H. R., and Wing, A. J. Simultaneous ^{51}Cr edetic acid, inulin, and endogenous creatinine clearances in 20 patients with renal disease. *Br. Med. J.* 1:84, 1968.
14. Friedman, E. A. *Strategy in Renal Failure.* New York: Wiley, 1978. P. 22.
15. Garnett, E. S., Parsons, V., and Veall, N. Measurement of glomerular filtration-rate in man using a ^{51}Cr/edetic acid complex. *Lancet* 1:818, 1967.
16. Goldring, W. Clinical application of current tests of renal function. *J.A.M.A.* 153:1245, 1953.
17. Hosain, F., Reba, R. C., and Wagner, H. N., Jr. Measurement of glomerular filtration rate using chelated ytterbium-169. *Int. J. Appl. Radiat. Isot.* 20:517, 1969.
18. Israelit, A. H., Long, D. L., White, M. G., et al. Measurement of glomerular filtration rate utilizing a single subcutaneous injection of ^{125}I-iothalamate. *Kidney Int.* 4:346, 1973.
19. Jones, J. D., and Burnett, P. C. Creatinine metabolism in humans with decreased renal function: Creatinine deficit. *Clin. Chem.* 20:1204, 1974.
20. Kim, K. E., Onesti, G., Ramirez, O., et al. Creatinine clearance in renal disease: A reappraisal. *Br. Med. J.* 4:11, 1969.
21. Lavender, S., Hilton, P. J., and Jones, N. F. The measurement of glomerular filtration-rate in renal disease. *Lancet* 2:1216, 1969.
22. Levin, D. M., and Cade, R. Influence of dietary sodium on renal function in patients with chronic renal disease. *Ann. Intern. Med.* 62:231, 1965.
23. Levinsky, N. G. Measurement of Renal Function in the Diseased Kidney. In A. N. Brest and J. H. Moyer (Eds.), *Renal Failure.* Philadelphia: Lippincott, 1967. P. 95.
24. Lubowitz, H., Slatopolsky, E., Shankel, S., et al. Glomerular filtration rate determination in patients with chronic renal disease. *J.A.M.A.* 199:252, 1967.

25. Milutinovic, J., Cutler, R. E., Hoover, P., et al. Measurement of residual glomerular filtration rate in the patient receiving repetitive hemodialysis. *Kidney Int.* 8:185, 1975.
26. Milutinovic, J., Strand, M., Casaretto, A., et al. Clinical impact of residual glomerular filtration rate (GFR) on dialysis time—a preliminary report. *Trans. Am. Soc. Artif. Intern. Organs* 20:410, 1974.
27. Nelp, W. B., Wagner, H. N., Jr., and Reba, R. C. Renal excretion of vitamin B_{12} and its use in measurement of glomerular filtration rate in man. *J. Lab. Clin. Med.* 63:480, 1964.
28. Nickel, J. F., Lowrance, P. B., Leifer, E., et al. Renal function, electrolyte excretion and body fluids in patients with chronic renal insufficiency before and after sodium deprivation. *J. Clin. Invest.* 32:68, 1953.
29. Ott, N. T., and Wilson, D. M. A simple technique for estimating glomerular filtration rate with subcutaneous injection of [^{125}I] iothalamate. *Mayo Clin. Proc.* 50:664, 1975.
30. Pauze, J. A., and Gilmore, J. P. Influence of volume expansion on sodium excretion during parabiotic dialysis. *Proc. Soc. Exp. Biol. Med.* 151:126, 1976.
31. Perillie, P. E., and Epstein, F. H. Sickling phenomenon produced by hypertonic solutions: A possible explanation for hyposthenuria of sicklemia. *J. Clin. Invest.* 42:570, 1963.
32. Pitts, R. F. *Physiology of the Kidney and Body Fluids: An introductory Text.* Chicago: Year Book, 1963.
33. Rowe, J. W., Andres, R., Tobin, J. D., et al. The effect of age on creatinine clearance in men: A cross-sectional and longitudinal study. *J. Gerontol.* 31:155, 1976.
34. Schwartz, W. B., and Polak, A. Electrolyte disorders in chronic renal disease. *J. Chronic Dis.* 11:319, 1960.
35. Shaffer, P. The excretion of kreatinin and kreatin in health and disease. *Am. J. Physiol.* 23:1, 1908.
36. Skov, P. E. Glomerular filtration rate in patients with severe and very severe renal insufficiency: Determined by simultaneous inulin, creatinine and ^{125}iothalamate clearance. *Acta Med. Scand.* 187:419, 1970.
37. Sziklas, J. J., Hosain, F., Reba, R. C., et al. Comparison of ^{169}Yb-DTPA, ^{113m}In-DTPA, ^{14}C-inulin and endogenous creatinine to estimate glomerular filtration. *J. Nucl. Biol. Med.* 15:122, 1971.
38. Thorn, G. W., Koepf, G. F., and Clinton, M., Jr. Renal failure simulating adrenocortical insufficiency. *N. Engl. J. Med.* 231:76, 1944.
39. Tobias, G. J., McLaughlin, R. F., Jr., and Hopper, J., Jr. Endogenous creatinine clearance: A valuable clinical test of glomerular filtration and a prognostic guide in chronic renal disease. *N. Engl. J. Med.* 266:317, 1962.
40. Ulvila, J. M., Kennedy, J. A., Lamberg, J. D., et al. Blood pressure in chronic renal failure: Effect of sodium intake and furosemide. *J.A.M.A.* 220:233, 1972.
41. Young, J. A., Cooke, H., and Freedman, B. Clearance and microperfusion studies of EDTA-^{51}Cr by rat kidney. *Abstracts of the Fourth International Congress of Nephrology*, 1969. P. 296.

6. Disorders of Hydration

Tomas Berl and William L. Henrich

Disorders of hydration are among the most common problems encountered in clinical medicine. Under normal physiological conditions, both the volume of extracellular fluid (ECF) and its osmolality are maintained within very narrow ranges despite large variations in sodium and water intake. This fine control is ultimately made possible by the ability of the kidney to adjust its sodium and water excretion in such a way as to return to the environment amounts of these substances commensurate with those taken in, thereby leaving constant what Claude Bernard called the "milieu intérieur." Although the control of volume and that of osmolality are necessarily interdependent, it is useful to consider the factors that affect the volume of ECF separately from those that control its tonicity. This chapter will deal primarily with the evaluation of patients with disturbed tonicity. However, since the approach to these patients also involves an assessment of their ECF volume status, we will briefly discuss the physiological control of both volume and osmolality.

The tonicity (osmolality) of body fluids in man is maintained remarkably constant between 285 and 295 mOsm/kg H_2O. This constancy is made possible by the very close regulation of the renal excretion of water, which in turn is primarily dependent on the circulating levels of the posterior pituitary hormone vasopressin (antidiuretic hormone). The secretion of this hormone, as well as the sensation of thirst, is exquisitely sensitive to minute alterations in the osmolality of plasma; thus even a 1- to 2-percent change in plasma osmolality will either suppress or stimulate thirst and vasopressin secretion [61]. In normal man, this mechanism allows for an enormous flexibility in the volume of water that can be taken in (from as little as 0.5 to as much as 25 L/day). An increase in electrolyte-free water intake brings about a small decrease in the tonicity of body fluids which, by suppressing the release of vasopressin, results in the excretion of a urine that is more dilute than plasma. The excretion of such urine then restores the osmolality of plasma to normal. Conversely, if water intake is limited, a slight increase in the osmolality of body fluids will activate the water-conserving mechanisms by increasing thirst and causing vasopressin secretion. The action of vasopressin on the renal collecting duct then results in the formation of a concentrated urine. Disturbances in either the urinary diluting or concentrating mechanisms markedly limit the flexibility in water intake and, when these limits are exceeded, can culminate in abnormalities in body tonicity. Since sodium is the most abundant electrolyte in serum, the concentration of sodium will reflect this abnormal osmolality and is thus the most common means by which disorders of tonicity come to the attention of the clinician.

Although the serum sodium concentration provides a good index of the tonicity of body fluids, it is not a measure of the volume of the ECF. Sodium is actively extruded from the cell to the ECF, and more than 90 percent of this cation resides in this space. Since the concentration of sodium is closely controlled by the mechanisms described above, it follows that the body's total sodium content will be the primary determinant of the volume of ECF. The regulation of this volume is therefore dependent on the balance between the intake and the excretion of sodium. Mechanisms that control the renal excretion of sodium have been the subject of intensive investigation but have not yet been fully defined [19]. There is considerable evidence to suggest that receptors located in the atria, in the arterial tree, and perhaps even in the kidney itself sense alterations in circulating volume and can regulate, through neural or humoral pathways (or both), the renal excretion of sodium. Under normal conditions the daily excretion of sodium closely matches and reflects the intake of the cation. The renal excretory mechanism can adjust to large variations in sodium intake. Therefore, under conditions of volume expansion or generous sodium intake, abundant amounts of sodium will appear in the urine. Conversely, in the face of volume contraction or with marked dietary sodium restriction, the mechanisms involved in sodium conservation will be called into play, resulting in its virtual absence from the urine.

Disturbances either in the pathways that sense the integrity of ECF and circulatory volume or in the renal excretory mechanisms can lead to inappropriate sodium losses or retention. Urinary sodium losses culminate in volume contraction and renal sodium retention in edema. ECF volume alterations are best detected by physical examination; laboratory assessment of serum sodium concentration does not provide diagnostic information of ECF expansion or contraction.

Serum Sodium Concentration and Osmolality

Laboratory Measurement and Interpretation

The routine determination of serum (as well as urine) sodium concentration is performed by emission flame photometry [31, 59, 60]. In this technique, an aliquot of sample is diluted, atomized, and passed into a flame. The resultant combustion emits a characteristic wavelength, which is registered by a photo cell. The intensity of the light emitted by the combustion is proportional to the concentration of the sodium in the measured sample. Standardization is performed with aqueous solutions of known concentrations of sodium. The amount of sodium in any given sample is expressed as a concentration term, milliequivalents per liter (mEq/L). In most laboratories, the normal range of serum sodium is 135 to 145 mEq/L. It is important to stress that since the measurement of serum sodium is a concentration term, any given value of sodium is expressed relative to the amount of water in the sample; thus low serum sodium concentration values denote an excess of water relative to the amount of sodium present and, conversely, high serum sodium concentrations denote a lack of water relative to the amount of sodium present. The serum sodium concentration is not, therefore, a reflection of total body sodium content, since a low serum sodium may accompany conditions in which total body sodium is either low, normal, or even increased. Rather, the serum sodium concentration is a laboratory test of both water and sodium balance and depends on a clinical evaluation of the patient's ECF volume status for precise interpretation. An isolated serum sodium value is therefore devoid of clinical relevance without knowledge of the clinical setting in which it was obtained.

Osmolality is a measure of one of the colligative properties of water and therefore depends on the number of solute particles in solution. The addition of solute to a volume of water changes the colligative properties of water, which include freezing point depression, melting point depression, vapor pressure lowering, boiling point elevation, and osmotic pressure. The most frequently employed method for clinical measurement of osmolality is freezing point depression [30]. The test is performed by placing an aliquot of the sample to be measured in a refrigerated bath and monitoring the temperature. The temperature at which the water in the sample begins to freeze is the endpoint and may be directly converted to osmolality. The preferred means of expressing concentration of water is milliosmoles per kilogram of water (mOsm/kg H_2O). A concentration of 1 mOsm/kg H_2O denotes that 6×10^{20} solute particles (1/1000 of Avogadro's number) are present in each kilogram of water in the solution.

The normal osmolality of human plasma is between 285 and 295 mOsm/kg. Since sodium is the main extracellular cation, it and its accompanying anions account for most of the osmolality. In fact, in most circumstances the osmolality of plasma can be derived simply by doubling the serum sodium. Thus, hypernatremia reflects a relative lack of water and hyperosmolality; and hyponatremia, a relative water excess of hypoosmolality. The measurement of serum osmolality is clinically most useful, however, in the circumstances in which the serum sodium concentration does not accurately reflect the tonicity of serum. Conditions in which the serum sodium concentration underestimates the osmolality of serum are as follows:

1. Severe hyperlipemia or hyperproteinemia
2. Hyperglycemia
3. Mannitol infusion
4. Azotemia (elevated blood urea)
5. Ingestion of ethanol, methanol, ethylene glycol

One instance in which the serum sodium concentration is reported by the laboratory as being low despite a normal plasma osmolality is one in which either plasma lipids or plasma proteins are markedly elevated and thereby occupy a significant volume of plasma [27, 62]. In this setting the sodium concentration would be normal if measured in plasma water but is decreased when determined, as is done in the laboratory, in the total volume now increased by the lipids or proteins.

Another situation in which the serum sodium concentration does not reflect the osmolality of serum is one in which osmotically active substances are present in the circulation. Water moves freely across cell membranes in order to maintain osmotic equilibration between cellular and extracellular fluid. Therefore, the effect that an osmotically active substance will have on the measured serum sodium concentration will largely depend on its own ability to move across cell membranes. If the substance is one that does not diffuse freely across cell membranes (such as glucose or mannitol), it will draw water from the intracellular space to the ECF, thereby lowering the serum sodium concentration. Since both mannitol and glucose have a molecular weight of 180, their contribution to the plasma osmolality can be obtained by dividing their concentration in milligrams per deciliter by 18 [9]. It must be noted that in this circumstance hyponatremia may not reflect an abnormality in total body water balance but rather a simple shift of water between two body compartments. In contrast, if the osmotically active substance present in the circulation crosses cellular membranes freely (e.g., urea, ethanol, methanol, ethylene glycol) it will itself enter the cell, it will not establish a force for water movement to the ECF, and the serum sodium concentration will be normal as serum osmolality is elevated [41].

Urinary Sodium Concentration

As was the case with the serum sodium concentration, the measurement of this parameter in the urine also reflects simply the amount of sodium relative to water in the sample. As such, it may be of limited value in the assessment of the total sodium excretion rate over a 24-hour period. For example, when urine flow rates are very high, a low concentration of sodium may translate itself into a large amount of sodium excretion; conversely, a high urinary sodium concentration may correspond to a low 24-hour excretion rate if urine flow is extremely low. However, except for these extreme situations, the concentration of sodium in a sample of urine does provide an index as to the general rate of sodium excretion, and in particular as to whether or not renal sodium conservation is taking place. Since, as described previously, the excretion of sodium is exquisitely sensitive to the status of ECF volume and the sodium intake of an individual, its measurement can be used as an adjunct to the assessment of ECF volume as well as in the discrimination between renal and extrarenal losses of sodium. Thus in the presence of ECF volume contraction, as assessed by the presence of poor skin turgor, dry mucous membranes, absent sweating, orthostatic decrease in blood pressure, and increase in pulse and flat neck veins, the urine should be virtually free of sodium. The presence of sodium in the urine of such a patient should raise the possibility that the kidney itself is the source of the sodium depletion or that some other factor impedes maximal conservation of the cation. Clinical conditions that are associated with a high urinary sodium excretion despite ECF volume depletion are given in the following list.

1. Diuretic use
2. Adrenal insufficiency
3. Renal insufficiency of any cause [53], but in particular with the following:
   a. Medullary cystic disease [58]
   b. Diuretic phase of acute renal failure [34]
   c. After relief of urinary tract obstruction [64]
   d. After renal transplantation [39]
4. With any osmotic diuresis—glucose, urea, mannitol [18]
5. Severe vomiting with bicarbonaturia [54]
6. Proximal renal tubular acidosis with bicarbonaturia [46]

As noted previously, the use of diuretics, adrenal insufficiency, and various forms of intrinsic renal disease can limit the ability of the kidney to lower urinary sodium concentration maximally [34, 39, 53, 58, 64]. Likewise, in the presence of an osmotic diuresis [18] or when large amounts of bicarbonate appear in the urine, as in severe vomiting [54] and proximal renal tubular acidosis [46], a sodium-rich urine may be excreted. Such an inability to lower the excretion of the cation despite ECF depletion perpetrates and further aggravates the disturbance in volume.

Conversely, in a number of pathological conditions urinary sodium excretion is low despite ECF expansion. These conditions are usually disorders characterized by the accumulation of interstitial fluid (i.e., edema) and include among others congestive heart failure, cirrhosis, and the nephrotic syndrome [51]. The questions of why the kidney retains sodium so avidly in this state despite ECF expansion and whether this is a primary renal disorder or one in which the kidney simply responds to sensing an ineffective blood volume remain thus far largely unanswered [19].

Urinary Osmolality: Disorders of Urinary Dilution and Concentration

The osmolality of urine is measured by the same method described previously for plasma. However, in contrast to plasma, no "normal" urinary osmolality can be defined, since it may vary widely depending on the water intake of the individual. Thus the urine can be much more dilute than plasma (urinary osmolality below 100 mOsm/kg H_2O) when water intake is high, or it can be four times as concentrated as plasma (urinary osmolality approximately 1200 mOsm/kg) in the presence of water deprivation.

The ability of normal man to excrete large volumes of dilute urine and there-

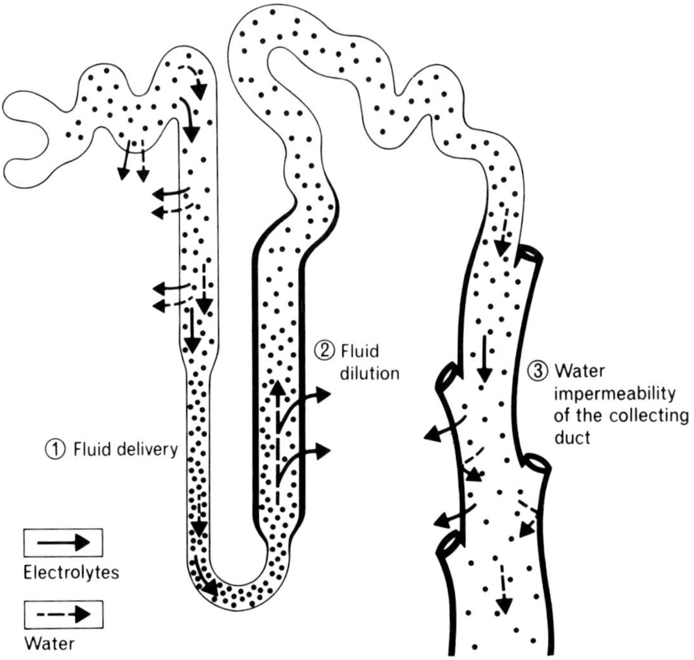

Figure 6–1
Components of the normal renal diluting mechanism. (Reprinted, by permission, from T. Berl, and R. W. Schrier, Water Metabolism and the Hypo-osmolar Syndromes. In B. Brenner and J. Stein (Eds.), *Contemporary Issues in Nephrology,* Vol. 1. New York: Churchill Livingstone, 1978.)

fore to drink as much as 25 liters of free water per day is contingent on the normal operation of the renal diluting mechanism. The components of this mechanism are illustrated schematically in Figure 6–1 and involve the following factors:

1. Normal delivery of fluid to the diluting segment of the nephron (i.e., normal glomerular filtration rate and proximal reabsorption). Although tubular fluid remains isotonic in the proximal tubule, this factor is primarily one of quantitative importance. Thus when proximal delivery is markedly curtailed and the urine can be normally diluted, the total volume of urine that can be excreted will be limited.
2. Normal sodium chloride reabsorption in the diluting segment of the nephron. Urine is diluted in the water-impermeable ascending limb of Henle by the active reabsorption of chloride.
3. Absence of vasopressin or any other substance that could render the collecting duct permeable to water. This factor is of primary importance be-

cause the medullary interstitium is always isotonic or hypertonic, and if the collecting duct were water-permeable, tubular fluid would equilibrate with the interstitium and thus become increasingly concentrated.

Failure of the diluting mechanism limits the amount of free water an individual can ingest without running the risk of retaining it and diluting his body fluids [6]. The ability of the kidney to dilute the urine may be tested with an oral or intravenous water load test. From a historical perspective, it should be noted that water loading tests were formerly performed to aid in the diagnosis of adrenal insufficiency. However, water loading in modern clinical practice is performed primarily in a clinical research context, since the development of a hypotonic state with a less than maximally dilute urine is in itself prima facie evidence of a diluting disorder. The test is performed by having the patient ingest 20 ml/kg of water orally within 30 minutes. A normal result is obtained when the subject urinates greater than 80 percent of the water load over 4 hours and produces a urine with an osmolality of less than 100 mOsm/kg following the test.

The ability of the kidney to concentrate the urine maximally to approximately 1200 mOsm/kg H_2O enables the individual to maintain water balance with an intake of as little as 0.5 L/day. This normal function of the concentrating mechanism is also dependent on various factors [35], as listed below:

1. The generation of a concentrated medullary interstitium. The anatomical arrangement of the loop of Henle allows it to act as a countercurrent multiplier whose energy source is the aforementioned active reabsorption of sodium chloride in the ascending limb of Henle. This process dilutes tubular fluid and concentrates the medullary interstitial space with a gradient of increasing tonicity from the cortex to the inner medulla.
2. The presence of antidiuretic hormone in the circulation. This hormone renders the collecting duct permeable to water and allows the dilute fluid delivered from the distal tubule to equilibrate with the concentrated interstitium. Failure of antidiuretic hormone secretion occurs in hypothalamic diabetes insipidus.
3. Normal collecting duct responsiveness to vasopressin. In a number of pathological states (to be discussed later), the renal responsiveness to antidiuretic hormone is impaired and thus urine cannot be concentrated despite maximal circulating levels of the hormone (nephrogenic diabetes insipidus).

Disorders in the renal concentrating mechanism obligate a large volume of urine (polyuria) and subsequent water intake (polydipsia). Clinically, the concentrating mechanism and antidiuretic hormone secretory ability can best be tested by fluid deprivation and the exogenous administration of antidiuretic hormone [42]. After 12 to 16 hours of fluid deprivation or after the patient loses 3 to 5 percent of his body weight, the normal urinary osmolality is greater than 800 mOsm/kg H_2O. If the osmolality does not achieve this level, 3 to 5 units of aqueous vasopressin should be given subcutaneously (or 0.5 to 1 unit may be given intravenously), and urinary osmolality should be monitored during the next 1 to 2 hours. The subcutaneous method of injection is preferred because it is associated with fewer hemodynamic changes. An increase in urinary osmolality of more than 10 percent would suggest failure of endogenous antidiuretic hormone release (hypothalamic diabetes insipidus), whereas no change suggests a renal defect (nephrogenic diabetes insipidus).

In addition to the water restriction test, two other diagnostic tests are available to assess release of antidiuretic hormone from the pituitary gland. The infusion of hypertonic saline (300 ml of 5% sodium chloride) will increase plasma osmolality and cause an antidiuresis within 30 to 60 minutes in normal subjects but not in patients with diabetes insipidus [47]. It is important to document an increase in plasma osmolality when using this test and to calculate a negative change in free water clearance. The test cannot be used in patients who are intolerant of ECF volume expansion (e.g., patients with congestive heart failure). Nicotine is also known to stimulate vasopressin release [13] and has occasionally been used to assess pituitary function. However, intravenous administration of the drug may produce troublesome nausea and syncope and can alter systemic and renal hemodynamics, thus changing urine flow independently of any vasopressin secretion. For these reasons, fluid deprivation is the preferred test in the diagnosis of diabetes insipidus.

It is clear from the foregoing discussion that the absence or presence of antidiuretic hormone in the circulation plays a pivotal role in allowing both normal dilution and concentration of the urine. Although the control of antidiuretic hormone release is primarily determined by the osmolality of body fluids, a number of nonosmolar factors can affect antidiuretic hormone as well [52]. The most important of these factors is the volume of ECF. Therefore, in an attempt to maintain circulating volume, the water-retaining mechanisms (i.e., antidiuretic hormone release and thirst) are activated even in the presence of serum hypotonicity. The nonosmolar factors affecting renal water excretion are summarized in the following list:*

1. Changes in blood volume—volume receptors
2. Changes in systemic arterial pressure—baroreceptors
3. Hormonal factors
   a. Catecholamines
   b. Prostaglandins
   c. Adrenocortical hormones
   d. Renin-angiotensin system
   e. Thyroid hormone
4. Physical and emotional stress

* Reprinted, by permission, from R. W. Schrier and T. Berl, Non-osmolar factors affecting renal water excretion. *N. Engl. J. Med.* 292:81–88, 1975.

5. Pharmacological agents
   a. Oxytocin
   b. Chlorpropamide
   c. Clofibrate
   d. Carbamazepine
   e. Cyclophosphamide
   f. Vincristine

The ability to measure the levels of circulating vasopressin would permit the delineation of the pathogenesis of many of the disorders discussed in this section. Initially, bioassay techniques were employed [16]; these techniques used ethanol-anesthetized rats. Alterations in urine flow in response to standard amounts of vasopressin and unknown samples were used to extrapolate the antidiuretic activity of the latter. Unfortunately, bioassay data have yielded sometimes conflicting results as to the role of vasopressin in various disorders [2, 38], and the reproducibility of these data has been questioned. More recently, a number of laboratories have developed a radioimmunoassay for vasopressin [33, 48, 49, 55]. Since there are a number of difficulties involved in the iodination of the antigen, the development of the antibody, the extraction of serum, and so forth, any laboratory that wants to set up such an assay is strongly urged to obtain direct advice from the authors cited above. Despite these difficulties, these investigators have measured vasopressin levels in a variety of physiological and pathological settings. It appears that arginine vasopressin levels rise by approximately 0.34 pg per milliliter per every milliosmole rise in plasma osmolality, which results in a change in urinary osmolality of 100 mOsm. Since very small changes in arginine vasopressin levels cause large changes in urinary concentration, it is clear that a very sensitive assay is needed to help in the evaluation of disorders in the urinary concentrating and diluting mechanisms. Whether or not such an assay will find widespread clinical use remains to be determined.

Etiologies of Hypernatremia and Hyperosmolality

The development of hypernatremia (and, therefore, hyperosmolality) implies that water has been lost from body fluids. Since water is freely permeable across nearly all membranes in the body, an increase in ECF volume osmolality also indicates an increase in intracellular fluid osmolality. Therefore, an increase in the serum sodium concentration connotes intracellular desiccation. Loss of water from the body may occur via renal or extrarenal routes. However, as little as a 1 percent increase in plasma osmolality triggers the thirst mechanism, so that severe hypernatremia is not observed unless the patient has a neurological disease associated with hypodipsia or does not have access to water. As shown in Figure 6–2, hypernatremia may develop in the setting of low, normal, or, rarely, high body sodium; thus an accurate assessment of the ECF volume status is essential to both the diagnosis and the treatment of such patients.

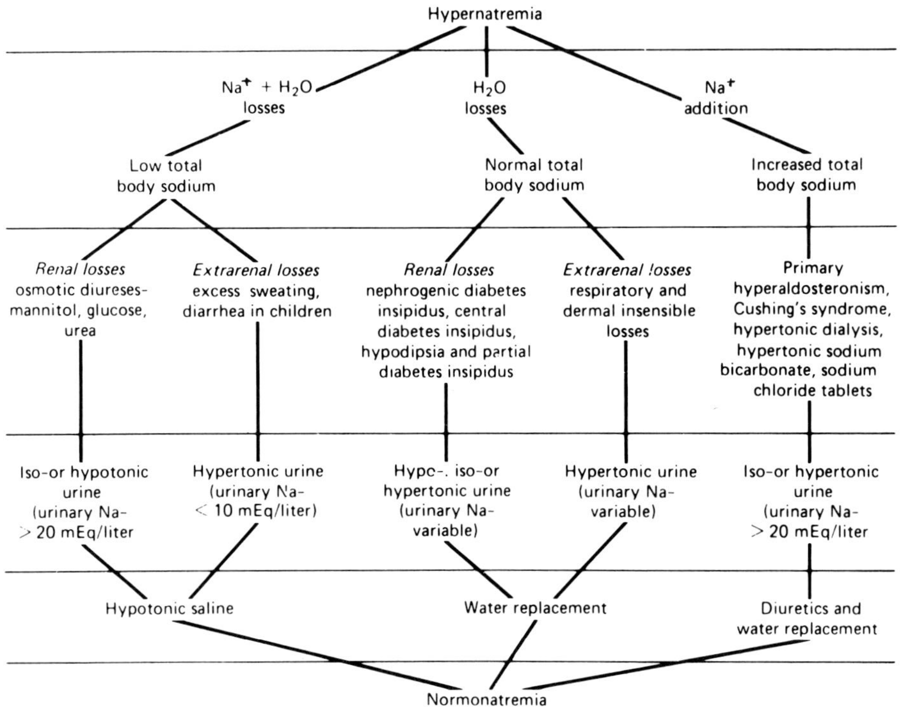

Figure 6–2
Approach to the hypernatremic patient. (Reprinted from *Kidney International* [6] with permission.)

Hypernatremia and Low Total Body Sodium

Patients with low total body sodium and hypernatremia have sustained losses of both sodium and water, but a relatively greater loss of water. These hypotonic fluid losses may occur through the skin secondary to profuse sweating or from diarrhea. With these extrarenal losses urinary osmolality is high (usually greater than 800 mOsm/kg H_2O), reflecting the secretion of antidiuretic hormone as part of the body's attempt to conserve water and minimize further losses. Urinary sodium concentration in such cases is usually low (less than 10 mEq/L), indicating that active renal conservation of sodium is present. Alternatively, the source of fluid loss may be through the kidney itself, in which case urinary osmolality will be low (isotonic or hypotonic) and urinary sodium concentration will be greater than 20 mEq/L despite ECF volume depletion. Such renal loss of salt and water may result from osmotic diuresis (glucosuria, urea, mannitol). As noted earlier in the chapter, increased concentrations of glucose and mannitol will increase serum osmolality but will remove water from cells so that plasma sodium concentration may be only slightly increased or even normal. Treatment of this disorder includes extracellular volume repletion with isotonic saline initially, followed by hypotonic fluid infusions.

Hypernatremia and Normal Body Sodium

Hypernatremia may occur without sodium losses and significant volume depletion. Such a disturbance ensues when water is lost from the organism without sodium. Insensible water is lost through the skin and the respiratory tract at all times, but when the environmental temperature is high or when a patient is in febrile or hypermetabolic states, these losses can be considerable. If these conditions are not accompanied by appropriate water intake, the patient becomes hypernatremic. In this setting, the hypothalamic-renal concentrating mechanism is normal and the urinary osmolality is high. Likewise, since sodium balance is normal, urinary sodium will simply reflect sodium intake and thus is variable.

More frequently, however, in euvolemic hypernatremic patients the losses of water are renal in origin. This situation occurs in either complete or partial failure of vasopressin secretion (hypothalamic diabetes insipidus) when accompanied by a blunted thirst response [40]. Alternatively, renal water losses may occur as a consequence of a failure of the kidney to respond to vasopressin (nephrogenic diabetes insipidus). The laboratory differentiation between hypothalamic and nephrogenic diabetes insipidus was described in the discussion of the concentrating mechanism. The causes of nephrogenic diabetes insipidus are given in the following list.

1. Congenital [10, 15, 24]
2. Acquired
   a. Renal insufficiency of any cause, but in particular due to disease of medulla or papilla [9, 11, 14, 21, 32, 37]
   b. Protein starvation [23]
   c. Marked and prolonged sodium restriction [28]
   d. Increased water intake [3]
   e. Hypercalcemia [35]
   f. Hypokalemia [50]
   g. Sickle cell disease [57]

Congenital diabetes insipidus is a rare genetic disorder that may occur initially in infants [8, 10, 15, 24]. Acquired nephrogenic diabetes insipidus refers to a heterogeneous group of disorders that reflect the kidney's inability to concentrate the urine maximally. Acquired nephrogenic diabetes insipidus may occur in some forms of chronic renal insufficiency, particularly parenchymal diseases affecting the medulla and papilla regions of the kidney (e.g., medullary cystic disease [32], polycystic kidney disease [32], obstructive uropathy [21], amyloidosis [11], pyelonephritis [37], radiation nephritis [14], sickle cell disease [9], and light chain nephropathy [56]). Extreme dietary alterations in protein, sodium chloride, and water intake may affect maximal concentrating capacity by affecting the renal medullary environment [3, 23, 28]. Finally, hypercalcemia [35] and hypokalemia [50] are two common electrolyte abnormalities that diminish renal concentrating ability by impairing the renal response to endogenous vasopressin. In sickle cell disease, urinary concentration is impaired as a result of medullary infarcts [57].

Hypernatremia and High Total Body Sodium

Hypernatremia with high total body sodium is less frequently observed than the two previous categories, primarily because of the ability of the kidney to excrete excess ingested sodium. Mild increases in the serum sodium concentration may occur in Cushing's syndrome or in hyperaldosteronism. Other causes of hypernatremia and volume expansion are either iatrogenic (e.g., sodium bicarbonate administration during resuscitation) or inadvertent (e.g., administration of hypertonic sodium chloride during therapeutic abortion or a dialysis with high dialysate sodium bath). Finally, salt tablet ingestion without water may lead to severe hypernatremia. Treatment of hypernatremia consists of removal of excess total body sodium with diuretics or with dialysis if renal function is impaired. Water losses may be replaced either parenterally or orally.

Etiologies of Hyponatremia and Hypoosmolality

As discussed earlier, hyponatremia is a condition in which an excess of water relative to sodium exists, resulting in a decreased sodium concentration. Hyponatremia thus implies a relative defect in water excretion and may occur under conditions of total body sodium depletion or excess as well as under conditions of normal total body sodium. The circumstances in which hyponatremia may develop are discussed in the following sections (Fig. 6–3).

Hyponatremia and Hypoosmolality with Increased Total Body Sodium

Patients with congestive heart failure, cirrhosis, and the nephrotic syndrome may have an increase in total body sodium but a larger increase in total body water. The precise mechanism responsible for impaired diluting ability in these conditions is unknown but is related to a decrease in effective blood volume. Elevated antidiuretic hormone-like material has been identified in some but not all patients with these conditions [6]. The decrease in effective arterial blood volume may also result in a decrease in glomerular filtration rate (GFR) and enhanced proximal reabsorption of fluid, thus further impairing the ability of the kidney to excrete water. Therefore, persistent antidiuretic hormone secretion and intrarenal mechanisms combine to impair water excretion in patients with heart failure, cirrhosis, and the nephrotic syndrome. Since sodium reabsorption is stimulated in these conditions, urinary sodium concentrations will usually be less than 10 mEq/L unless the patient has been receiving diuretics.

Patients with advanced chronic renal insufficiency have a more limited capacity to excrete water than normals. A reduction in GFR limits the delivery of

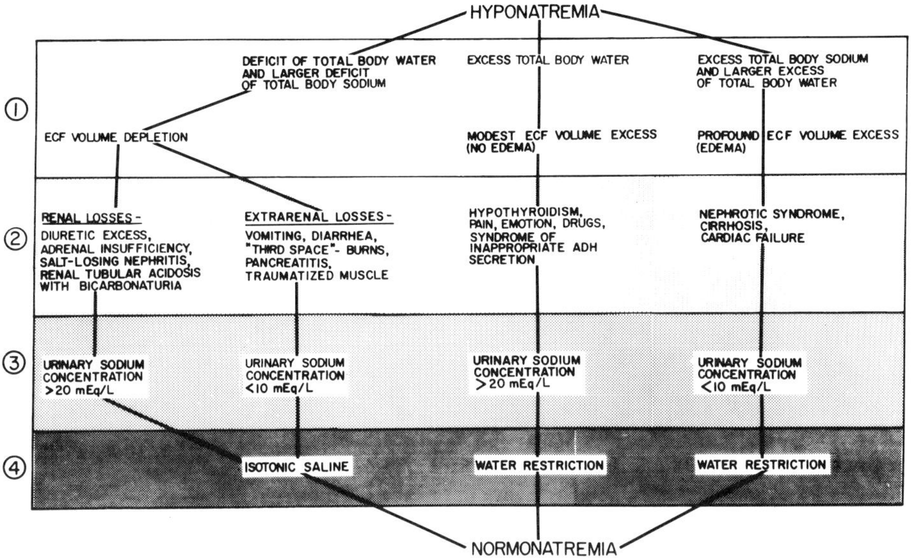

Figure 6–3
Approach to the hyponatremic patient. (Reprinted from *Kidney International* [6] with permission.)

filtrate to diluting sites in the nephron. Thus with a GFR of 5 ml/min (7 L/day) and an estimated 20 percent of the filtrate reaching the diluting segment of the nephron, a maximum of 1.4 L/day may be excreted. An intake of water in excess of this amount may result in hyponatremia. In contrast to the group of patients with cardiac failure, cirrhosis, or the nephrotic syndrome, patients with advanced renal failure often have urinary sodium concentrations greater than 20 mEq/L.

Treatment of patients with hyponatremia and increased total body sodium is directed at improving the cardiac output (in heart failure), improving hepatic function (in cirrhosis), or reducing proteinuria (in the nephrotic syndrome). Water restriction is appropriate to increase serum sodium concentration. Diuretics and sodium restriction are also used to reduce total body sodium excess. The use of saline infusions to improve the sodium concentration is frankly dangerous and contraindicated, since it will result in greater overexpansion of the ECF volume in these sodium-overloaded subjects.

Hyponatremia Associated with Decreased Total Body Sodium

As mentioned previously, hypovolemia is probably the most potent nonosmolar stimulus for vasopressin release (see list on p. 108). Given the alternatives of hypoosmolality versus hypovolemia, the body elects to protect ECF volume at the expense of hypoosmolality and hyponatremia by secreting vasopressin.

Therefore, persistent vasopressin secretion prevents excretion of water. Patients with hyponatremia in the context of decreased total body sodium have deficits in both total body sodium and water, but a greater deficit in total body sodium.

Fluid losses may take place through extrarenal or renal routes. Extrarenal losses may occur via the gastrointestinal tract or through "third space" fluid accumulation (as in burns, pancreatitis, and peritonitis). The kidney will respond to hypovolemia by maximally conserving sodium and water so that the urine sodium concentration is normally below 10 mEq/L.

The finding of a urinary sodium concentration greater than 20 mEq/L in the setting of volume contraction suggests that the patient's loss of sodium has occurred via the kidney. These losses may be due to intrinsic renal disease (particularly with some tubulointerstitial diseases, such as medullary cystic disease or polycystic kidney disease). Diuretics and mineralocorticoid deficiency may also result in renal losses of sodium. Finally, some patients with proximal renal tubular acidosis (type II) have significant bicarbonaturia, which obligates sodium loss. If hypovolemia is severe enough in any of these conditions the GFR may be decreased, further lowering the kidney's ability to excrete water.

Treatment of these disorders is directed at prompt expansion of the ECF volume with isotonic sodium chloride. This maneuver will ablate the hypovolemic stimulus to vasopressin release; hypotonicity will turn off vasopressin release, and a water diuresis can occur. In the case of diuretic-induced hypovolemia and hyponatremia, diuretics should be discontinued and any potassium deficit corrected. Patients with mineralocorticoid or glucocorticoid deficiency should receive therapeutic doses of the appropriate hormone or hormones.

Hyponatremia with Undetectable Alterations in Total Body Sodium

This category of hyponatremia and hypoosmolality is characterized by clinical euvolemia (i.e., no edema or evident volume contraction). However, in many patients with euvolemia and hyponatremia a small amount of ECF volume expansion may be present.

The etiology of this type of hyponatremia includes glucocorticoid deficiency [1], which is partly due to persistent secretion of vasopressin. The exact mechanism by which glucocorticoid hormones affect vasopressin synthesis, release, or action is unknown. Patients with hypothyroidism without hypovolemia may also be unable to dilute their urine maximally, possibly secondary to subtle decreases in renal hemodynamics [17, 22]. A number of drugs may either stimulate vasopressin release (see list on p. 108) or potentiate its peripheral action; these drugs are discussed in detail in a recent complete review [43]. Finally, some patients who are taking diuretics may drink enough water to obscure any evident reduction in ECF volume. These patients appear to be euvolemic and recover with cessation of diuretic therapy [25]. Persistent secretion of vasopressin may occur in patients experiencing pain [45] or emotional stress [20].

When all the factors mentioned above have been ruled out as the cause of hyponatremia in an apparently euvolemic patient, the syndrome of inappropriate antidiuretic hormone secretion (SIADH) should be considered. Neoplasms and abnormalities of the central nervous system and lung [4, 5, 12] have been associated with this syndrome. Since their ECF volume is essentially normal, patients with SIADH have a urinary sodium concentration that parallels dietary intake and therefore usually exceeds 20 mEq/L.

Water restriction is usually adequate therapy in hyponatremic patients with euvolemia. In patients who are severely symptomatic, however, a combination of furosemide and replacement of urinary electrolyte losses with 3% sodium chloride will result in rapid correction of hyponatremia [29]. Finally, lithium and demeclocycline have been shown to inhibit the peripheral action of antidiuretic hormone and thus may have a potential role in the management of some patients [26, 63]. However, demeclocycline may be associated with nephrotoxicity in a high percentage of treated patients [44], particularly those with liver disease, and its use for this purpose must be in selected patients while under meticulous observation.

References

1. Agus, Z. S., and Goldberg, M. Role of antidiuretic hormone in the abnormal water diuresis of anterior hypopituitarism in man. *J. Clin. Invest.* 50:1478, 1971.
2. Ahmed, A. B. J., George, B. C., Gonzalez-Auvert, C., et al. Increased plasma arginine vasopressin in clinical adrenocortical insufficiency and its inhibition by glucosteroids. *J. Clin. Invest.* 46:111, 1967.
3. Barlow, E. D., and de Wardener, H. E. Compulsive water drinking. *Q. J. Med.* 28:235, 1959.
4. Bartter, F. C. The syndrome of inappropriate secretion of antidiuretic hormone (SIADH). *D.M.; Disease-a-Month,* pp. 3–47, November 1973.
5. Bartter, F. C., and Schwartz, W. B. The syndrome of inappropriate secretion of antidiuretic hormone. *Am. J. Med.* 42:790, 1967.
6. Berl, T., Anderson, R. J., McDonald, K. M., et al. Clinical disorders of water metabolism. *Kidney Int.* 10:117, 1976.
7. Blotner, H. Primary or idiopathic diabetes insipidus: A system disease. *Metabolism* 7:191, 1958.
8. Bode, H. H., and Crawford, J. D. Nephrogenic diabetes insipidus in North America: The Hopewell hypothesis. *N. Engl. J. Med.* 280:750, 1969.
9. Buckalew, V., Jr., and Someren, A. Renal manifestations of sickle cell disease. *Arch. Intern. Med.* 133:660, 1974.
10. Cannon, J. F. Diabetes insipidus: Clinical and experimental studies with consideration of genetic relationships. *Arch. Intern. Med.* 96:215, 1955.
11. Carone, F. A., and Epstein, F. H. Nephrogenic diabetes insipidus caused by amyloid disease: Evidence in man of role of collecting ducts in concentrating urine. *Am. J. Med.* 29:539, 1960.
12. Carter, N. W., Rector, F. C., and Seldin, D. W. Hyponatremia in cerebral disease resulting from inappropriate secretion of antidiuretic hormone. *N. Engl. J. Med.* 264:67, 1961.
13. Cater, J. E., and Garrod, O. The effect of nicotine on urine flow in diabetes insipidus. *Clin. Sci.* 10:145, 1951.

14. Coburn, J. W., Kleeman, C. R., and Rubin, H. E. Hyposthenuria in radiation nephritis in dogs: A specific tubular defect (abstract). *Clin. Res.* 12:249A, 1964.
15. Cutler, R., Kleeman, C. R., Maxwell, M. H., et al. Physiologic studies in nephrogenic diabetes insipidus. *J. Clin. Endocrinol.* 22:827, 1962.
16. Czaczkes, J. W., Kleeman, C. R., and Koenig, M. Physiologic studies of antidiuretic hormone by its direct measurement in human plasma. *J. Clin. Invest.* 43:1625, 1964.
17. Derubertis, F. R., Jr., Michellis, M. F., Bloom, M. E., et al. Impaired water excretion in myxedema. *Am. J. Med.* 51:41, 1971.
18. De Wardener, H. E., and del Greco, F. Influence of solute excretion rate on production of hypotonic urine in man. *Clin. Sci.* 14:715, 1955.
19. Dirks, J. H., Seely, J. F., and Levy, M. Control of Extracellular Fluid Volume and the Pathophysiology of Edema Formation. In B. M. Brenner and F. C. Rector, Jr. (Eds.), *The Kidney,* Vol. 1. Philadelphia: Saunders, 1976.
20. Dubovsky, S. L., Groban, S., Berl, T., et al. Syndrome of inappropriate secretion of antidiuretic hormone with exacerbated psychosis. *Ann. Intern. Med.* 79:551, 1973.
21. Earley, L. E. Extreme polyuria in obstructive uropathy: Report of case of "water-losing nephritis" in infant with discussion of polyuria. *N. Engl. J. Med.* 255:600, 1956.
22. Emmanouel, D. S., Lindheimer, M. D., and Katz, A. I. Mechanism of impaired water excretion in the hypothyroid rat. *J. Clin. Invest.* 54:926, 1974.
23. Epstein, F. H., Kleeman, C. R., Pursel, S., et al. The effect of feeding protein and urea on the renal concentrating process. *J. Clin. Invest.* 36:635, 1957.
24. Fichman, M. P., and Brooker, G. Deficient renal cyclic adenosine 3′,5′-monophosphate production in nephrogenic diabetes insipidus. *J. Clin. Endocrinol. Metab.* 35:35, 1972.
25. Fichman, M. P., Vorherr, H., Kleeman, C. R., et al. Diuretic-induced hyponatremia. *Ann. Intern. Med.* 75:853, 1971.
26. Forrest, J. N., Jr., Cox, M., Hong, C., et al. Demeclocycline versus lithium for inappropriate secretion of antidiuretic hormone. *N. Engl. J. Med.* 298:173, 1978.
27. Frick, P. G., Schmid, J. R., Kestler, J. H., et al. Hyponatremia associated with hyperproteinemia in multiple myeloma. *Helv. Med. Acta* 33:317, 1966.
28. Goldsmith, C., Beasly, H. K., Whalley, P. J., et al. Effect of salt deprivation on urinary concentrating mechanism in dog. *J. Clin. Invest.* 40:2043, 1961.
29. Hantman, O., Rossier, B., Zohlman, R., et al. Rapid correction of hyponatremia in the syndrome of inappropriate secretion of antidiuretic hormone. *Ann. Intern. Med.* 78:870, 1973.
30. Hendry, E. B. Osmolarity of human serum and of chemical solutions of biologic importance. *Clin. Chem.* 7:156, 1961.
31. Henry, R. J., Cannon, D. C., and Winkelman, J. W. *Clinical Chemistry: Principles and Technics* (2nd ed.). Hagerstown, Md.: Harper & Row, 1974.
32. Holliday, M. A., Egar, T. J., Morris, C. R., et al. Vasopressin-resistant hyposthenuria in chronic renal disease. *Am. J. Med.* 42:378, 1967.
33. Husain, M. K., Fernando, N., Shapiro, M., et al. Radioimmunoassay of arginine vasopressin in human plasma. *J. Clin. Endocrinol. Metab.* 37:616, 1973.
34. Iseri, L. T., Batchelor, T. M., Boyle, A. J., et al. Studies of fluid, electrolyte and nitrogen balance in acute renal insufficiency. *Arch. Intern. Med.* 89:188, 1952.
35. Jamison, R. L., and Maffly, R. H. The urinary concentrating mechanism. *N. Engl. J. Med.* 295:1059, 1976.

36. Katz, M. A. Hyperglycemia-induced hyponatremia—calculation of expected serum sodium depression. *N. Engl. J. Med.* 289:843, 1973.
37. Kaye, D., and Rocha, H. Urinary concentrating ability in early experimental pyelonephritis. *J. Clin. Invest.* 49:1427, 1970.
38. Kleeman, C. R., Czaczkes, J. W., and Cutler, R. Mechanisms of impaired water excretion in adrenal and pituitary insufficiency: IV. Antidiuretic hormone in primary and secondary adrenal insufficiency. *J. Clin. Invest.* 43:1641, 1964.
39. Kramer, H. J., Goldman, R., and Gonick, H. C. Salt-losing syndromes following renal transplantation. *Am. J. Med.* 53:368, 1972.
40. Lascelles, P. T., and Lewis, P. D. Hypodipsia and hypernatremia associated with hypothalamic and suprasellar lesions. *Brain* 95:249, 1972.
41. Loeb, J. N. The hyperosmolar state. *N. Engl. J. Med.* 290:1184, 1974.
42. Miller, M., Dalakos, T., Moses, A. M., et al. Recognition of partial defects in antidiuretic hormone secretion. *Ann. Intern. Med.* 73:721, 1970.
43. Miller, M., and Moses, A. M. Drug induced states of impaired water excretion. *Kidney Int.* 10:96, 1976.
44. Miller, P. D., Linas, S. L., Anderson, R. J., et al. Nephrotoxic and natriuretic effects of demeclochlorotetracycline (DMC) in hyponatremic cirrhotic subjects (HCS) (abstract). *Clin. Res.* 25(3):274A, 1977.
45. Moran, W. H., Jr., Miltenberger, F. W., Shuayb, W. A., et al. The relationship of antidiuretic hormone secretion to surgical stress. *Surgery* 56:99, 1964.
46. Morris, R. C., Sebastian, A., and McSherry, C. Renal acidosis. *Kidney Int.* 1:322, 1972.
47. Moses, A. M., and Streeten, D. H. T. Differentiation of polyuric states by measurement of responses to changes in plasma osmolality induced by hypertonic saline infusions. *Am. J. Med.* 42:368, 1967.
48. Robertson, G. L. Immunoassay of plasma vasopressin in man. *Proc. Natl. Acad. Sci. U.S.A.* 66:1298, 1970.
49. Robertson, S. L., Mahr, E. A., Athar, S., et al. Development and clinical application of a new method for the radioimmunoassay of arginine vasopressin in human plasma. *J. Clin. Invest.* 52:2340, 1973.
50. Rubini, M. E. Water excretion in potassium-deficient man. *J. Clin. Invest.* 40:2215, 1961.
51. Schrier, R. W. Renal Sodium Excretion, Edematous Disorders, and Diuretic Use. In R. W. Schrier (Ed.), *Renal and Electrolyte Disorders.* Boston: Little, Brown, 1976.
52. Schrier, R. W., and Berl, T. Non-osmolar factors affecting renal water excretion. *N. Engl. J. Med.* 292:81, 1975.
53. Seldin, D. W., Carter, N. W., and Rector, F. C., Jr. Consequences of Renal Failure and Their Management. In M. B. Strauss and L. G. Welt (Eds.), *Diseases of the Kidney* (2nd ed.), Vol. 1. Boston: Little, Brown, 1971.
54. Seldin, D. W., and Rector, F. C., Jr. The generation and maintenance of metabolic alkalosis. *Kidney Int.* 1:306, 1972.
55. Skowsky, W. R., Rosenbloom, A. A., and Fisher, D. A. Radioimmunoassay measurement of arginine vasopressin in serum: Development and application. *J. Clin. Endocrinol. Metab.* 38:278, 1974.
56. Smithline, N., Kassirer, J., and Cohen, J. J. Light-chain nephropathy, tubular dysfunction and light-chain proteinuria. *N. Engl. J. Med.* 294:71, 1976.
57. Statius Van Eps, L. W., Pinedo-Veels, C., de Vries, G. H., et al. Nature of concentrating defect in sickle cell nephropathy. *Lancet* 1:450, 1970.
58. Strauss, M. B. Clinical and pathological aspects of cystic disease of the renal medulla: Analysis of eighteen cases. *Ann. Intern. Med.* 57:373, 1962.

59. Sunderman, F. W., and Sunderman, F. W., Jr. *Clinical Pathology of the Serum Electrolytes.* Springfield, Ill.: Thomas, 1966.
60. Tietz, N. W. *Fundamentals of Clinical Chemistry.* Philadelphia: Saunders, 1970.
61. Verney, E. B. Croonian lecture: The antidiuretic hormone and the factors which determine its release. *Proc. R. Soc. Lond.* [*Biol.*] 135:25, 1947.
62. Waugh, W. H. Utility of expressing serum sodium per unit of water in assessing hyponatremia. *Metabolism* 18:706, 1969.
63. White, M. G., and Fetner, C. D. Treatment of the syndrome of inappropriate secretion of antidiuretic hormone with lithium carbonate. *N. Engl. J. Med.* 292:390, 1975.
64. Witte, M. G., Short, F. A., and Hollander, W., Jr. Massive polyuria and natriuresis following relief of urinary tract obstruction. *Am. J. Med.* 37:320, 1964.

7. The Renin-Angiotensin System

David C. Manahan, J. Carlos Romero, and Cameron G. Strong

Renin is a proteolytic enzyme that is synthesized, stored, and released by the juxtaglomerular cells (JG cells) in the kidney. Through a series of catalytic reactions, renin produces angiotensin I, II, and III (Fig. 7–1). Renin and renin-like substances have been found in various extrarenal sources, including the brain [16, 26], uterus [21, 22], amniotic fluid [20], and adrenal glands [27]. This chapter will deal principally with renal renin and with the description of methods to measure plasma renin activity (PRA). The concluding portion of the chapter describes a method for the measurement of renin substrate.

Renin-Angiotensin Biochemistry

Renin, with a molecular weight of approximately 38,000, cleaves its substrate angiotensinogen (an α_2-globulin synthesized in the liver) to produce the decapeptide angiotensin I (Fig. 7–1). Converting enzyme, a dipeptidylcarboxypeptidase found mainly in the lung, removes the carboxyl terminal histidine-leucine amino acids from angiotensin I to produce the octapeptide angiotensin II. Angiotensin II is a potent vasoconstrictor, and the vasopressor action is exerted primarily by direct stimulation of the smooth muscle of resistance vessels and by secondary stimulation of the adrenergic activity at the level of the central nervous system. Angiotensin II also stimulates the production of aldosterone by acting on the adrenal cortex [4]. Angiotensin III, the des-Asp^1 7-amino-acid derivative of angiotensin II, has also been shown to stimulate aldosterone production in adrenal cell suspensions in vitro [6, 48] and in vivo in the dog and rat [23, 58]. In turn, the aldosterone that is secreted controls the amount of sodium reabsorbed and the amount of potassium secreted by the distal nephron. Thus, the kidney, through the renin-angiotensin-aldosterone system, plays an important role in blood pressure regulation and in sodium-potassium homeostasis.

Renin Secretion

As already mentioned, renin is synthesized and stored in the JG cells of the kidney. These specialized cells are located in the afferent arteriole of the glomerulus. The JG cells and the macula densa portion of the distal convoluted tubule comprise the juxtaglomerular apparatus (Fig. 7–2). The control of renin release involves three main mechanisms: (1) afferent arteriole stretch receptors, (2) the macula densa, and (3) the sympathetic nervous system. The baroreceptor theory states that renin-releasing cells in the afferent arteriole can detect the degree of wall tension, which in normal circumstances is altered primarily by changes in blood pressure [5]. An increase in blood pressure will

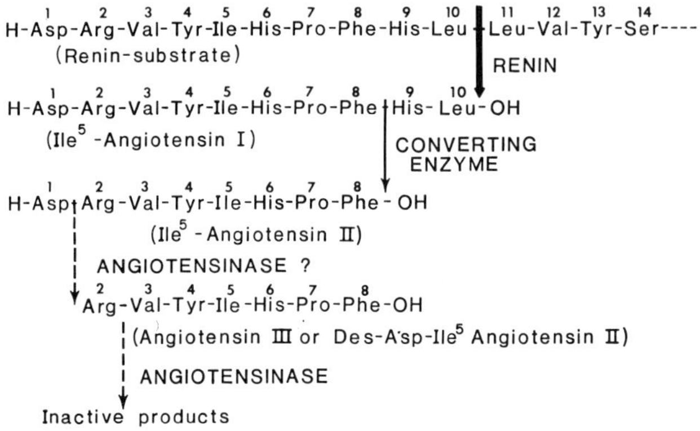

Figure 7–1
Renin-angiotensin biochemistry. The 14-amino-acid renin substrate is cleaved by renin to produce an 8-amino-acid angiotensin I. Converting enzyme then cleaves the two end amino acids from angiotensin I to form angiotensin II. Angiotensin III may be formed by the action of aminopeptidase A in removing the number 1 position amino acid (Asp) from angiotensin II, or it may be produced directly from angiotensin I. (Reprinted, by permission, from C. G. Strong, The Renin-Angiotensin-Aldosterone System. In F. G. Knox (Ed.), *Textbook of Renal Pathophysiology*. Hagerstown, Md.: Harper & Row, 1978.)

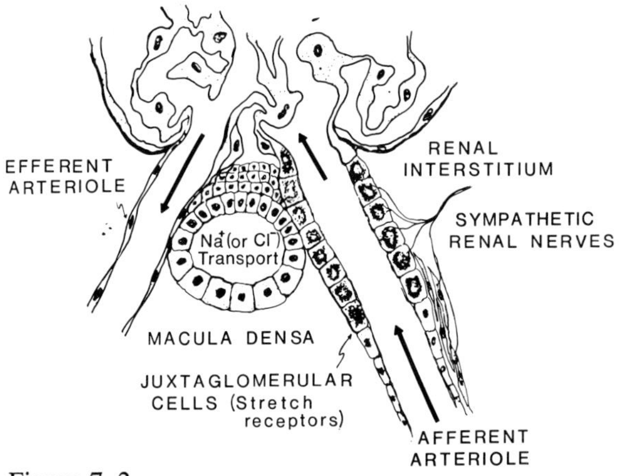

Figure 7–2
The juxtaglomerular apparatus. The relationship between macula densa cells and renin-releasing JG cells of the afferent arteriole enables the transport of sodium or chloride into macula densa cells to stimulate release of renin. The JG cells are stretch receptors that monitor afferent arteriolar pressure. (Modified from J. O. Davis, What signals the kidney to release renin? *Circ. Res.* 28:301, 1971. Reprinted by permission of the American Heart Association, Inc.)

inhibit renin release and, conversely, a decrease in blood pressure will stimulate renin production and release. The macula densa theory maintains that a group of specialized cells of the distal tubule is capable of detecting changes in distal tubular sodium load or chloride transport [3, 62]; thus an increase in sodium or chloride transport by the cells of the macula densa portion of the distal tubule will inhibit renin release. This mechanism is believed to be of major importance in mediating the release of renin elicited by the administration of furosemide and the restriction of salt intake.

On electrical stimulation, the renal sympathetic nerves have been shown to elicit renin release [36, 61]. This type of release is most likely mediated by beta-adrenergic receptors of the renal arteriolar walls [2]. Similarly, the release of renin can be inhibited by blocking these receptors. Recent evidence indicates that the neural-mediated release of renin can be triggered by changes in decreasing pressure in both atria. These pressure changes are sensed by the cardiopulmonary receptors [41] and are blocked by vagotomy, which suggests mediation by vagal afferents.

In summary, the release of renin is controlled by several stimuli, including the sympathetic nervous system, systemic pressure, and the composition of fluid entering the distal tubule of the macula densa. Other factors such as plasma potassium concentration, osmolarity, antidiuretic hormone, and catecholamines have been shown to influence renin release [17], but the physiological significance of these influences remains to be determined. Determinations of PRA are clinically important in the diagnosis of renovascular hypertension and of primary and idiopathic *hyperaldosteronism,* as well as in the evaluation of several conditions such as essential hypertension with high and low PRA levels, Bartter's syndrome, and the Robertson-Kihara syndrome. Measurement of PRA is also used in evaluating hypertension in women taking contraceptive pills and in preeclampsia. Therefore, it is relevant to describe briefly the involvement of renin in each of these entities.

Clinical Applications of Plasma Renin Measurement

Renovascular Hypertension

Renovascular hypertension, which is caused by stenosis of the main renal artery or its primary branches, is found in approximately 4 percent of the hypertensive population. Previous studies have shown that patients with renal arterial stenosis can be divided into two main groups: one group consists of older persons (mean age, 47 years) in whom the major cause of stenosis is an atherosclerotic plaque at the origin of the artery or in its proximal one-third; the second group consists of younger persons (mean age, 37 years) in whom the most frequent cause of stenosis is fibromuscular dysplasia, generally in the distal portion of the main renal artery or its primary branches.

In most patients with renovascular hypertension, the stenosis of the renal artery produces a hypersecretion of renin. This increase in renin secretion in turn produces an abnormal increase in circulating angiotensin II. Angiotensin II not only causes vasoconstriction but also stimulates the production of aldosterone, which in turn promotes sodium retention. These two factors, vasoconstriction and volume expansion through sodium retention, produce the increased blood pressure associated with renovascular hypertension.

The measurement of PRA levels in peripheral blood has proved to be of little clinical use in the management of renovascular hypertension. Studies have shown that many patients with renovascular hypertension do not have increased levels of peripheral renin but rather have values within the normal range [60]. However, the so-called normal range of renin frequently found in patients with renovascular hypertension could be interpreted as being inappropriately high with respect to the existing levels of blood pressure and sodium balance [49].

Renin-dependent renovascular hypertension is associated with an increase in renin activity from the affected kidney and often may be detected by the use of angiotensin II antagonists. Clinical studies by Brunner and colleagues [9], Streeten and co-workers [59], and others have shown that intravenous infusion of an angiotensin II antagonist, 1-sar-8-ala-angiotensin II (saralasin), has produced a significant decrease in blood pressure in patients with renovascular hypertension. The existence of a non-renin-dependent form of renovascular hypertension has also been reported [42, 49]. In this form, angiotensin antagonists do not alter the blood pressure but, as in the renin-dependent form, the affected kidney secretes more renin than does the contralateral kidney; therefore, it is important to determine renal vein renin activity (RVRA) in order to assess the significance of the arterial lesion.

Clinical procedures used in the diagnosis of renal artery stenosis may include tests such as rapid-sequence intravenous pyelography or isotopic renography. Indications of possible renal artery stenosis on intravenous pyelography include (1) a delayed appearance of the contrast medium on the affected side, (2) a difference of more than 1.5 cm in pole-to-pole diameters of the kidneys, and (3) a delayed excretion of the contrast medium on the affected side.

The isotopic renogram is derived by plotting the uptake and excretion rate of radiolabeled iodohippurate sodium (Hippuran). Results suggesting renal stenosis include delayed uptake and delayed excretion of the labeled Hippuran on the affected side.

Renal arteriography is probably the most accurate method of diagnosing renal artery stenosis. By means of femoral artery catheterization and the injection of contrast medium into the aorta above the origin of the renal arteries, both renal arteries and their branches may be visualized simultaneously. In many instances of distal renal disease, selective catheterization of the renal arteries with manual injections of small amounts of contrast medium will permit the delineation in greater detail, especially if this method is combined with the technique for obtaining magnified views. Through these series of films, the location and degree of the stenosis can be determined with great accuracy.

Differential measurement of PRA may be done on venous blood taken from each kidney before arteriography. A 1.5- to 2-fold higher renin activity measurement on the side of the affected or more severely affected kidney is indicative of correctable renovascular hypertension. With this criterion, the success of surgery may be predicted in 95 percent of patients, as reported by Hunt [33], Strong and associates [60], Amsterdam and colleagues [1], and others [28, 39, 56]. This is especially true in patients who are properly prepared for renin sampling by prior sodium depletion [60]. Lateralization of RVRA may be confirmed if the contralateral kidney is shown not to be secreting renin; this is the case if the contralateral RVRA is the same as or less than the PRA in the low inferior vena cava below the entrance of the renal veins (PRA here is the same as that in arterial blood entering the kidneys).

Hypertension with Mineralocorticoid Excess

PRIMARY ALDOSTERONISM. Primary aldosteronism is the prototype of hypertension caused by mineralocorticoid excess. It is the result of the presence of an adenoma or, rarely, carcinoma of the adrenal cortex, which causes the secretion of excessive amounts of aldosterone. The aldosterone excess increases the amount of sodium reabsorption by the distal tubules and increases potassium excretion, which results in hypokalemia. The hypokalemia may produce polyuria, muscle weakness, and excessive urinary loss of H^+, which results in hypokalemic alkalosis. The increase in intravascular volume associated with excessive sodium retention by the distal tubule will result in a suppression of renin secretion by the JG cells. Thus, suppressed renin secretion caused by sodium retention and hypertension mediated by volume expansion are early manifestations of primary aldosteronism. Indications of the presence of primary aldosteronism are hypokalemia, high aldosterone levels in plasma and urine that are not suppressible by administration of fluorocorticosterone, and suppressed PRA levels after stimulation attempts by low sodium intake and upright posture.

IDIOPATHIC HYPERALDOSTERONISM. Idiopathic hyperaldosteronism is a syndrome that manifests the same hormonal symptoms as those described for primary aldosteronism with adrenal adenoma such as hypertension, suppression of PRA, and hyperaldosteronism. The major difference is that the hypersecretion of aldosterone is produced by a functional hyperplasia of the adrenal gland and not by an adenoma. This distinction is important because Hunt and colleagues [34] have shown a good surgical prognosis in patients having adenoma but not in those with adrenal hyperplasia. In 1976, Schambelan and co-workers [51] reported that the secretion of renin is not completely suppressed in patients with adrenal hyperplasia, inasmuch as it can be enhanced by the assumption of upright posture. In contrast, this maneuver is not as effective in increasing PRA levels in patients with adenomas. Recently, a detailed study of the angiotensin-aldosterone relationship in idiopathic hyperaldosteronism was conducted by Wisgerhof and associates [65]. These investigators have shown that intravenous infusion of angiotensin II (0.5 ng/kg/min) is followed by a significant increase in the plasma aldosterone level in patients with idiopathic hyperaldosteronism, whereas an increase of this magnitude was not seen with infusion of angiotensin II in control patients or in patients with adrenal adenoma.

Essential Hypertension

Essential hypertension is found in 90 to 95 percent of the hypertensive population. Although the cause of this disease is unknown, several factors such as increased renin-angiotensin activity, mineralocorticoid excess, increased plasma volume, and increased cardiac output have been implicated. The relative participation of these factors in the production of essential hypertension, however, has not been defined. The issue is further obscured by the possibility that different causes could trigger the same pathogenetic constellation. Nevertheless, PRA and its role in essential hypertension are subjects of disagreement and controversy. Various groups have emphasized the importance of classifying patients with essential hypertension into subgroups based on the PRA level; these groups have reported that the risks of myocardial infarction and stroke are closely related to PRA levels [10–12]. Other investigative groups [18, 29, 37] have been unable to substantiate the theory that cardiovascular complications are less common in patients with low PRA levels. It is obvious that further studies are needed in order to assess the importance of high and low renin levels in patients with essential hypertension.

Special Conditions

BARTTER'S SYNDROME. Bartter's syndrome is a disease characterized by vascular insensitivity to angiotensin II, overproduction of renin and aldosterone, diminished chloride reabsorption by the distal tubule of the kidney, and normal blood pressure.

Recent studies have shown that prostaglandins stimulate the release of renin [40, 50, 63]. In addition, the administration of indomethacin, a known prostaglandin inhibitor, reportedly decreases PRA [24, 25, 40]. Other studies have shown that patients with Bartter's syndrome have increased levels of prostaglandins as well as hyperreninemia and hyperaldosteronism [30]. The administration of indomethacin has decreased urinary prostaglandins and partially or completely corrected the high renin and aldosterone levels in patients with Bartter's syndrome [30]. Blood pressure was not changed considerably by the indomethacin therapy.

ROBERTSON-KIHARA SYNDROME. The Robertson-Kihara syndrome is a rare clinical disorder characterized by hypertension, hyperaldosteronism, and hyperreninemia caused by a renin-producing tumor (hemangiopericytoma) of the kidney. In most patients, the tumor is smaller than 4 cm in diameter and may be difficult to detect by arteriography. RVRA clearly lateralizes to the kidney with the renin-producing tumor. After surgical removal of the renin-producing tumor in patients with this disease, blood pressure returned to normal, as did PRA and aldosterone levels [14, 52].

USE OF CONTRACEPTIVE PILLS. The use of contraceptive pills produces an appreciable increase in PRA, which is believed to be mediated by an increase in renin substrate. Skinner and colleagues [57] have suggested that in these circumstances, the actual concentration of renin is decreased because of the negative feedback effect of angiotensin and aldosterone on renin release. Furthermore, they have provided evidence that the failure of such a feedback loop to decrease renin release results in hypertension.

ECLAMPSIA. Eclampsia is a syndrome characterized by the presence of proteinuria, edema, hypertension, convulsions, and encephalopathy during pregnancy. The first three of these symptoms—proteinuria, edema, and hypertension—may be seen initially (preeclampsia). Chemical studies have demonstrated that PRA is increased during normal pregnancy but is decreased with eclampsia. PRA may be measured in pregnant women with the preeclamptic syndrome to rule out other causes of hypertension that have their onset during pregnancy.

Measurement of Plasma Renin Activity

PRA is determined by measuring the amount of angiotensin I generated by the activity of endogenous renin under controlled laboratory conditions.

Radioimmunoassay

Radioimmunoassay (RIA) for angiotensin I has the advantages of simplicity, specificity, and rapidity. In RIA, the concentration of angiotensin in plasma is calculated by comparing the ability of angiotensin I to displace radioactive angiotensin from the angiotensin antibody with the displacement produced by progressive concentrations of synthetic angiotensin I in a standard curve. In this method, angiotensin I antibody is the specific antiserum, [^{125}I] angiotensin I is the labeled antigen, and synthetic angiotensin I is the unlabeled antigen used as the reference standard.

PRODUCTION OF ANGIOTENSIN I ANTIBODY. Three important factors involved in the production of angiotensin I antibodies are titer, specificity, and affinity. *Titer* is the concentration of the antibody in the rabbit plasma and is expressed as the final dilution used in the assay system. *Specificity* is the property by which the antibody will react with only the substance that is intended to be measured —in this case, angiotensin I. *Affinity* describes how well the antibody and the antigen bind to each other. If we assume that the reaction between the antibody and the antigen follows the mass action law, it is possible to describe it by a dissociation constant, *K:*

$$K = \frac{(\text{Antigen})\ (\text{Antibody})}{(\text{Antigen}\quad \text{Antibody})}$$

The affinity may be expressed as the inverse of the dissociation constant; therefore, the lower the dissociation constant, the higher the affinity.

Angiotensin I, because of its low molecular weight (1295), elicits a poor immunogenic response. In order to achieve the "foreignness" needed to produce an antigenic effect, angiotensin must be coupled to a larger molecule. Bovine serum albumin (BSA), an excellent macromolecular carrier, is a protein frequently used for the conjugation step. The process of coupling angiotensin I to BSA is achieved by carbodiimide condensation [31]. The resulting angiotensin-BSA complex, together with Freund's adjuvant, is then injected intramuscularly into a group of rabbits. The Freund's adjuvant acts as a nonspecific carrier for the antigen and also enhances the immune response of the complex. The number of rabbits injected (usually three to five) should be sufficient to reduce the possible effects of a poor response from individual animals.

Satisfactory antibodies should be produced within 6 months. The antibodies to angiotensin I are generally very specific, but a cross-reactivity check against angiotensin II and other small peptide fragments should be performed to ensure maximum specificity (Fig. 7–3).

The titer of antibody from each bleeding of the animal should be determined by incubating small amounts of the [^{125}I] angiotensin I with serial dilutions of the antiserum. The dilution usually chosen is the one that yields at 1 : 1 ratio between the bound and the unbound [^{125}I] angiotensin I (the dilution that is required to bind 50 percent of the [^{125}I] angiotensin I). This dilution will produce the optimal sensitivity and precision needed for the RIA.

PRODUCTION OF LABELED ANGIOTENSIN I. Angiotensin I is readily iodinated with ^{125}I. Several methods for iodination and subsequent isolation of angiotensin have been reported [15, 35]. Iodinated angiotensin I can be obtained from various commercial sources (e.g., New England Nuclear, Boston, Mass., E. R. Squibb, Princeton, N.J., and Schwarz/Mann, Orangeburg, N.Y.).

ANGIOTENSIN I STANDARD. Synthetic angiotensin I (1-Asp-5-Ile-angiotensin I), which is used as the reference standard, can also be obtained from various commercial sources (e.g., Beckman, Palo Alto, Calif., Schwarz/Mann, Orangeburg, N.Y.).

SAMPLE COLLECTION. Blood samples for PRA should be collected in chilled tubes containing ethylenediamine tetra-acetic acid (EDTA). EDTA acts as an angiotensinase inhibitor as well as an anticoagulant. EDTA is essential for

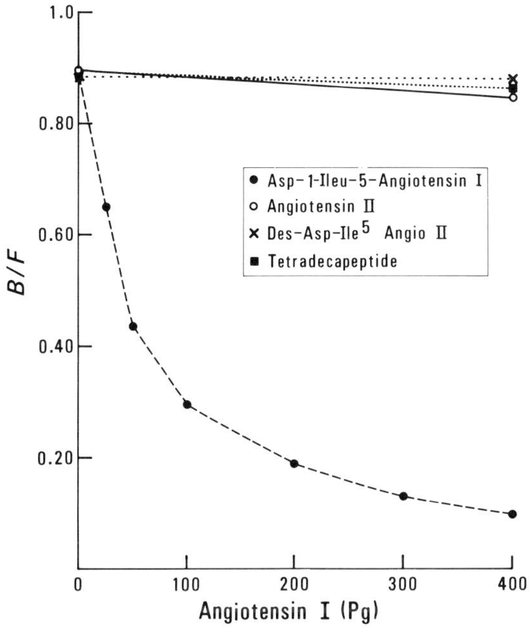

Figure 7–3
Angiotensin I antibody cross-reactivity. Angiotensin I, angiotensin II, des-Asp[1]-angiotensin II, and the tetradecapeptide are added separately to tubes containing [^{125}I] angiotensin I, angiotensin I antibody, and buffer. Displacement of the labeled angiotensin I from the angiotensin I antibody occurs when progressive concentrations of unlabeled angiotensin I are added, whereas no significant displacement is observed when higher doses (5 ng) of angiotensin II and the peptide fragments are added. This result is an indication of high specificity and low-reactivity for the angiotensin I antibody being tested.

sample collection; heparin should not be used because of its interference in the renin-substrate reaction when used in high concentrations [53]. Plasma is then separated by cold centrifugation and should be stored frozen at −20° C if not assayed within 24 hours.

Sealey and colleagues [54] have shown that a cryoactive form of renin called *prorenin* exists in human plasma. Osmond and co-workers [46] have reported that PRA values are appreciably increased when plasma is allowed to remain at 4° C for three days. The degree of activation is apparently time-dependent, and an increased duration during which the sample remains between −5° C and +4° C is associated with an increase in activity. The partial activation of prorenin may occur when blood samples are chilled during processing for PRA determinations. It is therefore recommended that blood samples for PRA be centrifuged, separated, and frozen (at −20° C) as soon as possible after the blood has been withdrawn.

PLASMA INCUBATION. The generation of angiotensin I in human plasma at 37° C is dependent on the choice of angiotensinase and converting enzyme inhibitors and the pH of the incubation mixture. Commonly used inhibitors include EDTA with dimercaprol and 8-hydroxyquinoline at pH 7.4, and EDTA with diisopropylfluorophosphate (DFP) at pH 5.5 to 6.0. More recently, phenylmethylsulfonylfluoride (PMSF) has been substituted for DFP because of the toxicity of the latter.

Previous studies with the human renin–renin substrate reaction have shown the optimal pH to be 5.5 to 6.0 [8]. There is no agreement about the optimal pH level for PRA measurement. It has been reported that the incubation of human plasma at pH 5.7 yields a twofold to fourfold increase in PRA over the pH 7.4 method [13]. It has also been reported that the generation of angiotensin I does not appear to be uniformly increased by decreasing the pH to 6.0 [44]. Since no technical advantage has been demonstrated with either pH, the choice of pH for angiotensin generation seems to be one of individual preference. If the objective is to generate angiotensin under optimal enzymatic conditions, a pH of 6.0 would seem to be the choice. However, if the major concern is to define the velocity of the renin-substrate reaction within its normal physiological setting, then pH 7.4 should be used.

The length of the incubation period and the buffering of the incubation mixture are elements of possible variation. In many procedures, the incubation period continues for 3 hours or longer. To report results in nanograms of angiotensin per hour of generation, the amount of angiotensin formed must be divided by the number of hours during which the sample has been incubated. Therefore, if the reaction velocity is not linear and the angiotensin formation decreases with time, the angiotensin formed expressed as an hourly concentration will be underestimated with long incubations [45].

An appropriate buffering method used to prevent pH changes during incubation is also highly relevant in maintaining a constant reaction velocity. At the optimal pH of angiotensin I formation (pH 5.5 to 6.0), small changes in pH are unlikely to produce considerable variations in the product formation (Fig. 7–4). At pH 7.4, however, because of the steepness of the slope, small changes in pH can greatly influence changes in reaction velocity. In order to prevent these errors in the incubation step, a suitable buffer should be used to avoid pH changes, and PRA should be measured at frequent intervals to determine an area of linearity for the reaction. In our experience, 1-hour incubation periods have been sufficient to measure relatively low levels of PRA and at the same time have fulfilled the requirements for linearity.

Another cause of variation is in the termination of the angiotensin I generation step, which is achieved either by placing the samples in ice water to lower the temperature rapidly or by placing the samples in a boiling water bath, which terminates the reaction and also precipitates plasma proteins that may interfere with the RIA. When results obtained from the two methods (chilling versus

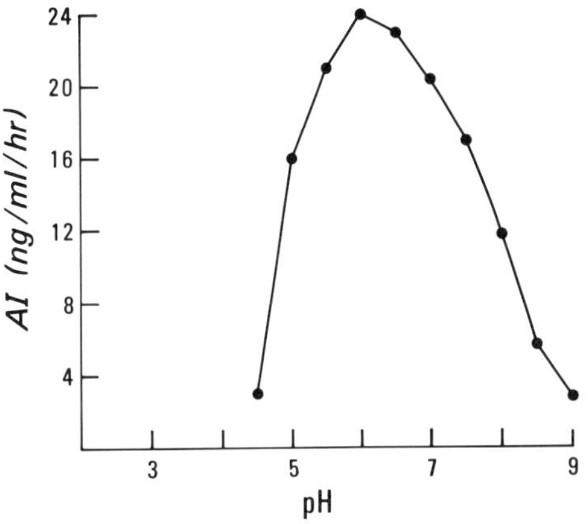

Figure 7–4
Human renin–renin substrate pH optimum. The amount of angiotensin I formation is largest at pH 5.5 to 6.0. A sharp decline in generation is seen between pH 6.5 and pH 8.5, which indicates the need for an appropriate buffering system to prevent pH changes during angiotensin formation.

boiling) are compared, there is poor agreement between the PRA values. This issue seems to be of importance because PRA values obtained by the boiling method correlate well for distinguishing primary from idiopathic aldosteronism, whereas such a distinction is not evident when values obtained by the chilling method are used [64]. The reasons underlying these observations are not clear and need to be investigated further.

Because of these variations in methods, comparisons of PRA values between individual laboratories are quite difficult. At present, the College of American Pathologists is attempting to standardize the renin method in such a way that results would be reported as renin in absolute units (Goldblatt units per milliliter of plasma) rather than angiotensin I activity (nanograms per milliliter per hour). This method was pioneered by Hass and Goldblatt [32].

COMPETITIVE PROTEIN BINDING AND CHARCOAL SEPARATION. The next step in the measurement of PRA is the analysis of the samples by RIA. The procedure follows the principle of saturation analysis, in which PRA is calculated by comparing the displacement of [^{125}I] angiotensin I from the angiotensin I antibody with the displacement produced by known amounts of unlabeled angiotensin I.

A standard curve consisting of increasing concentrations of synthetic angiotensin I is prepared (Table 7–1); the plasma samples are then assayed (Table 7–2). The first tube of each sample receives 50 μl of plasma that has been incubated at 4° C for 1 hour. This tube represents the measurement of endogenous angiotensin I and will be subtracted from the amount of angiotensin

Table 7–1. Standard Curve for Radioimmunoassay of Plasma Renin Activity

Tube [a]	Angiotensin I Standard (μl)	[^{125}I] Angiotensin I (μl) [b]	Antibody (μl)	Buffer (μl) [c]
1, 2	—	50	—	900
3, 4	—	50	—	900
5, 6	—	50	50	900
7, 8	25 (2 ng/ml)	50	50	900
9, 10	25 (4 ng/ml)	50	50	900
11, 12	25 (8 ng/ml)	50	50	900
13, 14	25 (12 ng/ml)	50	50	900
15, 16	25 (20 ng/ml)	50	50	900

[a] Tubes 1 and 2 indicate total counts and should not be charcoaled; tubes 3 and 4 represent nonspecific binding.
[b] Angiotensin I label concentration = 5 pg/5000 counts.
[c] Buffer = 0.1 M tris-acetate buffer.

Table 7–2. Plasma Sample Pipetting for Radioimmunoassay

Tube	Plasma Added (μl)	Temperature	[^{125}I] Angiotensin I (μl)	Antibody (μl)	Buffer (μl)
19	50	4°C	50	50	900
20, 21	50	37°C	50	50	900
22, 23	25	37°C	50	50	900

formed at 37° C. The next four tubes receive, in duplicate, 50 μl and 25 μl of plasma that has been incubated at 37° C for 1 hour. After the addition of the plasma and required reagents, the contents of the tubes are mixed well and allowed to equilibrate for 20 hours at 4° C. After completion of the equilibration period, the bound and free portions of the mixture are separated by the addition of a charcoal suspension to all tubes. On centrifugation, the charcoal will retain the free angiotensin I in the precipitate, and the bound portion will remain in the supernatant. Finally, the supernatant is separated from the charcoal precipitate, and the radioactivity is determined by counting in a gamma counter.

COUNTING AND CALCULATING. Either the supernatant or the charcoal precipitate may be counted. After subtraction of background radioactivity, the percent of [^{125}I] angiotensin I bound (B%) is calculated by the following method:

$$\text{Supernatant counted} = \frac{\text{Sample or standard counts}}{\text{Total counts}} \times 100$$

$$\text{Charcoal counted} = \frac{\text{Total counts} - \text{Sample or standard counts}}{\text{Totals counts}} \times 100$$

The standard curve is used to determine sample concentrations by comparing the amount of labeled angiotensin I bound in a sample with the amount bound in the standard (B%), and the concentrations are then corrected for known dilutions. If a sample concentration is too high to read on the standard curve, the sample must be diluted and reassayed. Final results are expressed as nanograms of angiotensin I generated per milliliter of plasma per hour of incubation (ng/ml/hour).

QUALITY CONTROL. For a continuous check of accuracy and reproducibility of the RIA, two control samples are analyzed with every assay. When these two samples are appropriately diluted, the concentrations cover the entire span of the standard curve. The calculated results of both control samples must be within ± 20 percent of the true mean, or the entire assay must be repeated.

Bioassay

In 1898, Tigerstedt and Bergman reported that crude saline extracts of rabbit kidney injected into anesthetized rabbits produced a substantial increase in blood pressure. This observation suggested to other investigators that after appropriate extractions, concentrations of renin in blood could be measured by bioassay. However, attempts to bioassay renin have proved to be very difficult, tedious, and highly irreproducible. With relatively large doses of renin, the pressor action persists up to 30 minutes, which severely limits the number of injections per assay. Furthermore, if injections of renin are made before the blood pressure returns to basal levels, the pressor response becomes progressively less (tachyphylaxis), until no response is obtained [7]. At present, there is no satisfactory explanation to account for renin tachyphylaxis, and this has seriously limited the development of a renin bioassay. These difficulties can be overcome by estimating renin activity indirectly, that is by bioassaying the concentration of angiotensin formed after incubation of plasma. Several methods for angiotensin bioassay have been developed, including determination of the vasoconstrictor activity in isolated smooth muscle [38] and measurement of the increase in systemic blood pressure in the total animal [43]. In measuring PRA by the total-animal method, the Sprague-Dawley rat is the most sensitive species, although the Wistar rat has also been used.

The rat is anesthetized with sodium pentobarbital (40 mg/kg) given intraperitoneally. Atropine (0.8 mg subcutaneously) is also given to avoid obstruction of the respiratory tract. After induction of the anesthesia, the rat is placed on a small operating board with the four extremities secured. The head is then immobilized by placing a small metal clip over the upper teeth of the animal and securing it to the board. The trachea and one carotid artery (either right or left) are then exposed through a medial neck incision, and the trachea is cannulated with a 3-cm PE-90 tubing to facilitate respiration. The carotid artery is cannulated with a PE-50 tubing and is connected to either a mercury manometer or a transducer to measure blood pressure. Subsequently, a PE-10 tubing is inserted into the femoral artery for the injections of angiotensin. An initial injection of heparin (1000 units/kg) is given to prevent blood coagulation in the catheters.

Before beginning the assay, a ganglionic blocking agent such as pentolinium tartrate (1 to 40 mg/kg) should be given. The administration of the ganglionic blocking agent will result in a decrease in systemic pressure by 40 to 50 mm Hg. The injection of this drug will prevent baroreceptor reflex compensation that would tend to minimize the pressor effect of the angiotensin. Ganglionic blocking agents increase the sensitivity of vasopressor responses to angiotensin [47].

A dose-response curve to three doses of angiotensin II should then be made; this should be done at least twice to ensure reproducibility. Under these conditions, the angiotensin I formed will yield constant pressor dose-response curves because most, if not all, angiotensin I is quantitatively transformed to angiotensin II through the pulmonary circulation in the assay animal. In order to bioassay angiotensin, however, it is advisable to avoid undesirable hemodynamic reactions produced by other vasoactive substances contained in plasma. To a large extent, this is achieved by following simple procedures to extract angiotensin or by precipitating in plasma most proteins and high-molecular-weight polypeptides by boiling the plasma after incubation [43].

The sensitivity of a rat to angiotensin varies from twofold to fourfold. In low doses (1, 2, and 3 ng per rat), a linear response is usually obtained. When higher doses are required because of low sensitivity, however, the response is proportional to the logarithm of the dose. Once the desired reproducibility of the dose-response curve has been obtained, the unknowns are assayed to determine the relative concentrations. Unknowns producing pressor responses greater than that of the highest standard must be diluted and reassayed. The standards and unknowns are then assayed a second time. The standard producing the smallest response is assayed first, followed by the unknowns whose pressor responses are between the first and second standards. This process, known as bracketing, is then repeated for the remaining standards and unknowns.

At present, numerous comparisons show that PRA levels measured by bioassay correlate well with those measured by RIA. The bioassay method may even offer some financial advantages over the RIA procedure in that there is no need to purchase expensive equipment such as gamma counters and automatic pipetting devices. This is an important factor to consider when the total sample throughout is relatively small.

Measurement of Renin Substrate

The measurement of renin substrate is of interest because changes in substrate concentration in plasma can affect the formation of angiotensin I. Renin substrate is calculated indirectly by measuring the final concentration of angiotensin I formed in the presence of excess renin. This large concentration of renin will cleave its substrate to form angiotensin I until the substrate is completely exhausted, at which time no further increase in product formation will be seen.

This method assumes that the formation of angiotensin I is stoichiometric and therefore that the production of angiotensin I is proportional to the substrate concentration. Renin from the same animal species (homologous renin) should be used to ensure maximum angiotensin I production because the total production of angiotensin I has been reported to be decreased when plasma is incubated with heterologous renin [55].

Sample Collection

Blood samples should be collected in chilled tubes containing EDTA. The samples should then be processed as described in the PRA procedure.

Plasma Incubation

Angiotensinase and converting enzyme inhibitors are added to the plasma, as described in the procedure for PRA. An excess of renin is then added to the plasma samples, and they are incubated at 37° C for a length of time that is sufficient to consume all of the substrate. The amount of angiotensin I formed is then measured by RIA.

Calculations

The amount of angiotensin I formed is plotted against the time of incubation. It is assumed that hydrolysis is virtually complete and will be indicated by a plateau in angiotensin I formation. The point in time at which this plateau is reached represents the substrate concentration of the plasma sample. This concentration is reported as nanograms of angiotensin I equivalents.

A method for the direct measurement of human renin substrate has recently been reported [19]. This method describes the procedures of substrate purification, antibody and label production, and RIA.

References

1. Amsterdam, E. A., Couch, N. P., Christlieb, A. R., et al. Renal vein renin activity in the prognosis of surgery for renovascular hypertension. *Am. J. Med.* 47:860, 1969.
2. Assaykeen, T. A., Clayton, P. L., Goldfien, A., et al. Effect of alpha- and beta-adrenergic blocking agents on the renin response to hypoglycemia and epinephrine in dogs. *Endocrinology* 87:1318, 1970.
3. Barajas, L. Renin secretion: An anatomical basis for tubular control. *Science* 172:485, 1971.
4. Biron, P., Koiw, E., Nowaczynski, W., et al. The effects of intravenous infusions of valine-5 angiotensin II and other pressor agents on urinary electrolytes and corticosteroids, including aldosterone. *J. Clin. Invest.* 40:338, 1961.
5. Blaine, E. H., Davis, J. O., and Prewitt, R. L. Evidence for a renal vascular receptor in control of renin secretion. *Am. J. Physiol.* 220:1593, 1971.
6. Blair-West, J. R., Coghlan, J. P., Denton, D. A., et al. The effect of the hepta-

peptide (2–8) and hexapeptide (3–8) fragments of angiotensin II on aldosterone secretion. *J. Clin. Endocrinol. Metab.* 32:575, 1971.
7. Bock, K. D., and Gross, F. Renin and angiotensin tachyphylaxis. *Circ. Res.* 9:1044, 1961.
8. Boucher, R., Veyrat, R., de Champlain, J., et al. New procedures for measurement of human plasma angiotensin and renin activity levels. *Can. Med. Assoc. J.* 90:194, 1964.
9. Brunner, H. R., Gavras, H., Laragh, J. H., et al. Hypertension in man: Exposure of the renin and sodium components using angiotensin II blockade. *Circ. Res.* 34(Suppl. 1):35, 1974.
10. Brunner, H. R., Laragh, J. H., Baer, L., et al. Essential hypertension: Renin and aldosterone, heart attack and stroke. *N. Engl. J. Med.* 286:441, 1972.
11. Brunner, H. R., Sealey, J. E., and Laragh, J. H. Renin as a risk factor in essential hypertension: More evidence. *Am. J. Med.* 55:295, 1973.
12. Christlieb, A. R., Gleason, R. E., Hickler, R. B., et al. Renin: A risk factor for cardiovascular disease? *Ann. Intern. Med.* 81:7, 1974.
13. Cohen, E. L., Grim, C. E., Conn, J. W., et al. Accurate and rapid measurement of plasma renin activity by radioimmunoassay: Results in normal and hypertensive people. *J. Lab. Clin. Med.* 77:1025, 1971.
14. Conn, J. W., Cohen, E. L., Lucas, C. P., et al. Primary reninism: Hypertension, hyperreninemia, and secondary aldosteronism due to renin-producing juxtaglomerular cell tumors. *Arch. Intern. Med.* 130:682, 1972.
15. Damkjaer Nielsen, M., Jørgensen, M., and Giese, J. ^{125}I-labelling of angiotensin I and II. *Acta Endocrinol.* (*Kbh.*) 67:104, 1971.
16. Daul, C. B., Heath, R. G., and Garey, R. E. Angiotensin-forming enzyme in human brain. *Neuropharmacology* 14:75, 1975.
17. Davis, J. O., and Freeman, R. H. Mechanisms regulating renin release. *Physiol. Rev.* 56:1, 1976.
18. Doyle, A. E., Jerums, G., Johnston, C. I., et al. Plasma renin levels and vascular complications in hypertension. *Br. Med. J.* 2:206, 1973.
19. Eggena, P., Barrett, J. D., Hidaka, H., et al. A direct radioimmunoassay for human renin substrate and identification of multiple substrate types in plasma. *Circ. Res.* 41(Suppl. 2):34, 1977.
20. Eskildsen, P. C. Renin in different tissues, amniotic fluid and plasma of pregnant and non-pregnant rabbits. *Acta Pathol. Microbiol. Scand* [*A*] 81:263, 1973.
21. Ferris, T. F., and Mulrow, P. J. The uterus as a source of renin (abstract). *Clin. Res.* 13:206, 1965.
22. Ferris, T. F., Stein, J. H., and Kauffman, J. Uterine blood flow and uterine renin secretion. *J. Clin. Invest.* 51:2827, 1972.
23. Freeman, R. H., Davis, J. O., Lohmeier, T. E., et al. Evidence that des-asp^{1}-angiotensin II mediates the renin-angiotensin response. *Circ. Res.* 38(Suppl. 2):99, 1976.
24. Frolich, J., Hollifield, J., Wilkinson, G., et al. Effect of indomethacin on furosemide stimulated renin and sodium excretion (abstract). *Circ. Res.* 52(Suppl. 2):99, 1975.
25. Frolich, J. C., Hollifield, J. W., and Oates, J. A. Effect of indomethacin on isoproterenol induced renin release (abstract). *Clin. Res.* 24:9, 1976.
26. Ganten, D., Boucher, R., and Genest, J. Renin activity in brain tissue of puppies and adult dogs. *Brain Res.* 33:557, 1971.
27. Ganten, D., Hutchinson, J. S., Schelling, P., et al. The iso-renin angiotensin systems in extrarenal tissue. *Clin. Exp. Pharmacol. Physiol.* 3:103, 1976.
28. Genest, J. The Renin-Angiotensin-Aldosterone System. In A. N. Brest and

J. H. Moyer (Eds.), *Cardiovascular Disorders*. Philadelphia: Davis, 1968. Pp. 144–160.
29. Genest, J., Boucher, R., Kuchel, O., et al. Renin in hypertension: How important as a risk factor? *Can. Med. Assoc. J.* 109:475, 1973.
30. Gill, J. R., Jr., Frölich, J. C., Bowden, R. E., et al. Bartter's syndrome: A disorder characterized by high urinary prostaglandins and a dependence of hyperreninemia on prostaglandin synthesis. *Am. J. Med.* 61:43, 1976.
31. Goodfriend, T. L., Levine, L., and Fasman, G. D. Antibodies to bradykinin and angiotensin: A use of carbodiimides in immunology. *Science* 144:1344, 1964.
32. Haas, E., and Goldblatt, H. Indirect assay of plasma-renin. *Lancet* 1:1330, 1972.
33. Hunt, J. C. Diagnosis of renovascular hypertension. *Bull. N. Y. Acad. Med.* 45:877, 1969.
34. Hunt, T. K., Schambelan, M., and Biglieri, E. G. Selection of patients and operative approach in primary aldosteronism. *Ann. Surg.* 182:353, 1975.
35. Hunter, W. M., and Greenwood, F. C. Preparation of iodine-131 labelled human growth hormone of high specific activity. *Nature* 194:495, 1962.
36. Johnson, J. A., Davis, J. O., and Witty, R. T. Effects of catecholamines and renal nerve stimulation on renin release in the nonfiltering kidney. *Circ. Res.* 29:646, 1971.
37. Kaplan, N. M. The prognostic implications of plasma renin in essential hypertension. *J. A. M. A.* 231:167, 1975.
38. Khairallah, P. A., and Page, I. H. Mechanism of action of angiotensin and bradykinin on smooth muscle in situ. *Am. J. Physiol.* 200:51, 1961.
39. Laragh, J. H., Sealey, J. E., Bühler, F. R., et al. The renin axis and vasoconstriction volume analysis for understanding and treating renovascular and renal hypertension. *Am. J. Med.* 58:4, 1975.
40. Larsson, C., Weber, P., and Änggård, E. Arachidonic acid increases and indomethacin decreases plasma renin activity in the rabbit. *Eur. J. Pharmacol.* 28:391, 1974.
41. Mancia, G., Romero, J. C., and Shepherd, J. T. Continuous inhibition of renin release in dogs by vagally innervated receptors in the cardiopulmonary region. *Circ. Res.* 36:529, 1975.
42. Marks, L. S., Maxwell, M. H., and Kaufman, J. J. Non-renin-mediated renovascular hypertension: A new syndrome? *Lancet* 1:615, 1977.
43. Nasjletti, A., and Masson, G. M. C. A method for the measurement of plasma renin in the rat. *Proc. Soc. Exp. Biol. Med.* 136:344, 1971.
44. Oparil, S., Koerner, T. J., and Haber, E. Effects of pH and enzyme inhibitors on apparent generation of angiotensin I in human plasma. *J. Clin. Endocrinol. Metab.* 39:965, 1974.
45. Osmond, D. H., McFadzean, P. A., and Scaiff, K. D. Renin activity by radioimmunoassay: The plasma incubation step. *Clin. Biochem.* 7:52, 1974.
46. Osmond, D. H., Ross, L. J., and Scaiff, K. D. Increased renin activity after cold storage of human plasma. *Can. J. Physiol. Pharmacol.* 51:705, 1973.
47. Page, I. H., and Olmsted, F. Hemodynamic mechanisms of increased cardiovascular response resulting from ganglioplegics and atropine. *Am. J. Physiol.* 204:582, 1963.
48. Peach, M. J., and Chiu, A. T. Stimulation and inhibition of aldosterone biosynthesis in vitro by angiotensin II analogs. *Circ. Res.* 34(Suppl. 1):7, 1974.
49. Romero, J. C., Holmes, D. R., and Strong, C. G. The effect of high sodium intake and angiotensin antagonist in rabbits with severe and moderate hyper-

tension induced by constriction of one renal artery. *Circ. Res.* 40(Suppl. 1):17, 1977.
50. Romero, J. C., and Strong, C. G. Hypertension and the interrelated renal circulatory effects of prostaglandins and the renin-angiotensin system. *Mayo Clin. Proc.* 52:462, 1977.
51. Schambelan, M., Brust, N. L., Chang, B. C. F., et al. Circadian rhythm and effect of posture on plasma aldosterone concentration in primary aldosteronism. *J. Clin. Endocrinol. Metab.* 43:115, 1976.
52. Schambelan, M., Howes, E. L., Jr., Stockigt, J. R., et al. Role of renin and aldosterone in hypertension due to a renin-secreting tumor. *Am. J. Med.* 55:86, 1973.
53. Sealey, J. E., Gerten, J. N., Ledingham, J. G. G., et al. Inhibition of renin by heparin. *J. Clin. Endocrinol. Metab.* 27:699, 1967.
54. Sealey, J. E., Moon, C., Laragh, J. H., et al. Plasma prorenin in normal, hypertensive, and anephric subjects and its effect on renin measurements. *Circ. Res.* 40(Suppl. 1):41, 1977.
55. Sen, S., Hirasawa, K., Smeby, R. R., et al. Measurement of plasma renin substrate using homologous and heterologous renin. *Am. J. Physiol.* 221:1476, 1971.
56. Simmons, J. L., and Michelakis, A. M. Renovascular hypertension: The diagnostic value of renal vein renin ratios. *J. Urol.* 104:497, 1970.
57. Skinner, S. L., Lumbers, E. R., and Symonds, E. M. Alteration by oral contraceptives of normal menstrual changes in plasma renin activity, concentration and substrate. *Clin. Sci.* 36:67, 1969.
58. Spielman, W. S., Davis, J. O., and Freeman, R. H. Des-asp-1-angiotensin II: Possible role in mediating the renin-angiotensin response in the rat. *Proc. Soc. Exp. Biol. Med.* 151:177, 1976.
59. Streeten, D. H. P., Anderson, G. H., Freiberg, J. M., et al. Use of an angiotensin II antagonist (saralasin) in the recognition of "angiotensinogenic" hypertension. *N. Engl. J. Med.* 292:657, 1975.
60. Strong, C. G., Hunt, J. C., Sheps, S. G., et al. Renal venous renin activity: Enhancement of sensitivity of lateralization by sodium depletion. *Am. J. Cardiol.* 27:602, 1971.
61. Vander, A. J. Effect of catecholamines and the renal nerves on renin secretion in anesthetized dogs. *Am. J. Physiol.* 209:659, 1965.
62. Vander, A. J. Control of renin release. *Physiol. Rev.* 47:359, 1967.
63. Werning, C., Vetter, W., Weidmann, P., et al. Effect of prostaglandin E_1 on renin in the dog. *Am. J. Physiol.* 220:852, 1971.
64. Wisgerhof, M., and Brown, R. D. Personal communication, 1977.
65. Wisgerhof, M., Carpenter, P. C., and Brown, R. D. Increased adrenal sensitivity to angiotensin II in idiopathic hyperaldosteronism (abstract). *Clin. Res.* 25:568, 1977.

8. Serum Angiotensin Converting Enzyme

Michael S. Rohrbach

Angiotensin converting enzyme (peptidyldipeptide hydrolase EC 3.4.15.1) is the terminal proteolytic enzyme in the renin-angiotensin system. This system is responsible for the generation of angiotensin II, a potent vasoconstricting polypeptide hormone, from circulating alpha globulin (for a review of this system, see reference [32]). The enzyme functions by cleaving dipeptides from the free carboxyl terminus of peptides. In vivo, it generates angiotensin II from angiotensin I, a decapeptide with little or no vasoconstricting activity, by removing the carboxyl terminal histidylleucine. It also degrades and thereby inactivates the vasodilator bradykinin by sequentially cleaving the dipeptides, phenylalanylarginine and serylproline, from the carboxyl terminus of the hormone.

In vitro, the enzyme exhibits a broad substrate specificity. In addition to hydrolyzing angiotensin I and bradykinin, it also hydrolyzes higher homologues of both peptides. The bradykinin homologues, Lys-bradykinin, Met-Lys-bradykinin, and Lys-Lys-bradykinin, are cleaved by the enzyme, although at a slower rate than bradykinin itself [7]. The angiotensin homologue, tetradecapeptide renin substrate (angiotensin I with the extended amino acid sequence Leu-Val-Tyr-Ser at the carboxyl terminus) is also cleaved by the enzyme in sequential steps to yield angiotensin II and three dipeptides. As discussed by Dorer and co-workers [6], the ability of angiotensin converting enzyme to hydrolyze this substrate makes it a poor choice for the detection and quantitation of renin activity. In addition to these homologues of its natural substrates, the enzyme will also hydrolyze a wide variety of other peptides ranging in size from N-blocked tripeptides [3, 8, 20] to the beta chain of insulin [12]. The ability of the enzyme to hydrolyze N-blocked tripeptides has proved to be particularly useful in the development of simplified assays for the enzyme, since these small peptides can be easily synthesized and designed to contain readily detectable reporter groups. The only constraints on the design of synthetic substrates are the enzyme's requirement for a free carboxyl terminus and its inability to cleave peptides that contain either glutamic acid in the C-terminal position or proline in the penultimate C-terminal position [8].

Forms of the Enzyme

Although angiotensin converting enzyme was first detected in serum [33], it soon became apparent both from kinetic studies with semipurified serum enzyme [13] and from angiotensin I tracer studies with excised lungs [18] that the biologically important in vivo conversion of angiotensin I was carried out

Portions of this work were supported by grant HL-21894 from the National Institutes of Health.

by a particulate rather than a soluble form of the enzyme. This discovery led to an effort in a number of laboratories to identify the subcellular location of the particulate enzyme. Sanders and Huggins [27] and Ryan and co-workers [26] independently described capillary endothelial plasma membrane fractions that possessed angiotensin converting enzyme activity. The endothelial plasma membrane was confirmed as the site of the immobilized form of the enzyme, using microperoxidase-coupled angiotensin converting enzyme antibody [25], where the antibody was found to be localized on the luminal surface of lung capillaries and venules. Studies on other tissue demonstrated that the enzyme was widespread throughout the vascular system [2].

The relationship between the serum and membrane-bound forms of the enzyme has been examined by Soffer and co-workers [4, 5], who have purified both forms of the enzyme from rabbit. The catalytic properties of the two forms with respect to hydrolysis of angiotensin I, bradykinin, and hippurylhistidylleucine were similar. Immunologically they were identical, and they were physically comparable. Both were metalloglycoproteins of 130,000 to 140,000 molecular weight, with the carbohydrate composing 25 to 30 percent of the total weight. The serum enzyme, however, had three times more sialic acid than the membrane-bound enzyme. Soffer [34] has speculated that the serum enzyme arises from membrane-bound enzyme that has been sloughed off into the bloodstream, and that the increase in sialic acid is due to the clearance of sialic acid–deficient enzyme by normal plasma glycoprotein clearance mechanisms. Although the serum form of the enzyme does not appear to be of significant physiological importance in the regulation of angiotensin or bradykinin, quantitation of the serum activity does appear to have useful diagnostic potential.

Serum Angiotensin Converting Enzyme as a Diagnostic Index

In 1975, Lieberman [14] reported an investigation of the relationship between blood pressure and serum angiotensin converting enzyme (SACE) activity in patients with chronic obstructive lung disease. Although he found no correlation between blood pressure and SACE activity, he did discover that SACE activity was elevated in patients with sarcoidosis. This rather serendipitous discovery was shortly confirmed in a number of other laboratories [1, 9, 19, 23, 31]. At present, quantitation of SACE activity represents a simple, potentially valuable test for the differential diagnosis of sarcoidosis. Sarcoidosis is an ill-defined systemic disease of unknown etiology and pathogenesis; it is characterized by noncaseating granulomas with the histological appearance of epithelioid tubercles and, in 90 percent of the patients, by roentgenograms showing bilateral hilar adenopathy or parenchymal infiltrates, or both [28]. At present, its diagnosis is considered established in patients who have the appropriate clinical and radiographic features by biopsy evidence of noncaseating granulomas and in whom other diseases with similar clinical features, such as fungal infections, tuberculosis, and beryllium disease, have been eliminated. The great potential utility of SACE quantitation for the differential diagnosis of sarcoidosis is that it is not significantly elevated in these other disease states [14, 15, 31].

Although there is unanimous agreement among all studies on the general observation that SACE activity is elevated in sarcoidosis, there is considerable disagreement on the specifics of the observation and on the limitations of the test. Table 8–1 gives the values obtained by various investigators for SACE activity in normal controls, in patients with inactive or corticosteroid-suppressed sarcoidosis, and in patients with active sarcoidosis. As would be expected, SACE values for normal controls are very dependent on the substrate used, and even with the same substrate, the mean SACE values vary by greater than a factor of 2 among the studies. In addition to this variability of mean SACE activity in normal controls, the effects of age and sex on SACE activity are also widely in dispute. Lieberman [14] noted a slow decrease in SACE activity with age, whereas Ashutosh and Keighley [1] reported a slow increase in mean activity levels with age. This author has found no age dependence in adults aged 20 or older [23], a finding that is in agreement with a study by Fanburg and colleagues [9], who found no statistical difference in SACE activity in normal controls older than 40 as compared to those younger than 40. In our study of normal subjects younger than 20, however, we found markedly elevated SACE activity. Children 6 to 10 years old had levels that in many instances equaled the highest activity seen in patients with active sarcoidosis. The SACE activity fell with age until at age 20, as described above, it was no longer age-dependent.

The relationship between sex and SACE activity has been examined in three studies. Fanburg and colleagues [9] and this author [23] have noted no sex dependence on SACE activity, whereas Lieberman [14] found females had lower activity at all ages.

Although mean SACE activity and those factors that affect activity in normal subjects vary among the various studies, there is even more uncertainty about the usefulness of elevated SACE activity for the diagnosis of sarcoidosis and the effect of corticosteroids on SACE activity in these patients. The mean SACE activity for patients with active sarcoidosis was higher than the normal control mean activity in all the studies reported to date. The extent of the elevation in the disease state ranged from 59 percent to 129 percent. However, the usefulness of elevated activity as a diagnostic test for sarcoidosis is still unclear. If one considers SACE activity greater than 2 standard deviations above the mean activity observed in normal subjects as being significantly elevated, the percentage of patients who had significantly elevated activity has varied from 100 percent to 34 percent among the various studies (Table 8–2). The cause for such a wide variation in significantly elevated activity is not readily apparent.

The effect of corticosteroid treatment on SACE activity is perhaps the most disputed question about the relationship between SACE activity and sarcoidosis. The data relating to this question are about equally divided between studies showing that corticosteroids have no effect on SACE activity [9, 19, 31] and

Table 8–1. SACE Activity in Normal Subjects, Patients with Inactive or Steroid-Suppressed Sarcoidosis, and Active Sarcoidosis

Study	Substrate [b]	Method [c]	Normal [d]	Active [d]	Inactive [d]
Lieberman [14] [a]	HHL	SP	22.8 ± 6.0 (172)	41.0 ± 6.8 (17)	21.3 ± 7.0 (11)
Lieberman [15] [a]	HHL	SP	22.8 ± 6.0 (172)	47.3 ± 22.2 (64)	20.6 ± 7.2 (17)
Fanburg et al. [9]	HHL	SP	28.2 ± 11.3 (84)	52.7 ± 25.3 (56)	46.6 ± 20.3 (9)
Ashutosh and Keighley [1] [a]	HHL	SP	17.6 ± 5.6 (21)	40.5 ± 7.6 (12)	20.6 ± 7.4 (9)
Silverstein et al. [31]	HHL	SF	28.6 ± 7.5 (63)	48.3 (58)	—
Friedland and Silverstein [10]	HHL	SF	32.2 ± 9.9 (58)	—	—
Friedland and Silverstein [11]	AI	SF	4.7 ± 1.3 (45)	17.3 ± 6.5 (4)	—
Rohrbach and DeRemee [23]	HHL	R	40.3 ± 8.5 (60)	71.8 ± 17.3 (37)	44.9 ± 9.9 (24)
Rohatgi et al. [21]	HGG	R	89.2 ± 28.4 (15)	171.4 ± 63.5 (14)	98.9 ± 24.0 (15)

[a] Corrected for a threefold calculation error noted by Silverstein et al. [31].
[b] HHL = hippuryl-L-histidyl-L-leucine, AI = angiotensin I, HHG = hippurylglycylglycine.
[c] SP = spectrophotometric, SF = spectrofluorometric, R = radiochemical.
[d] The values shown are nanomoles of substrate hydrolyzed per minute per milliliter of serum ± 1 SD. The number of sera analyzed are shown in parentheses.

Table 8–2. Prevalence of SACE Activity Greater than 2 Standard Deviations above the Control Mean for Patients with Active Sarcoidosis

Study	No. of Patients	Percent
Lieberman [14]	15/17	88.2
Lieberman [15]	53/64	82.8
Ashutosh and Keighley [1]	12/12	100.0
Silverstein et al. [31]	20/58	34.5
Fanburg et al. [9]	27/56	48.2
Friedland and Silverstein [11]	4/4	100.0
Rohrbach and DeRemee [23]	32/37	86.5

studies showing that corticosteroids lower activity to normal or near-normal levels [1, 14, 15, 23, 24]. While it is difficult to see the cause of these contradictory experimental findings, it may be due to differences in the corticosteroid dose administered or to individual differences in the response to corticosteroid. In our study, we found that prednisone treatment generally lowered SACE levels to normal values. However, we encountered one patient who, although showing clinical improvement, had no change in SACE activity, and a second patient whose SACE activity dropped by a factor of 2 but stabilized at a value greater than 2 standard deviations above the normal mean value. The second patient presents a possible explanation for the studies that found no effect of corticosteroids on SACE activity. A single measurement of the patient's activity after corticosteroid treatment would reveal elevated activity. Without knowledge of the patient's pretreatment activity, one would arrive at the erroneous conclusion that corticosteroids had no effect on SACE activity.

Subsequent to the discovery of elevated levels of SACE activity in sarcoidosis, elevated levels have also been found in patients with Gaucher's disease and patients with leprosy. Lieberman and Beutler [16] reported mean SACE activity of 121 $\pm$ 73 units per milliliter in patients with Gaucher's disease. One hundred percent of these patients had activity greater than 2 standard deviations above the normal mean activity. A similar finding was reported by Silverstein and Friedland [29], who found mean activity levels of 93.3 $\pm$ 14.8 units per milliliter, with 73 percent of the patients having significantly elevated activity. In a study of SACE activity in leprosy, Lieberman and Rea [17] found mean SACE activity of 35.3 $\pm$ 12 units per milliliter in patients with untreated leprosy; 48 percent of these patients had significantly elevated activity.

The common factor among these three diseases is the occurrence of monocytic phagocytes that have been transformed into nonphagocytic storage or secretory cells [17]. Since it has been shown that the epithelioid cells in sarcoidosis are producing angiotensin converting enzyme [30], Lieberman has hypothesized that elevated SACE activity may be common to other diseases characterized by proliferation of transformed nonphagocytic monocytic cells [16, 17].

Assay Methods

A number of assay procedures are currently available for the determination of serum angiotensin converting enzyme concentrations. These assays employ either small synthetic substrates or angiotensin I and use spectrophotometric, spectrofluorometric, or radiochemical techniques to quantitate hydrolysis. While each of the assay methods has features that recommend its use, each method is subject to intrinsic limitations, which will be discussed below. In light of the diversity of assay methods available and their individual limitations, investigators should choose a method that fulfills their own particular needs.

Assays Employing Angiotensin I

Two assay methods have been developed that use angiotensin I as the substrate.

METHOD OF OPARIL AND COLLEAGUES. Oparil and colleagues [19] have used (tyrosyl-^{125}I) angiotensin I in a radiochemical assay in which the conversion of (tyrosyl-^{125}I) angiotensin I to (tyrosyl-^{125}I) angiotensin II is followed either by high-voltage paper electrophoresis or ion-exchange chromatography.

Materials. The following materials are used in this method:

(Tyrosyl-^{125}I) angiotensin (New England Nuclear Corp., Boston, Mass.)
100 mM tris-acetate (pH 7.4), 100 mM NaCl
100 mM sodium phosphage (pH 7.4)
0.14 M 8-hydroxyquinoline
Pyridine-acetate (pH 3.55)
DEAE-Sephadex A-25
Whatman 3 MM electrophoresis paper

Method. Dilute 1 ml of heparinized plasma to 4.5 ml with 100 mM tris-acetate (pH 7.4), 100 mM NaCl buffer. Add 30 pmol of (tyrosyl-^{125}I) angiotensin I to this solution, and then incubate it at 37° C. Aliquots (250 μl) are withdrawn at 0, 2.5, 5.0, 7.5, 10, 15, and 30 minutes for quantitation of hydrolysis. This quantitation is performed by two methods. A portion (50 μl) of each aliquot is immediately spotted on Whatman 3 MM paper and subjected to electrophoresis at 4000 v for 1 hour in pyridine-acetate buffer. Following electrophoresis, the paper is dried and cut into 1-cm strips. Location and quantitation of angiotensin I, angiotensin II, and their metabolites are performed by gamma radiation counting of the electrophoresis strips. To the remainder of each aliquot (200 μl), 5 μl of 8-hydroxyquinoline is added, and the sample is subjected to chromatography on a 0.9 × 100 cm column of DEAE-Sephadex A-25. Elution is carried out at room temperature with 100 mM sodium phosphage (pH 7.4) buffer. Then 3-ml fractions are collected, and 1-ml samples of each fraction are counted to quantitate hydrolysis.

For both methods of analysis, angiotensin I and angiotensin II are located by comparison to standard samples of these two peptides run under identical conditions. Activity is calculated as percent conversion of each time point as follows:

$$\text{Percent conversion} = \frac{\text{dpm Angiotensin II} \times 100}{\text{dpm Angiotensin I} + \text{dpm Angiotensin II}}$$

Comments. The major advantages of this assay method are that it employs the native substrate for the enzyme, and both the substrate and its hydrolysis products are detected. However, because plasma contains a number of proteolytic enzymes, angiotensin II is not the limit product of digestion. Oparil and co-workers [19] also noted the time-dependent appearance of [^{125}I] tyrosine and [tyrosyl-^{125}I] Asp-Arg-Val-Tyr. The appearance of these peptides could pose some difficulties in the quantitation of hydrolysis if, for example, they represent the action of other serum proteases competing with angiotensin converting enzyme for the available angiotensin I. This situation will result in an underestimation of activity, as defined above. Even if these peptides arise only from proteolysis of angiotensin II, their presence will result in an underestimation of activity. In addition, both the electrophoresis and the chromatography methods of quantitation are more time-consuming than the other assay methods described below and are therefore less suitable for processing large numbers of samples.

METHOD OF FRIEDLAND AND SILVERSTEIN. The second assay method using angiotensin I as the substrate was developed by Friedland and Silverstein [11] and is based on the spectrofluorometric quantitation of histidylleucine released during hydrolysis.

Materials. The following materials are used in this method:

Serum
0.2 mM angiotensin I in 0.104 M potassium phosphate (pH 7.5), 31.25 mM NaCl
2% (200 mg/10 ml) *o*-phthalaldehyde in methanol
0.516 mM L-histidyl-L-leucine in 0.104 M potassium phosphate (pH 7.5), 31.25 mM NaCl
0.28 M NaOH
3 M HCl
0.104 M potassium phosphate (pH 7.5), 31.25 mM NaCl

Method. Add 10 μl of serum to 240 μl of the buffered angiotensin I solution and incubate the reaction mixture for 1 hour at 37° C. The reaction is terminated by the addition of 1.45 ml of 0.28 M NaOH. Then 100 μl of 2% *o*-phthalaldehyde is added and mixed by vortexing. Ten minutes after the addition of the *o*-phthalaldehyde, 200 μl of 3 N HCl is added. The resulting precipitate is cleared by centrifugation at 1000 × *g* for 10 minutes. The fluorescence of the cleared solution is read 30 to 90 minutes after the addition of HCl. The excitation wavelength for this measurement is 360 mm, and the emission wavelength is 500 nm.

Several blanks and controls are run with each assay. An assay blank consisting of 240 μl of buffered angiotensin is incubated at 37° C for 1 hour. Then 1.45 ml of 0.28 M NaOH is added, followed by 10 μl of serum. This sample is treated with *o*-phthalaldehyde, as described above. As controls, 10 μl of buffered L-histidyl-L-leucine is added to 230 μl of 0.104 M potassium phosphate (pH 7.5), 31.25 mM NaCl; 10 μl of serum is then added and incubated for 1 hour at 37° C. The reaction is terminated by the addition of 1.45 ml of 0.28 M NaOH. Fluorescence is measured after treatment with *o*-phthalaldehyde, as described above. An unincubated control blank consisting of 10 μl of buffered L-histidyl-L-leucine solution and 230 μl of 0.104 M potassium phosphate (pH 7.5), 31.25 mM NaCl is prepared. Then 1.45 ml of 0.28 M NaOH is added, followed by 10 μl of serum. This solution is immediately treated with *o*-phthalaldehyde, and the fluorescence is measured as described above. Activity is calculated as nanomoles of histidylleucine produced per minute per milliliter of serum, as follows:

$$\text{Activity} = \frac{5.16 \text{ nmol His-Leu} \times (\text{FI}_{\text{assay}} - \text{FI}_{\text{assay blank}})}{60 \text{ min} \times 0.01 \text{ ml} \times (\text{FI}_{\text{control}} - \text{FI}_{\text{control blank}})}$$

Comments. Like the preceding assay, a major advantage of this assay is its use of the native enzyme substrate, angiotensin I. Unlike the radiochemical assay of Oparil and colleagues [19], it is based on quantitation of the His-Leu rather than the angiotensin II formed from the hydrolysis of angiotensin. Since Friedland and Silverstein have not detected significant L-histidyl-L-leucine peptidase activity in the serum, this assay has the additional advantage of not being affected by other serum proteases. The use of spectrofluorometric techniques for quantitation of hydrolysis results in a very sensitive assay, and the design of the assay is such that it is well suited for the processing of a significant number of samples at one time. The drawbacks to the assay arise from the general nature of fluorescence labeling. Since *o*-phthalaldehyde reacts with free amino groups, proteins and small molecules containing amino groups which are present in serum will be labeled in addition to the generated His-Leu. Acid precipitation removes some of these components, but any acid-soluble, *o*-phthalaldehyde-labeled molecules will contribute to the observed fluorescence. This reduces the sensitivity of the assay and necessitates the running of several assay blanks for each serum.

Assays Employing Synthetic Substrates

Four assay methods have been developed using synthetic substrates. Three of the assays use hippuryl-L-histidyl-L-leucine (Hip-His-Leu).

METHOD OF LIEBERMAN. Lieberman [14] has adapted the spectrophotometric assay of Cushman and Cheung [3] for the determination of SACE. The assay is based on the spectrophotometric quantitation of the hippuric acid released on hydrolysis.

Materials. The following materials are used in this method:

Serum
12.5 mM hippuryl-L-histidyl-L-leucine in 500 mM potassium phosphate (pH 8.3), 750 mM NaCl
1 N HCl
1 M NaCl
Ethyl acetate

Method. First, 150 μl of serum is added to 100 μl of buffered Hip-His-Leu solution and incubated at 37° C for 1 hour. The reaction is then stopped by the addition of 250 μl of 1 N HCl. After 5 minutes, 1.5 ml of ethyl acetate is added and vortexed vigorously for 15 seconds. The two phases are separated by centrifugation at 3000 × *g* for 10 minutes, and then 1 ml of the upper ethyl acetate phase is transferred to a clean test tube and heated to 120° for 15 minutes in a heating block to evaporate the ethyl acetate. It is important that the ethyl acetate extract be completely evaporated, since it absorbs strongly in the ultraviolet region used to quantitate the hippuric acid. Following evaporation to dryness, 3 ml of 1 M NaCl are added and vortexed to solubilize the hippuric acid; the absorbance at 228 nm is then read to quantitate the hippuric acid. An assay blank in which the HCl is added prior to the addition of serum is also carried through this procedure. Activity, expressed as nanomoles of hippuric acid liberated per minute per milliliter of serum, is calculated as follows:

$$\text{Activity} = \frac{(A_{228}\text{ assay} - A_{228}\text{ blank} \times 10^3 \times 3}{9.8 \times 0.91 \times .67 \times 60 \times 0.15}$$

where 9.8 = the millimolar extinction coefficient of hippuric acid,
0.91 = the fraction extracted,
0.67 = the faction of ethyl acetate extract transferred,
60 = the incubation time,
0.15 = the milliliter of serum,
10^3 = the conversion to nanomols,
3 = the dilution correction

Comments. This assay is the most widely used method at the present time. Its advantages are the ease with which the quantitation can be performed and, because Hip-His-Leu is much more rapidly hydrolyzed than angiotensin I, the number of samples that can be analyzed in a given time period. In addition, since Hip-His-Leu is considerably less costly than angiotensin I, the cost per analysis is much lower with this assay. The disadvantages of the assay are the use of a synthetic rather than the natural substrate for the assay and problems of sensitivity arising both from the wavelength used for quantitation of hippuric acid and from its low extinction coefficient. The use of a synthetic rather than the natural substrate for quantitation of an enzyme is always subject to some criticism. Unless it can be shown that the synthetic and natural substrates behave in an identical manner, it is hard to estimate the significance of any observations obtained with the synthetic substrate. However, based on comparative serum assays using angiotensin I and Hip-His-Leu [11], the use of the synthetic substrate does not appear to be a significant problem in this particular instance. Since these considerations hold for all the following assays, they will not be discussed again for each specific assay.

A more significant problem arises from the coextraction of serum lipids with the hippuric acid. Since lipids absorb strongly at 228 nm, the wavelength used to quantitate the hippuric acid, they can contribute a substantial background absorbance. This phenomenon, coupled with the low extinction coefficient, decreases the sensitivity of the assay. In addition, the extent of this problem will vary from one patient to another, introducing more variability in SACE activity measurements than is found with the other assay methods. In addition to the problem introduced by the presence of lipids, erroneous readings can also arise from incomplete removal of the ethyl acetate, since this substance also absorbs strongly at 228 nm.

METHOD OF FRIEDLAND AND SILVERSTEIN. The second assay method using Hip-His-Leu as the substrate was developed by Friedland and Silverstein [10] and is based on the fluorometric quantitation of the His-Leu liberated after reaction with *o*-phthalaldehyde.

Materials. The following materials are used in this method:

Serum
25 mM Hip-His-Leu in 25 mM NaOH
0.5 M potassium phosphate buffer (pH 9.3), 1.5 M NaCl
0.28 M NaOH
3 M HCl
0.516 mM His-Leu in water
2% *o*-phthalaldehyde (200 mg/100 ml methanol)

Method. An assay stock solution is prepared by mixing substrate, buffer, and water in a 1 : 1 : 2.8 ratio. To 240 μl of this solution, 10 μl of serum is added and incubated at 37° C for 15 minutes. The reaction is terminated by the addition of 1.45 ml of 0.28 M NaOH followed by vortexing. Then 100 μl of 2% *o*-phthalaldehyde is added and mixed by vortexing, and after 10 minutes, 200 μl of 3 N HCl is added. The resulting precipitate is cleared by centrifugation at 1000 × *g* for 10 minutes. The fluorescence of the clarified solution is measured 30 to 90 minutes after the addition of HCl, with the excitation at 360 nm and the emission at 500 nm.

Several blanks and controls are run with each assay. A substrate buffer blank is treated as above except that 10 μl is added after termination by NaOH. Three control solutions (10 μl 0.516 mM His-Leu, 50 μl buffer, and 180 μl H_2O) are incubated as above. Following termination by NaOH, 10 μl of serum is added, and the fluorescence is developed and measured as above. Since these values do not vary greatly among sera, three different sera are added and the average value is used. An unincubated control blank consisting of 10 μl 0.516 mM His-Leu, 50 μl buffer, and 180 μl H_2O is mixed with 1.45 ml 0.28 M NaOH. Then 10 μl of serum is added, and the fluorescence is immediately developed as above. Activity is calculated as follows:

$$\text{Activity} = \frac{5.16 \text{ nmol His-Leu} \times (FI_{\text{assay}} - FI_{\text{assay blank}})}{15 \times 0.01 \text{ ml} \times (FI_{\text{control}} - FI_{\text{control blank}})}$$

Comments. The major advantages of this method are its speed and sensitivity. Because the method of analysis is fluorometric, as little as 1 to 2 nmol of product can be reliably determined; this in turn shortens the incubation time by a factor of 4 compared to the spectrophotometric technique. The disadvantages of this assay are the same as those described for the fluorometric assay employing angiotensin I.

METHOD OF ROHRBACH. The final method using Hip-His-Leu was developed by Rohrbach [22] and is based on the radiometric quantitation of [^{14}C] hippuric acid released from [^{14}C] Hip-His-Leu.

Materials. The following materials are used in this method:

12.5 mM [glycine-1-^{14}C] Hip-His-Leu (pH 8.3)
0.25 M borate buffer (pH 8.3), 0.75 M NaCl
1 N HCl
Ethyl acetate
Toluene-based scintillator fluid

Method. A grand assay cocktail consisting of equal volumes of substrate and buffer is prepared. To 40 μl of this solution, 10 μl of serum is added and incubated at 37° C for 30 minutes. The reaction is then terminated by the addition of 50 μl of 1 N HCl. Next, 300 μl of ethyl acetate is added, and the solution is vortexed for 15 seconds. The two phases are separated by centrifugation at 1000 × g for 5 minutes; then 200 μl of the upper ethyl acetate solution is placed directly in 5 ml of toluene-based scintillation fluid, and the disintegrations per minute is determined. With each series of assays, blanks in which 10 μl H_2O is added in lieu of serum are carried out as above. To test for proper hydrolysis, triplicate 10-μl samples of pooled sera of known activity are also carried out as above. Activity is calculated as follows:

$$\text{Activity} = \frac{(\text{dpm}_{\text{sample}} - \text{dpm}_{\text{blank}})}{\text{SA} \times 0.91 \times 0.67 \times 0.01 \text{ ml} \times 30 \text{ min}}$$

where SA = the specific activity of the substrate,
0.91 = the extraction coefficient of hippuric acid,
0.67 = the fraction counted

Comments. The major advantages of this method are its sensitivity, speed, and lack of interference by other serum components. The sensitivity of the assay is determined only by the specific activity of the substrate and approaches the sensitivity of the fluorometric assay [10]. The use of borate buffer rather than phosphate buffer increases the rate of hydrolysis by approximately 25 percent. These conditions permit the processing of a large number of samples in a relatively short time. Because the reaction is followed by the appearance of a radiolabeled product, this assay is not subject to the interference by lipids and ethyl acetate seen in the spectrophotometric assay [14] nor to the labeling of other serum proteins and peptides encountered in the spectrofluorometric assay [10].

The disadvantages of the assay are twofold. First, it is possible that successive cleavages by a serum carboxypeptidase could produce the hippuric acid, thereby giving a false activity estimate. This problem is equally true for all the above assays. Second, at present the [^{14}C] substrate is not commercially available and must be synthesized [22]. However, a [^{3}H]-labeled form is presently available (Ventrex Labs., Portland, Me.).

METHOD OF RYAN AND COLLEAGUES. The final assay using synthetic substrate to measure SACE activity was developed by Ryan and colleagues [24] and is based on the radiometric quantitation of [^{3}H] hippuric acid cleaved from [^{3}H] hippurylglycylglycine.

Materials. The following materials are used in this method:

Serum
0.05 M hepes buffer (pH 8.0), 0.1 M NaCl, 0.6 M Na_2SO_4
16 mM [^{3}H] Hip-Gly-Gly in buffer
Ethyl acetate
0.1 N HCl
Scintillator containing a water solubilizer

Method. Serum is diluted 1 : 4 with the Hepes buffer, and 50 μl of the diluted serum is added to 50 μl of buffered substrate to initiate the reaction. After incubation at 37° C for 60 minutes, the reaction is terminated by the addition of 1 ml of 0.1 N HCl. The solution is then extracted with 1 ml of ethyl acetate by vortexing for 15 seconds. Following 10 minutes of centrifugation at 2000 × g to separate the two phases, 500 μl of the upper ethyl acetate phase is transferred to a scintillation vial containing 10 ml of scintillation fluid and is then counted. Reaction blanks containing 50 μl of Hepes buffer in place of diluted serum are treated in the same manner. The specific activity of the substrate is measured by counting 50 μl of the buffered substrate. Activity is calculated as follows:

$$\text{Activity} = \frac{CPM_{sample} - CPM_{blank}}{CPM_{substrate}/(60 \text{ min} \times 0.01 \text{ ml} \times 0.5)} \times 800 \text{ nmol} \times \frac{1}{1 - (CPM_{blank}/CPM_{substrate})}$$

where 0.5 corrects for the fraction of ethyl acetate counted and

$$\frac{1}{1 - (CPM_{blank}/CPM_{substrate})}$$

corrects for the extraction of unhydrolyzed substrate.

Comments. The advantages of this assay are the same as those described for the radiochemical assay employing [^{14}C]-Hip-His-Leu. The use of Hip-Gly-Gly has one additional advantage over all the other substrates described. Because glycylglycine bonds are resistant to known carboxypeptidases, it is extremely unlikely that serum carboxypeptidases will interfere with this assay. The disadvantage of the assay is that approximately 7 percent of the unhydrolyzed substrate coextracts with the generated hippuric acid. Since the assay is linear only up to 10 percent hydrolysis, the blanks can comprise up to 50 percent of the total counts per minute for normal serum. The radiolabeled substrate can either be synthesized [24] or purchased (Ventrex Labs., Portland, Me.).

References

1. Ashutosh, K., and Keighley, J. F. H. Diagnostic value of serum angiotensin converting enzyme activity in lung diseases. *Thorax* 31:552, 1976.
2. Caldwell, P. R. B., Seegal, B. C., Hsu, K. C., et al. Angiotensin-converting enzyme: Vascular endothelial localization. *Science* 191:1050, 1976.
3. Cushman, D. W., and Cheung, H. S. Spectrophotometric assay and properties of the angiotensin-converting enzyme of rabbit lung. *Biochem. Pharmacol.* 20:1637, 1971.
4. Das, M., Hartley, J. L., and Soffer, R. L. Serum angiotensin-converting enzyme: Isolation and relationship to the pulmonary enzyme. *J. Biol. Chem.* 252:1316, 1977.
5. Das, M., and Soffer, R. L. Pulmonary angiotensin-converting enzyme: Structural and catalytic properties. *J. Biol. Chem.* 250:6762, 1975.
6. Dorer, F. E., Kahn, J. R., Lentz, K. E., et al. Formation of angiotensin II from tetradecapeptide renin substrate by angiotensin-converting enzyme. *Biochem. Pharmacol.* 24:1137, 1975.
7. Dorer, F. E., Ryan, J. W., and Stewart, J. M. Hydrolysis of bradykinin and its

higher homologues by angiotensin-converting enzyme. *Biochem. J.* 141:915, 1974.
8. Elisseeva, Y. E., Orekhovich, V. N., Pavlikhina, L. V., et al. Carboxycathepsin—a key regulatory component of two physiological systems involved in regulation of blood pressure. *Clin. Chim. Acta* 31:413, 1971.
9. Fanburg, B. L., Schoenberger, M. D., Bachus, B., et al. Elevated serum angiotensin I converting enzyme in sarcoidosis. *Am. Rev. Respir. Dis.* 114:525, 1976.
10. Friedland, J., and Silverstein, E. A sensitive fluorometric assay for serum angiotensin-converting enzyme. *Am. J. Clin. Pathol.* 66:418, 1976.
11. Friedland, J., and Silverstein, E. Sensitive fluorometric assay for serum angiotensin-converting enzyme with the natural substrate angiotensin I. *Am. J. Clin. Pathol.* 68:225, 1977.
12. Igic, R., Erdös, E. G., Yeh, H. J. S., et al. Angiotensin I converting enzyme of the lung. *Circ. Res.* 31(Suppl. II):81, 1972.
13. Lee, H. J., Larue, J. N., and Wilson, I. B. Angiotensin-converting enzyme from porcine plasma. *Biochim. Biophys. Acta* 235:521, 1971.
14. Lieberman, J. Elevation of serum angiotensin converting enzyme (ACE) level in sarcoidosis. *Am. J. Med.* 59:365, 1975.
15. Lieberman, J. The specificity and nature of serum angiotensin-converting enzyme (serum ACE) elevations in sarcoidosis. *Ann. N.Y. Acad. Sci.* 278:488, 1976.
16. Lieberman, J., and Beutler, E. Elevation of serum angiotensin-converting enzyme in Gaucher's disease. *N. Engl. J. Med.* 294:1442, 1976.
17. Lieberman, J., and Rea, T. H. Serum angiotensin converting enzymes in leprosy and coccidioidomycosis. *Ann. Intern. Med.* 87:422, 1977.
18. Ng, K. K. F., and Vane, J. R. Conversion of angiotensin I to angiotensin II. *Nature* 216:762, 1967.
19. Oparil, S., Low, J., and Koerner, T. J. Altered angiotensin I conversion in pulmonary disease. *Clin. Sci. Mol. Med.* 51:537, 1976.
20. Piquilloud, Y., Reinharz, A., and Roth, M. Studies on angiotensin converting enzyme with different substrates. *Biochim. Biophys. Acta* 206:136, 1970.
21. Rohatgi, P. K., Massey, T. H., and Ryan, J. W. Serum angiotensin converting enzyme and sarcoidosis. *Clin. Res.* 26:62A, 1978.
22. Rohrbach, M. S. Glycine-1-^{14}C hippuryl-L-histidyl-L-leucine: A substrate for the radiochemical assay of angiotensin converting enzyme. *Anal. Biochem.* 84:272, 1978.
23. Rohrbach, M. S., and DeRemee, R. A. Serum angiotensin converting enzyme activity in sarcoidosis as measured by a single radiochemical assay. *Am. Rev. Resp. Dis.* 119:761, 1979.
24. Ryan, J. W., Chung, A., Ammons, C., et al. A simple radioassay for angiotensin-converting enzyme. *Biochem. J.* 167:501, 1977.
25. Ryan, J. W., Ryan, U. S., Schultz, D. R., et al. Subcellular localization of pulmonary angiotensin-converting enzyme (kininase II). *Biochem. J.* 146:497, 1975.
26. Ryan, J. W., Smith, U., and Niemeyer, R. S. Angiotensin I: Metabolism by plasma membrane of lung. *Science* 176:64, 1972.
27. Sanders, G. E., and Huggins, C. G. Subcellular localization of angiotensin I converting enzyme in rabbit lung. *Nature New Biology* 230:27, 1971.
28. Sharma, O. P. *Sarcoidosis: A Clinical Approach.* Springfield, Ill.: Thomas, 1975.
29. Silverstein, E., and Friedland, J. Elevated serum and spleen angiotensin converting enzyme (ACE) and serum lysozyme (L) in chronic Gaucher's disease. *Clin. Res.* 24:498A, 1976.

30. Silverstein, E., Friedland, J., and Ackerman, T. Elevation of granulomatous lymph-node and serum lysozyme in sarcoidosis and correlation with angiotensin-converting enzyme. *Am. J. Clin. Pathol.* 68:219, 1977.
31. Silverstein, E., Friedland, J., Lyons, H. A., et al. Elevation of angiotensin-converting enzyme in granulomatous lymph nodes and serum in sarcoidosis: Clinical and possible pathogenic significance. *Ann. N.Y. Acad. Sci.* 278:498, 1976.
32. Skeggs, L. T., Dorer, F. E., Kahn, J. R., et al. The Biological Production of Angiotensin. In I. H. Page and F. M. Bumpus (Eds.), *Angiotensin.* New York: Springer, 1974.
33. Skeggs, L. T., Marsh, W. H., Kahn, J. R., et al. The preparation and function of hypertension-converting enzyme. *J. Exp. Med.* 103:295, 1956.
34. Soffer, R. L. Angiotensin-converting enzyme and the regulation of vasoactive peptides. *Annu. Rev. Biochem.* 45:73, 1976.

9. Radioimmunoassay of Aldosterone

Ronald D. Brown and Max Wisgerhof

Aldosterone, the most potent natural mineralocorticoid, is secreted by cells located in the zona glomerulosa of the adrenal cortex. Aldosterone plays an important role in the homeostatic control of sodium and potassium. Excessive secretion of this hormone leads to the development of the syndromes of primary and secondary aldosteronism. Primary aldosteronism is usually caused by a benign adenoma of the adrenal cortex and is characterized by hypertension and potassium depletion. Secondary aldosteronism is a consequence of the stimulation of the adrenal gland by abnormally high levels of angiotensin II. This type of aldosteronism may or may not be associated with hypertension, depending on the underlying abnormality. Edema is common in secondary aldosteronism but is rare in primary aldosteronism. Insufficient secretion of aldosterone results in the loss of sodium and the retention of potassium by the kidney, which leads to hypotension and hyperkalemia.

Discovery

The presence of large amounts of sodium-retaining activity in the urine of edematous patients was first reported in 1950 [39]. After aldosterone was isolated from adrenal extracts and characterized [43, 60], it was demonstrated that the sodium-retaining activity in urine was due to aldosterone [38]. The first syndrome in man in which excess aldosterone was the cause was described by Conn in 1955 [10].

Physiology

The major effect of aldosterone is on the urinary excretion of electrolytes. Aldosterone acts on the distal tubule and collecting duct of the nephron to enhance the resorption of sodium and the excretion of potassium, hydrogen, and ammonium ions. Only a small percentage of the sodium that is filtered by the kidney reaches the distal tubule and collecting duct to be resorbed under the influence of aldosterone. This fraction is critical to life, however, as evidenced by the profound hypotension observed in patients who are unable to synthesize aldosterone. The effect of aldosterone on potassium secretion is dependent on the quantity of sodium reaching the ion exchange site in the distal portion of the nephron. Enhanced resorption of sodium by the proximal tubule, as occurs during periods of reduced intake of sodium, decreases the amount of sodium that is delivered to the distal portion of the nephron, which decreases the kaliuresis following administration of aldosterone.

After several days of administration of aldosterone, the kidney "escapes" from the sodium-retaining effect of aldosterone, but not from its potassium-secretory effect. In states of secondary aldosteronism associated with edema, exemplified by patients with congestive heart failure, cirrhosis of the liver, or the nephrotic syndrome, such escape does not occur. When aldosterone is administered to patients with these diseases, there is less of an effect on the secretion of potassium by the kidney than in normal individuals. In these diseases the proximal tubule resorbs a greater fraction of the filtered sodium so that less is available at the distal ion exchange site for exchange with potassium, and thus the kaliuretic effect of aldosterone is not prominent.

In addition to its renal effect, aldosterone affects electrolyte transport in the gastrointestinal tract by decreasing sodium excretion and increasing potassium excretion. Aldosterone also decreases the sodium concentration and increases the potassium concentration in both sweat and saliva. In contrast to the kidney, there is no "escape" of the gastrointestinal tract, salivary glands, or sweat glands from the effects of aldosterone during prolonged administration.

Aldosterone has no direct effect on renin production, but as a result of sodium retention by the kidneys there is expansion of the extracellular fluid volume and an increase in the effective blood volume. The increase in blood volume causes an increase in renal blood flow and in renal perfusion pressure, which suppresses the production of renin. Increases in the amount of sodium delivered to the distal tubule also suppress the production of renin. Prolonged administration of aldosterone depresses the production of renin, which results in atrophy of the zona glomerulosa and decreased secretion of aldosterone.

The mechanism of action of aldosterone is similar to that of all steroid hormones. Aldosterone passively enters all cells in the body but is active only in cells that have specific aldosterone-binding proteins in their cytoplasm. These cytoplasmic binding proteins have the characteristics of a hormone receptor (i.e., they bind aldosterone with high affinity, and the binding is specific and of limited capacity). The aldosterone-cytoplasmic receptor complex then enters the nucleus where, by mechanisms still not completely understood, the complex binds to chromatin and initiates the synthesis of new messenger RNA (mRNA). This new mRNA promotes the synthesis of cytoplasmic proteins, which in turn enhance the transport of sodium from the cell into the interstitial fluid bathing the cell. The mechanism by which this enhancement occurs is unknown. The regulation of potassium, ammonium, and hydrogen transport by the distal nephron is linked to the sodium transport mechanism. When sodium leaves the cell, these ions are exchanged for the sodium. There is evidence, however, for the existence of a potassium transport mechanism that is not linked to this sodium transport mechanism [17]. Other mineralocorticoids appear to act in a similar fashion and can, in fact, compete with aldosterone for its cytoplasmic receptor.

The regulation of the secretion of aldosterone is a complex process involving the renin-angiotensin system, potassium, ACTH, and sodium. The renin-angiotensin system is thought to be the dominant regulator of aldosterone, particularly during periods of sodium depletion, after hemorrhage, and in response to upright posture. Increases in serum potassium stimulate the secretion of aldosterone, and hypokalemia diminishes its secretion. Large increases in levels of serum potassium directly cause decreases in plasma renin activity, but the effect on aldosterone production through this mechanism is of less importance than the direct effect of potassium on the adrenal cortex. ACTH appears to play a permissive role in the production of aldosterone. In the prolonged absence of ACTH, levels of aldosterone are often normal but may not respond as briskly as normal to depletion of sodium or to changes in potassium or angiotensin II. When levels of renin are low, ACTH may assume a more important role in the regulation of aldosterone [70]. Profound lowering of the levels of serum sodium stimulates the secretion of aldosterone independent of any effects on the renin-angiotensin system.

Aldosterone secretion is episodic [32] and follows a circadian rhythm similar to that of cortisol [71]. However, the amplitude of these changes is less marked compared to those of cortisol. Aldosterone levels are higher during the luteal phase of the menstrual cycle than during the proliferative phase [31]. Aldosterone levels are high during pregnancy and the administration of estrogens. The urinary excretion of aldosterone declines with advancing age [13].

In healthy individuals, approximately 90 percent of the aldosterone secreted by the adrenal glands is metabolized by the liver, and the remainder is metabolized by the kidneys. The major metabolite formed by the liver is 3α, 5β-tetrahydroaldosterone 3β-glucosiduronic acid. The kidneys metabolize aldosterone to aldosterone 18β-glucosiduronic acid. These and other metabolites, together with a small amount (less than 1 percent) of hormone that is not metabolized, are excreted by the kidneys into the urine.

Disease States in Which Measurement of Aldosterone is Useful

Aldosteronism

Aldosteronism can be divided into primary and secondary forms. The primary forms are characterized by hypertension and hypokalemia without edema; the secondary forms may or may not be associated with hypertension or hypokalemia but are commonly associated with edema. The level of plasma renin activity is low in primary aldosteronism but is high in secondary aldosteronism. The classification of aldosteronism is summarized in the following outline.

- I. Primary aldosteronism
  - A. Aldosterone-producing adenoma
  - B. Idiopathic aldosteronism
    - 1. Glucocorticoid nonsuppressible
    - 2. Glucocorticoid suppressible
  - C. Aldosterone-producing carcinoma

II. Secondary aldosteronism
   A. Associated with hypertension
      1. Renin-secreting renal tumor
      2. Malignant hypertension
      3. Renovascular hypertension
      4. Oral contraceptive–induced hypertension
      5. Essential hypertension treated with diuretics
   B. Not associated with hypertension
      1. Congestive heart failure
      2. Cirrhosis of the liver
      3. Nephrotic syndrome
      4. Bartter's syndrome
      5. Sodium-wasting nephritis

Aldosterone should be measured in any hypertensive patient who, on the basis of unprovoked hypokalemia, is suspected of having primary aldosteronism. If levels of urinary or plasma aldosterone are elevated while the patient is ingesting liberal amounts of sodium, and if plasma renin activity is low and unresponsive to sodium depletion, the patient has primary aldosteronism. If plasma renin activity is elevated, the patient has secondary aldosteronism.

Aldosteronism resulting from an aldosterone-producing adenoma should be differentiated from idiopathic aldosteronism. The hypertension of the former condition responds well to surgical intervention, whereas the hypertension of the latter state often is not significantly improved by adrenalectomy, even when there is histological evidence of adrenal hyperplasia [21]. Measurements of aldosterone levels are helpful in making this distinction. Higher levels of aldosterone are found in the adrenal vein effluent of the adrenal gland containing the adenoma; in contrast, the levels of aldosterone in the venous effluents of the adrenal glands of patients with idiopathic aldosteronism are characteristically about equal. Recently a "postural response" test was developed to differentiate these two types of aldosteronism. When patients with aldosterone-producing adenomas are upright during the morning hours, their levels of peripheral plasma aldosterone decrease or remain unchanged. In contrast, the levels of plasma aldosterone of patients with idiopathic aldosteronism increase under these conditions [5, 22, 40, 56].

Several other syndromes characterized by hypertension and hypokalemia must be differentiated from primary aldosteronism. These syndromes include Cushing's syndrome, particularly when it is due to ectopic ACTH or adrenal carcinoma; the hypertensive forms of congenital adrenal hyperplasia (11β-hydroxylase deficiency and 17α-hydroxylase deficiency); licorice intoxication; and Liddle's syndrome. Cushing's syndrome is usually readily excluded by the clinical manifestations of glucocorticoid excess and the finding of elevated levels of cortisol in plasma and urine. The hypertensive forms of congenital adrenal hyperplasia can usually be excluded on clinical grounds by noting whether or not there are abnormalities in sexual development. Licorice intoxication is caused by a steroid-like substance (glycyrrhetinic acid) present in licorice, which causes sodium retention and hypertension. Liddle's syndrome is caused by an inherited renal tubular defect of sodium and potassium transport. Aldosterone levels are usually low rather than increased in these syndromes.

Measurement of aldosterone levels in the edematous forms of aldosteronism is of little diagnostic usefulness and is not routinely done.

Hypoaldosteronism

Hypoaldosteronism can be caused by destruction of the adrenal cortex, as in Addison's disease; surgical removal of the adrenal glands; chemical inhibitors of adrenal function; enzymatic defects in the aldosterone biosynthetic pathway; or following impairment or prolonged suppression of the renin-angiotensin axis. Measurement of aldosterone levels is useful in the diagnosis of these syndromes.

The clinical manifestations of aldosterone deficiency result from an inability of the kidneys to conserve sodium. Sodium loss leads to hypovolemia, which is manifested by tachycardia, hypotension, decreased renal blood flow with prerenal azotemia, and eventually shock. The impaired renal secretion of potassium and hydrogen ions leads to hyperkalemia and a metabolic acidosis. If hypoaldosteronism is caused by Addison's disease or the surgical removal of the adrenal glands, there are concomitant signs, symptoms, and laboratory abnormalities of cortisol deficiency. The administration of certain inhibitors of adrenal aldosterone biosynthesis, such as heparin, may lead to hypoaldosteronism.

Hypoaldosteronism is characteristic of several forms of congenital adrenal hyperplasia. In the 3β-ol-dehydrogenase deficiency, the 11β- and 21-hydroxylase deficiencies, and the 18-hydroxylase or the 18-dehydrogenase deficiency syndromes, the decrease in aldosterone secretion is a direct consequence of the deficient enzymatic processes. In contrast, the hypoaldosteronism of the 17α-hydroxylase deficiency syndrome is a secondary phenomenon. In this syndrome large amounts of mineralocorticoid, deoxycorticosterone, are secreted by the adrenal glands. These high levels of deoxycorticosterone lead to excessive resorption of sodium by the kidneys, which in turn leads to an increase in blood volume, a decrease in the activity of the renin-angiotensin axis, and secondary hypoaldosteronism. The 11β- and 17α-hydroxylase deficiency syndromes are characterized by hypertension, the other syndromes by hypotension.

A syndrome of hypoaldosteronism caused by a defect in the secretion of renin has recently been described [57]. Commonly, patients with this syndrome have mild diabetes mellitus and renal insufficiency, hyperkalemia, a tendency to waste sodium in the urine, and orthostatic hypotension. In general, they respond well to mineralocorticoid supplements.

Immediately after the removal of an aldosterone-producing adenoma, levels of aldosterone are low because the renin-angiotensin axis and the zona glomerulosa cells of the remaining adrenal tissue do not recover quickly from the suppressive effects of the presence of the adenoma. The deficiency of aldo-

Table 9–1. Differential Diagnosis of Disease States with Abnormal Levels of Aldosterone

Disease State	Serum or Urinary Aldosterone	Plasma Renin Activity	Serum Potassium
Primary aldosteronism	High	Low	Low or normal [a]
Secondary aldosteronism	High	High	Low or normal
Hypoaldosteronism			
Impaired or absent adrenal function			
Addison's disease, bilateral adrenalectomy, adrenal inhibitors	Low	High	High or normal
Congenital adrenal hyperplasia: 3β-ol-dehydrogenase, 11β- and 21-hydroxylase, 18-hydroxylase and 18-dehydrogenase deficiencies	Low	High	High or normal [b]
Impaired production of renin			
Hyporeninemic hypoaldosteronism	Low	Low	High
Suppressed production of renin			
Congenital adrenal hyperplasia: 17α-hydroxylase deficiency	Low	Low	Low
Pseudoaldosteronism (Liddle's syndrome)	Low	Low	Low
Licorice intoxication	Low	Low	Low
Immediately after removal of an aldosterone-producing adenoma	Low	Low	High or normal

[a] Rarely normal unless sodium intake is restricted.
[b] Low in the 11β-hydroxylase syndrome.

sterone may lead to hypovolemia during the postoperative period. Gradually, however, the renin-angiotensin axis recovers and levels of angiotensin II are increased. After a period of weeks to months the zona glomerulosa cells are able to respond to angiotensin II, and eventually they are able to secrete normal amounts of aldosterone.

As described earlier, ACTH plays a permissive role in the secretion of aldosterone. In patients with chronic hypopituitarism the adrenal cortex may not respond maximally to the other regulators of aldosterone, particularly angiotensin II. However, patients with hypopituitarism usually do not require mineralocorticoid replacement therapy.

The differential diagnosis of diseases characterized by abnormalities of aldosterone secretion is summarized in Table 9–1.

Interpretation of Aldosterone Levels

The interpretation of the results of measurements of aldosterone levels should take into consideration factors that might influence the levels of aldosterone independently of the disease being diagnosed. These factors include the activity of the normal regulators of aldosterone secretion, the metabolic clearance of aldosterone, the age of the patient, pregnancy, and treatment with estrogens or diuretic drugs. In addition, a change in the pattern of metabolism of aldosterone can lead to changes in the excretion rates of the metabolites even though the secretion rate of aldosterone is unchanged. Since the liver metabolizes most of the aldosterone secreted, a decrease in liver function may decrease the amount of aldosterone that is metabolized by the liver to the tetrahydro-metabolite. As a result, a greater percentage of aldosterone is metabolized by the kidneys to the 18β-glucosiduronic acid conjugate [12]. This can lead to measurements of increases in the urinary excretion of aldosterone by assays that measure the 18-conjugate of aldosterone, even though the adrenal secretion of aldosterone has not changed.

The temperature at which the blood sample is processed and the level of cortisol in the blood sample have been shown to influence the distribution of aldosterone between plasma and red cells in blood [9]. To avoid this problem, blood samples should always be processed at the same temperature.

The results of measurements of aldosterone in samples from patients should be interpreted by comparing them with the results from samples obtained from normal subjects under similar conditions. The most helpful conditions are those that keep constant the physiological factors that normally regulate aldosterone production. The effects of sodium balance and posture on aldosterone production can be controlled by instructing the patient to eat a diet that contains liberal amounts of sodium for 3 to 5 days and by keeping the patient in the recumbent position for several hours prior to obtaining blood samples. Since hypokalemia blunts aldosterone secretion, potassium supplementation should be given before aldosterone levels are measured if levels of serum potassium are low. To assess the responsiveness of the secretion of aldosterone to volume depletion, levels of aldosterone should be measured after severe dietary sodium restriction or after multiple doses of a diuretic, such as furosemide, and 4 hours of upright posture.

Former Techniques for Measurement of Aldosterone

The advent of radioimmunoassay methods made it feasible to measure aldosterone in both plasma and urine with relative ease. Prior to the development of radioimmunoassays, the techniques employed were too complex and expensive to allow measurement of aldosterone in a routine clinical laboratory. The earliest methods utilized the urinary excretion of sodium and potassium in adrenalectomized dogs or rats as an index of the aldosterone concentration in the extract being assayed. Chemical and radiochemical techniques subsequently improved both sensitivity and accuracy, but they were tedious and costly, and only a few were sufficiently sensitive to measure aldosterone accurately in plasma or serum. Successful gas-liquid chromatography techniques, employing very sensitive detectors, have been reported. Currently, however, aldosterone is measured by radioimmunoassay in most laboratories.

Radioimmunoassay of Aldosterone

The principle of the radioimmunoassay of aldosterone is the same as that of all other radioimmunoassays. Isotopically labeled aldosterone, either tritium-labeled or ^{125}I-labeled aldosterone, and an anti-aldosterone antiserum are incubated under standard conditions with the plasma or urine or an extract of the plasma or urine being assayed. The isotopically labeled aldosterone and the aldosterone in the extract compete for binding sites on the antiserum. The greater the amount of aldosterone in the extract, the lesser the amount of binding of the isotopically labeled aldosterone to the antiserum. The bound and unbound aldosterone are then separated, and the bound and/or unbound isotopically labeled aldosterone is counted with the use of a liquid scintillation spectrometer or a gamma spectrometer. Varying amounts of authentic aldosterone are measured in each assay, and a standard curve is constructed.

As in all radioimmunoassays, an antiserum is first developed (see Tables 9–2 through 9–4). Since aldosterone is a small molecule and is not antigenic, it is conjugated to a larger molecule, usually a protein, to increase its antigenicity. The steroid-protein antigen is then injected repeatedly into animals to induce the formation of the antiserum.

Two approaches have been used to conjugate aldosterone to proteins. In one approach, aldosterone-21-mono- or 18, 21-dihemisuccinate is synthesized and then conjugated to the protein; in the other, the aldosterone-3-carboxymethoxime (or aldosterone-18, 21-diacetate-3-carboxymethoxime) is prepared and conjugated to the protein. The proteins most commonly used have been bovine or rabbit serum albumin and bovine gamma globulin. Antisera have been produced in rabbits, guinea pigs, and sheep. The most widely used antiserum was prepared by Dr. R. Haning of the Worcester Foundation for Experimental Biology. This material is distributed to qualified investigators by the National Institutes of Health.

None of these antisera is entirely specific for aldosterone. The occurrence of even small amounts of cross-reaction with cortisol presents a problem, since cortisol levels in samples are usually 1000 times greater than aldosterone levels. Antibodies against the aldosterone-3-carboxymethoxime conjugates are generally more specific than those against the aldosterone hemisuccinate conjugates. This greater specificity has made it possible to develop assays that require very little preliminary purification, or in some instances no purification, prior to the radioimmunoassay (see Tables 9–2 through 9–4).

Specific or nonspecific binding of aldosterone to plasma proteins makes it difficult to perform direct radioimmunoassays of plasma aldosterone. To circumvent this problem, agents that inhibit the binding of aldosterone to plasma proteins, such as 8-anilino-1-naphthalene-sulfonic acid and thimerosal (Merthiolate), are added to the plasma prior to the radioimmunoassay. Cortisol has been used to prevent aldosterone from binding to transcortin. The use of low pH (pH 5.0) has also been suggested as a way to minimize plasma protein binding.

Tritium-labeled aldosterone has generally been used as the ligand. However, in several assays reported recently, [^{125}I] aldosterone was used rather than tritium-labeled aldosterone. The use of [^{125}I] aldosterone is less expensive, since a scintillation solvent is not required for counting. On the other hand, tritium-labeled aldosterone is more stable than [^{125}I] aldosterone, and highly purified material is available from several commercial sources. ^{125}I-labeled aldosterone is not available commercially and must be prepared and purified frequently.

As noted earlier, many different metabolites of aldosterone are excreted in the urine. At pH 1.0, aldosterone-18β-glucosiduronic acid undergoes hydrolysis to produce free aldosterone. It is the aldosterone that is liberated from the conjugate at pH 1.0 that is most commonly measured in the procedures published to date. A few methods, however, measure only the free aldosterone present (Table 9–2). Recently, methods to measure urinary tetrahydroaldosterone (after enzymatic hydrolysis) and a method for direct measurement of tetrahydroaldosterone glucosiduronic acid in urine have been published (Table 9–2).

Several methods are used to separate the aldosterone bound to the antiserum from the unbound or free aldosterone. A mixture of charcoal and dextran, so-called dextran-coated charcoal, and Florisil are the most common agents employed. The unbound aldosterone is adsorbed to the charcoal or Florisil, and the adsorbent is removed by centrifugation or allowed to sediment. The labeled aldosterone bound to the antiserum in the supernatant is then counted in a liquid scintillation spectrometer or a gamma spectrometer. Other separation methods include precipitation of the antibody-aldosterone complex with ammonium sulfate or polyethylene glycol, extraction of the unbound aldosterone into the toluene scintillator, and solid-phase techniques in which the antiserum is linked to a support material such as nylon.

There is reasonably close agreement on the normal range of urinary excretion rates of aldosterone (18-conjugate) and the levels of plasma aldosterone in normal subjects ingesting average amounts of sodium. Tables 9–2 and 9–3 summarize the urinary aldosterone excretion rates and the levels of plasma aldosterone that have been reported with the various methods. The range of urinary aldosterone excretion is 2 to 25 μg per 24 hours, with a mean of 9.1 μg per 24 hours. The range of levels of plasma aldosterone in recumbent, sodium-replete, normal subjects is 1.1 to 18 ng/dl (mean = 6.9 ng/dl), and in upright, sodium-replete, normal subjects the range is 3.4 to 40 ng/dl (mean = 17.6 ng/dl). Most of the new, direct radioimmunoassays give similar results (Table 9–4).

Radioimmunoassay of Aldosterone in Serum

MATERIALS. *Anti-Aldosterone Antiserum.* A very specific anti-aldosterone antiserum that was prepared by McKenzie and Clements [45] is used in this method.

Table 9–2. Methods for Radioimmunoassay of Excretion Rates of Urinary Aldosterone

Antiserum Development						
Developer or Source [a]	Antigen	Animal	Cortisol Cross-Reactivity (%)	Purification Steps	Normal Values (μg/24 hr)	Reference
Author	Aldo-CMO-RSA	Rabbit	0.01	Paper chromatography [2]	61 [b] (24–99)	3
Author	Aldo-21-hemisuccinate-BSA	Rabbit	0.50	Paper chromatography; silica gel column chromatography	8 (3–14)	66
Dr. W. Kelly	Aldo-21-hemisuccinate-BSA	Sheep	0.40	None	9 (6–13)	59
Author	Aldo(γ-lactone)-CMO-BSA	Sheep and rabbit	—	Benzene : water partition; oxidation; extraction into dichloromethane	—	20
NIH	Aldo-18, 21-dihemisuccinate-BSA	Sheep	—	None	7.1 (—)	15
Author	Aldo-CMO-BSA	Rabbit	0.05	Paper chromatography	—	19
NIH	Aldo-18, 21-dihemisuccinate-BSA	Sheep	—	LH-20 Sephadex column chromatography	9.5 (4–15)	69
Research plus Labs	Aldo-18, 21-dihemisuccinate-BSA	Sheep	0.36	Silica gel column chromatography	12.7 (6–25)	18
NIH	Aldo-18, 21-hemisuccinate-BSA	Sheep	—	Thin-layer chromatography	0.35 [c] (0–0.7)	16
Antibodies, Inc. (Davis, Calif.)	Aldo(γ-lactone)-CMO-BSA	—	—	Benzene : water partition; oxidation; extraction into chloroform	8.8 (4–14)	62
Author	Aldo-CMO-BGG	Rabbit	< 0.001	None	7.4 (4–13)	67

Author	Aldo-CMO-BSA	Rabbit	0.03	None	—	30
NIH	Aldo-18, 21-dihemisuccinate-BSA	Sheep	—	Paper chromatography	14.3 (5–20)	11
NIH	Aldo-18, 21-dihemisuccinate-BSA	Sheep	—	Paper chromatography; thin-layer chromatography	7.5 (2–16)	25
Isotopendienst West (Frankfurt, Germany)	Aldo-21-hemisuccinate-BSA	—	—	Thin-layer chromatography [2]	8.2 (2–17)	58
NIH	Aldo-18, 21-dihemisuccinate-BSA	Sheep	—	None	7.3 (2–12)	35
NIH	Aldo-18, 21-dihemisuccinate-BSA	Sheep	—	LH-20 Sephadex column chromatography	9.1 (2–15)	46
NIH	Aldo-18, 21-dihemisuccinate-BSA	Sheep	0.02	Celite column chromatography	—	8
Author	Aldo-CMO-BSA	Rabbit	< 0.002	None	—	7
NIH	Aldo-18, 21-dihemisuccinate-BSA	Sheep	—	None	7.9 (3–21)	34
NIH	Aldo-18, 21-dihemisuccinate-BSA	Sheep	—	None	10.2 (—)	49
Author	Aldo(γ-lactone)-CMO-BSA	Sheep	—	β-glucuronidase hydrolysis; extraction into dichloromethane	32 [d] (16–68)	53
Author	3α, 5β-tetrahydroaldo-20-carboxymethoxime-BSA	Rabbit	0.0	β-glucuronidase hydrolysis; paper chromatography	26 [d] (10–65)	33
Author	3α, 5β-tetrahydroaldo-20-carboxymethoxime-BSA	Rabbit	0.0	Pre-extraction with ethyl acetate	9 [e] (4–15)	33

[a] The antisera developed by the author(s) of the reference cited in the far right column may not be available to other laboratories.
[b] Aldosterone secretion rate.
[c] Free aldosterone excretion rate.
[d] Tetrahydroaldosterone excretion rate.
[e] Aldosterone-18-glucuronide excretion rate.
RSA = rabbit serum albumin; BSA = bovine serum albumin; BGG = bovine gamma globulin; BTG = bovine thyroglobulin; NIH = National Institutes of Health; Aldo = aldosterone; Aldo-CMO = Aldosterone-3-carboxymethoxime.

Table 9–3. Methods for the Radioimmunoassay of Serum or Plasma Aldosterone That Require Extraction

Antiserum Development			Cortisol Cross-Reactivity (%)	Purification Steps	Normal Values (ng/dl)		Reference
Developer or Source	Antigen	Animal			Recumbent	Upright	
Author	Aldo-CMO-BSA *	Rabbit	0.8	Paper chromatography; silica gel column chromatography [2]	7.4 (3–16)	13.2 (4–31)	44
Author	Aldo-CMO-RSA	Rabbit	0.01	Paper chromatography	1.4	12.2	4
Author	Aldo-CMO-BSA	Rabbit	< 0.5	Paper chromatography or LH-20 Sephadex column chromatography	—	—	28
NIH	Aldo-18, 21-dihemisuccinate-BSA	Sheep	0.01	Paper chromatography	7.0	—	63
NIH	Aldo-18, 21-dihemisuccinate-BSA	Sheep	0.03	Ethanol : petroleum ether partition; thin-layer chromatography	8.6	18.3	61
NIH	Aldo-18, 21-dihemisuccinate-BSA	Sheep	0.6	Fuller's earth adsorption; antibody (Mayes) adsorption; ammonium sulfate precipitation; extraction into dichloromethane	—	—	42

NIH	Aldo-18, 21-dihemisuccinate-BSA	Sheep	—	Toluene : water partition; oxidation; extraction into ether	8.0	11.2	64
Author	Aldo-CMO-BGG	Rabbit	0.001	None	6.9 (4–10.2)	21.2 (8.2–32.4)	68
NIH	Aldo-18, 21-dihemisuccinate-BSA	Sheep	—	Antibody adsorption; ammonium sulfate precipitation; extraction into dichloromethane	—	—	23
Author	Aldo-CMO-BSA	Rabbit	0.02	Paper chromatography	7.5 (3.3–14.4)	16.8 (5.9–26)	30
Author	Aldo-CMO-BSA	Rabbit	< 0.00003	None	—	13.4 (3.4–35)	45
Author	Aldo-CMO-BSA	Rabbit	0.000001	Paper chromatography	—	—	6
NIH	Aldo-18, 21-dihemisuccinate-BSA	Sheep	—	LH-20 Sephadex column chromatography	8.0 (2–18)	18.3 (4–32)	46
NIH	Aldo-18, 21-dihemisuccinate-BSA	Sheep	—	Charcoal-dextran adsorption; methanol : dichloromethane elution	—	—	65
Author	Aldo-CMO-RSA	Rabbit	< 0.005	LH-20 Sephadex column chromatography	3.8 (1.1–6)	—	14
NIH	Aldo-18, 21-dihemisuccinate-BSA	Sheep	0.01	LH-20 Sephadex column chromatography	8.2 (3.1–11.3)	10.6 (8.6–13.6)	27
Author	Aldo-CMO-BSA *	Rabbit	None	None	4.4 (1.4–7.1)	—	51

Table 9–3 (Continued)

Antiserum Development			Cortisol Cross-Reactivity (%)	Purification Steps	Normal Values (ng/dl)		Reference
Developer or Source	Antigen	Animal			Recumbent	Upright	
NIH	Aldo-18, 21-dihemisuccinate-BSA	Sheep	0.02	Celite column chromatography	—	—	8
rF Laboratories (Houston, Tex.)	—	Guinea pig	—	XAD-2 adsorption; oxidation; ethyl acetate elution	7.9 (4.0–12.5)	21.4 (7.0–27.5)	54
NIH	Aldo-18, 21-dihemisuccinate-BSA	Sheep	—	Paper chromatography	—	12 (3.3–22.3)	48
Author	Aldo-21-hemisuccinate-BSA	Rabbit	< 0.0001	None	7.2	20.8	26
NIH	Aldo-18, 21-dihemisuccinate-BSA	Sheep	—	Paper chromatography	—	19.7	37
NIH	Aldo-18, 21-dihemisuccinate-BSA	Sheep	—	Thin-layer chromatography	7.3	—	50
Author	Aldo(γ-lactone)-CMO-BSA	Sheep	—	Oxidation	6	—	2
Author	Aldo-CMO-BSA	Rabbit	< 0.001	None	6.5 (1.2–12.5)	17.2 (7–29.5)	41
NIH	Aldo-18, 21-dihemisuccinate-BSA	Sheep	—	Thin-layer chromatography	8.9 (4.5–18)	20 (11–40)	34
NIH	Aldo-18, 21-dihemisuccinate-BSA	Sheep	—	Silica gel column chromatography; LH-20 Sephadex column chromatography	5.9	11.2	49
Author	Aldo-18, 21-diacetate-CMO-BSA	Rabbit	0.0	None	—	(2–21)	36
Author	Aldo-3, 20-carboxydioxime-BGG	Rabbit	0.0000005	None	10.7	23.9	55

* The abbreviations used in this table are the same as those used in Table 9–2.

Table 9–4. Methods for the Radioimmunoassay of Serum or Plasma Aldosterone That Do Not Require Extraction or Chromatography

Antiserum Development			Cortisol Cross-Reactivity (%)	Normal Values (ng/dl)		Comment	Reference
Developer or Source	Antigen	Animal		Recumbent	Upright		
Author	Aldo-CMO-BGG *	Rabbit	< 0.00009	4.3	11.4	[^{125}I] aldosterone labeled antigen	47
Author	Aldo-CMO-BGG	Rabbit	—	—	—	[^{125}I] aldosterone labeled antigen	24
Author	Aldo-CMO-BGG	Rabbit	0.005	18.1	28.9	Overestimates levels of aldosterone	29
Author	Aldo-20, 21-diacetate-CMO-BTG	Rabbit	0.001– < 0.00001	—	—	Eight of nine rabbits provided good antisera	52
Author	Aldo-CMO-BSA	Rabbit	0.000001	7.8 (4–12)	17.0 (9–28)	[^{125}I] aldosterone labeled antigen	1

* The abbreviations used in this table are the same as those used in Table 9–2.

A concentrated solution of the antiserum in 0.05 M borate buffer pH 8.0 (1 : 100) is stored at −20° C.

Tritium-Labeled Aldosterone. Tritium-labeled aldosterone ([1,2-^{3}H] aldosterone; specific activity 50 Ci/mM) is stored in absolute ethanol at −20° C. Its purity is determined with the use of paper chromatography in a Bush-type solvent system of toluene : methanol : water in a ratio of 60 : 13 : 6. Most lots of tritium-labeled aldosterone are stable for at least 6 months. We recommend that purity be checked every 3 months.

Aldosterone. Aldosterone is dissolved in absolute ethanol at 0.1 μg/ml and stored at −20° C. Its purity is assessed by chromatography and melting-point determination. We have found that aldosterone is stable for several months when it is stored under these conditions. However, cupric ion contamination of the ethanol can cause aldosterone to decompose rapidly.

Solvents and Chemicals. The ethanol used is absolute ethanol (U.S.P.), and other solvents are reagent grade. Dichloromethane of spectrophotometric quality (Matheson, Coleman, and Bell, Norwood, Ohio) is purified by passage through activated silica gel in a 6 × 120 cm glass column. Deionized, distilled water is used to prepare the following solutions: 1 N, 0.2 N, and 20% sodium hydroxide; 1 N and 0.1 N hydrochloric acid; 0.1% acetic acid; and a 0.05 M borate buffer adjusted to pH 8.0 using 1 N sodium hydroxide. Fraction V bovine serum albumin (Sigma Chemical Co., St. Louis, Mo.), fraction II bovine gamma globulin (Schwarz/Mann, Orangeburg, N.Y.), and dextran T40 (Pharmacia Fine Chemicals, Piscataway, N.J.) are used as supplied. Norit A charcoal (American Norit Co., Jacksonville, Fla.) is washed six times with 4 volumes of 0.1 N hydrochloric acid, neutralized with 20% sodium hydroxide, washed two times with 4 volumes of water and two times with 2 volumes of acetone, and dried in a vacuum oven at 40° C. A stock charcoal-dextran solution is prepared by suspending 11.8 gm of the washed charcoal in 100 ml of water and dissolving 3 gm of the dextran T40 in 400 ml of water. The solutions are combined, mixed thoroughly, adjusted to pH 7.8, and stored at 4° C.

Glassware. Round-bottom glass culture tubes with screw caps, 25 × 200 mm, and 16 × 125 mm and 12 × 75 mm disposable borosilicate glass culture tubes are used. Reusable glassware is washed in chromic acid (sodium dichromate dissolved in sulfuric acid), rinsed with distilled water, and soaked in methanol.

METHODS. *Summary.* Aldosterone is extracted from serum into dichloromethane, the dichloromethane is evaporated, the dry extract is dissolved in a solution of gamma globulin, and the concentration of aldosterone in the solution is determined by radioimmunoassay. Varying amounts of standard aldosterone, dissolved in a buffered albumin solution, are processed in the same way as the serum and are used to construct a standard curve for each assay. Plasma can be used instead of serum in the assay without altering the results.

Assay Setup. Add 2 ml of each serum sample to a 25 × 200 mm tube. Add 2 ml of a serum pool, which is used to assess the variability between assays, to a

25 × 200 mm tube. Add 2 ml of water, which serves as a blank, to each of two 25 × 200 mm tubes.

Prepare a 1 ng/ml solution of aldosterone in borate buffer that contains 5% bovine serum albumin (BSA). Varying amounts of this solution are added to a series of 25 × 200 mm tubes, as summarized below. Borate buffer that contains 5% BSA is used to bring the volume to 2 ml in all the standard tubes.

Duplicate Extraction Tubes	Aldosterone in Borate Buffer with 5% BSA (1 ng/ml)	Borate Buffer with 5% BSA
S1, S2	2.0 ml	None
S3, S4	1.0 ml	1.0 ml
S5, S6	0.5 ml	1.5 ml
S7, S8	0.2 ml	1.8 ml
S9, S10	0.1 ml	1.9 ml
S11, S12	0.05 ml	1.95 ml
S13, S14	None	2.0 ml

Add 0.2 ml of 0.2 N sodium hydroxide to all the tubes.

Extraction. Add 20 ml of dichloromethane to all tubes and shake the tubes gently for 5 minutes. To avoid emulsions, do not shake the tubes vigorously.

Aspirate the top layer and discard it.

Wash each extract with 2 ml of 0.1% acetic acid and then with 2 ml of water.

Transfer 10 ml and 5 ml of the dichloromethane from the tubes that contain the samples, pool, and blanks and 10 ml of the dichloromethane from the tubes with the standards to 16 × 125 mm tubes and evaporate the dichloromethane under air in a 40° C water bath. We have not found it necessary to use nitrogen for this step.

Add 300 μl of 1% bovine gamma globulin in borate buffer to all tubes and agitate them gently.

Radioimmunoassay. Add 100 μl of the 300 μl of 1% bovine gamma globulin used to reconstitute the extracts to 12 × 75 mm tubes in duplicate for the samples, pool, and blanks. For each tube of standard, add 100 μl to 12 × 75 mm tubes.

Dilute the stock antiserum solution (1 : 100) with borate buffer containing 0.1% bovine gamma globulin to a titer that binds 35 to 50 percent of added tritium-labeled aldosterone. In our laboratory we dilute the stock solution to 1 : 2500, which results in a final titer of 1 : 6250 in the assay tubes.

Add 100 μl of dilute antiserum to all tubes except one set of the blanks; to this set add 100 μl of 0.1% bovine gamma globulin without antiserum. Shake the tubes briefly and incubate them at 4° C for 1 hour.

Dilute the concentrated tritium-labeled aldosterone to 20,000 dpm/0.05 ml with borate buffer that contains 0.1% bovine gamma globulin.

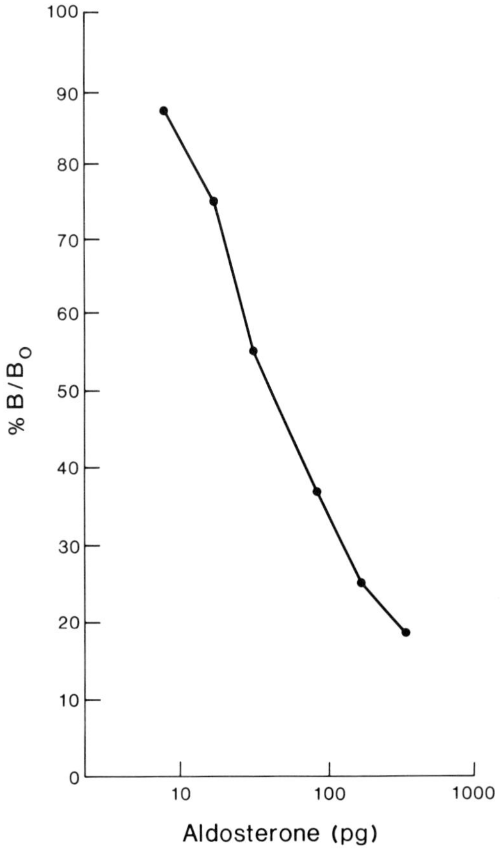

Figure 9–1
Example of a standard curve used in the radioimmunoassay of aldosterone in serum. The anti-aldosterone antiserum of McKenzie and Clements [45] was used at a dilution of 1 : 6250. B is the bound tritium (cpm) for each standard; B_0 is the bound tritium (cpm) in the tubes to which no aldosterone is added. The standard curve points are 9, 17, 33, 84, 167, and 333 pg of aldosterone.

Add 50 μl of the dilute tritium-labeled aldosterone to all tubes and to a counting vial to determine the amount of radioactivity added to each tube.

Shake the tubes briefly and incubate them for 2 hours at 4° C. The incubation may be extended up to 18 hours without altering the results. After the incubation, place the assay tubes in an ice bath.

Dilute the stock charcoal-dextran solution 1 : 2 with borate buffer, and stir the diluted solution in an ice bath with a magnetic stirrer for 20 minutes.

Add 0.5 ml of the dilute charcoal-dextran solution rapidly to the assay tubes. We add the solution, using a semiautomatic adjustable pipette, to tubes in batches of 40 or less. Briefly agitate the tubes in each batch and centrifuge them for 1 minute at 2000 rpm in a refrigerated centrifuge at 4° C. This method avoids disruption of the complex of antiserum and aldosterone due to prolonged contact of the complex with the charcoal. Centrifuge all the tubes for 20 minutes after completing the additions to all of the batches.

Decant the supernatants into vials that contain a counting cocktail suitable for counting aqueous samples and determine the amount of tritium in each vial in a liquid scintillation spectrophotometer. Accumulate 10,000 cpm to minimize the error of counting.

Calculations. Divide the mean counts per minute from the standard curve tubes with no aldosterone added (tubes 13 and 14) into the counts per minute from the standard, blank, pool, and sample tubes.

Construct a standard curve using these percentage results for the standards and the picograms of aldosterone added to the standard curve tubes. We use 2-cycle semilogarithmic paper (Fig. 9–1).

Convert the percentage results for the blanks, pool, and sample to picograms of aldosterone by using the standard curve.

Calculate the aldosterone in the 2-ml samples as follows:

$$A = M \times D \times \frac{20}{E} \times \frac{1}{V} \times \frac{1}{10}$$

where A = the aldosterone in the sample in nanograms per deciliter,
M = the picograms of aldosterone read from the standard curve,
D = the radioimmunoassay dilution factor, 3,
E = the volume of extract assayed, 10 ml or 5 ml,
20 = the volume of dichloromethane used for extraction, and
V = the volume of serum that was extracted.

Multiplication by 1/10 converts picograms per milliliter to nanograms per deciliter.

Normal Values. We found the following ranges of levels of serum aldosterone in normal subjects (1) after ad libitum sodium intake and 1 hour of recumbent posture and (2) after sodium depletion and 4 hours of upright posture. Sodium depletion was achieved by limiting sodium intake to 20 mEq of sodium daily for 3 days and administering a thiazide diuretic for 2 days.

Conditions	Serum Aldosterone
Ad libitum sodium intake—recumbent	$<$ 3–17 ng/dl
Sodium depletion—upright	5–209 ng/dl

Radioimmunoassay of Aldosterone in Urine

MATERIALS. The anti-aldosterone antiserum, the tritium-labeled aldosterone, the aldosterone, the solvents and chemicals, and the apparatus are used as described in the serum assay.

METHODS. This method measures aldosterone that is liberated by acid hydrolysis of the 18β-glucosiduronic acid conjugate of aldosterone [7]. Urine is extracted with ethyl acetate to remove unconjugated steroids. The urine is then incubated at pH 1.0 for 24 hours to liberate aldosterone. After incubation, a small amount of tritium-labeled aldosterone is added to the urine to estimate the loss of aldosterone during extraction. The urine is extracted with dichloromethane, the pH of the extract is adjusted to 8.0, and the dichloromethane is evaporated. The residue is dissolved in ethanol, and the radioactivity in an aliquot is counted to calculate the loss of aldosterone. A portion of the remaining solution is diluted, and aliquots are transferred to assay tubes. The ethanol is then evaporated, and the amount of aldosterone that is present is determined by radioimmunoassay.

Urine Collection. Collect urine for 24 hours into 3-liter bottles that contain 30 ml of 50% glacial acetic acid, which acts as a preservative.

Pre-extraction. Add approximately 10 ml of the urine, 10 ml of water, 10 ml of a high-aldosterone pool of urine, and 10 ml of a low-aldosterone pool of urine to 25 × 200 mm tubes.

Add 10 ml of ethyl acetate to each tube, shake the tubes gently for 1 minute, and then remove the top layer and discard it.

Acid Hydrolysis. Adjust the pH of the urine samples to 1.0 using 60% concentrated hydrochloric acid and incubate the samples in the dark at 24° C for 22 to 24 hours.

Extraction. Transfer aliquots of the samples to a second set of 25 × 200 mm tubes. Transfer 2 ml if the 24-hour urine volume was less than 1000 ml, and 5 ml if it was greater than 1000 ml.

Add 7 volumes of dichloromethane to each tube.

Add 50 μl of a solution of ethanol that contains approximately 3000 dpm of tritium-labeled aldosterone per 50 μl to each tube and to two counting vials for the determination of the amount of radioactivity added to each sample.

Shake all tubes, using a gentle rocking motion, for 1 minute. Aspirate the top layer and discard it.

Wash each extract with 2 ml of 0.2 N sodium hydroxide. Determine that the top layer is alkaline and remove it by aspiration. If it is not alkaline, add one to three drops of 20% sodium hydroxide and wash the extract again. Do not delay at this step because alkaline conditions can cause the inversion of the side chain of aldosterone.

Wash the extracts with 2 ml of water and then 2 ml of 0.1% acetic acid. Check to make sure that the top layer is acid; if it is not, wash the extract again with 2 ml of 0.1% acetic acid. Then wash with 2 ml of water and finally with 2 ml of the borate buffer.

Evaporate the dichloromethane to 5 to 10 ml, transfer the dichloromethane to 16 × 125 mm tubes, and evaporate the dichloromethane completely.

Radioimmunoassay. Add 1 ml of ethanol to each 16 × 125 mm tube.

Transfer 300 μl of the ethanol solution in each tube to a counting vial. Evaporate the ethanol from the recovery vials and count the radioactivity in them, using PPO (2,5-diphenyloxazole) and POPOP [1,4-bis-2-(5-phenyloxazolyl)-benzene] fluours dissolved in toluene. The amount of radioactivity in this aliquot will be used to estimate losses that occurred during the extraction step.

Remove a 100-μl aliquot from the 700 μl that remains in each 16 × 125 mm tube and dilute this aliquot fivefold with ethanol.

Transfer 100-μl, 50-μl, and 25-μl aliquots of the diluted ethanol solutions, in duplicate, to 12 × 75 mm tubes and bring the contents of each tube to 100 μl with ethanol.

Label 12 × 75 mm tubes for the standard curve as follows:

Duplicate Assay Tube	Aldosterone Standard Curve Point
S1, S2	1000 pg
S3, S4	500 pg
S5, S6	250 pg
S7, S8	125 pg
S9, S10	62 pg
S11, S12	31 pg
S13, S14	None

Add 100 μl of ethanol to each tube, and then add 100 μl of ethanol that contains 2 ng of aldosterone per 100 μl to tubes S1 and S2. Serially dilute the aldosterone in duplicate. Remove and discard 100 μl from tubes S11 and S12 at the end of the serial dilution.

Two tubes to which no antiserum is added are included in the assay to monitor the amount of nonspecific binding.

Evaporate the ethanol in all tubes in a vacuum oven at 40° C.

Prepare a solution in borate buffer that contains 2% ethanol, 1% human serum (obtained from a normal subject who received dexamethasone, 2 mg daily, for 2 days), and 30,000 dpm of tritium-labeled aldosterone per 0.5 ml of the solution.

Add 0.5 ml of this solution, which contains no antiserum, to the two tubes that are used to monitor nonspecific binding.

Then add an amount of stock antiserum (1 : 100) to the solution to obtain a titer that binds 35 to 50 percent of the added tritium-labeled aldosterone. In our laboratory this final titer is 1 : 20,000.

Add 0.5 ml of this solution to each 12 × 75 mm tube, except the two tubes used to monitor nonspecific binding. Also add 0.5 ml of this solution to two counting vials to determine the amount of radioactivity added to each tube.

Place the tubes in a 40° C water bath for 20 minutes.

Shake the tubes briefly and incubate them overnight at 4° C.

After incubation, place the assay tubes in an ice water bath and prepare a charcoal-dextran solution by diluting the stock charcoal-dextran solution 1 : 2 with borate buffer.

Add 0.5 ml of the diluted charcoal-dextran solution to each tube and centrifuge them, using the batch method as described for the serum assay. Count the radioactivity in the supernatant.

Calculations. To determine the recovery factor, divide the mean of the recovery total counts into the recovery counts of each sample, corrected for background radioactivity, and multiply by 3.33. Determine the percentage of tritium-labeled aldosterone that is bound to the antiserum, construct the standard curve, and calculate the picograms of aldosterone in the samples as in the serum method. Calculate the urinary excretion of aldosterone per 24 hours as follows:

$$A = \frac{M \times D \times Q \times TV}{R \times E} \times 10^{-6}$$

where A = the urinary excretion of aldosterone in micrograms per 24 hours,
M = the picograms of aldosterone read from the standard curve,
D = the radioimmunoassay dilution factor, 10, and
Q = the radioimmunoassay aliquot factor, determined as follows:

Aliquot Added to Assay Tube	Q
100 μl	5
50 μl	10
25 μl	20

TV = the total 24-hour urine volume in milliliters,
R = the recovery factor, usually 0.9 (90%), and
E = the aliquot of hydrolyzed urine that is assayed, 2 ml or 5 ml.

Multiplication by 10^{-6} converts picograms to micrograms.

Normal Values. We found the following ranges of rates of urinary aldosterone excretion in normal subjects (1) during ad libitum sodium intake and (2) during sodium loading, when their urinary sodium excretion rate was > 200 mEq/24 hours.

Conditions	Urinary Aldosterone Excretion Rate
Ad libitum sodium intake	2–16 μg/24 hours
Sodium loading	< 8 μg/24 hours

Assessment of Assay Results

Before the results of a radioimmunoassay are used, the specificity, sensitivity, accuracy, and precision of the method should be assessed.

SPECIFICITY. The specificity of an anti-aldosterone antiserum can be determined by incubating the antiserum, the tritium-labeled aldosterone, and increasing amounts of other steroids in an assay and calculating the cross-reactivity between these steroids and the antiserum. Cross-reactivity is the ratio of the masses of aldosterone and of the other steroids that displace 50 percent of the tritium-labeled aldosterone from the antiserum. The antiserum of McKenzie and Clements cross-reacts very minimally with 18-hydroxy-deoxycorticosterone (0.015%), 18-oxo-deoxycorticosterone (0.007%), and cortisone (0.0043%) and essentially not at all ($< 0.002\%$) with many C_{21}, C_{19}, and C_{18} steroids and steroidlike drugs [7, 45]. It does cross-react significantly (10%) with 3α, 5β-tetrahydroaldosterone-3β-glucosiduronic acid, which, however, is separated from aldosterone during the extraction procedure. The effect of purification by sequential chromatography steps on the results of the assay should be determined. If chromatography fails to alter the measured levels of the aldosterone, this is further evidence that the assay is specific for aldosterone. Specificity should also be assessed by determining the apparent increase in measured aldosterone after adding large amounts of other steroids or steroid-like drugs to control samples of urine or serum.

Assays are not specific if the values of aldosterone in the tubes containing water only (method blanks) are high. Problems with high blank measurements can be solved by testing each reagent as an unknown in an assay and purifying or obtaining a different supply of the interfering reagent. Measurements of dilutions of a sample and dilutions of the solution of standard aldosterone should be parallel. Nonparallelism can be caused by non-dose-dependent interference by a reagent, by substances in the sample, or by the use of inadequate amounts of charcoal-dextran to separate the bound and free steroids.

SENSITIVITY. The sensitivity of the assay should be quantitated by determining the least detectable concentration; this is the smallest concentration of aldosterone resulting in a response that is 2 standard deviations away from the zero dose response. In addition, sensitivity should be assessed by determining the slope of the standard curve. In our laboratory the average slope of the standard curve is minus 1.0.

ACCURACY. The accuracy of the assay should be validated by adding known amounts of standard aldosterone to urine or serum and determining that the concentration of aldosterone measured by radioimmunoassay equals the amount of aldosterone added plus the amount of aldosterone in the urine or serum prior to the addition of aldosterone. Losses of aldosterone are monitored in the urine method described in this chapter but not in the serum method, because in the latter method the standard curve and the samples are processed identically. In our laboratory the recovery of the tritium-labeled aldosterone added to urine is 87 ± 8.0 (SD) %.

PRECISION. The precision of the assay should be assessed using within-assay and between-assay variability of duplicate samples and pools. The average within-assay and between-assay coefficient of variations of aldosterone assays reported in the literature are 8 percent and 12 percent, respectively. These values are in close agreement with results in our laboratory. It should be remembered that precision depends on the position of the measurement on the standard curve. In general, values derived from the middle portion of the standard curve are more precise than the values derived from extremes of the curve.

Validation of the specificity and accuracy of an assay should also be obtained by demonstrating that an independent, proved method gives the same results.

Summary

The methods of radioimmunoassay discussed in the preceding sections can yield very accurate and precise measurements of aldosterone when attention is given to the purity of the reagents and the conditions of the assay. The new assays that measure plasma aldosterone directly, without isolation or purification steps, make it feasible for a clinical chemistry laboratory to assay aldosterone economically and with relative ease. Direct measurement of conjugates of the metabolites of aldosterone in urine will be a useful adjunct in the diagnosis of diseases of aldosterone secretion.

References

1. Al-Dujaili, E. A. S., and Edwards, C. R. W. The development and application of a direct radioimmunoassay for plasma aldosterone using ^{125}I-labeled ligand—comparison of three methods. *J. Clin. Endocrinol. Metab.* 46:105, 1978.
2. Antunes, J. R., Dale, S. L., and Melby, J. C. Simplified radioimmunoassay for aldosterone using antisera to aldosterone-γ-lactone. *Steroids* 28:621, 1976.
3. Bayard, F., Beitins, I. Z., Kowarski, A., et al. Measurement of aldosterone secretion rate by radioimmunoassay. *J. Clin. Endocrinol. Metab.* 31:507, 1970.
4. Bayard, F., Beitins, I. Z., Kowarski, A., et al. Measurement of plasma aldosterone by radioimmunoassay. *J. Clin. Endocrinol. Metab.* 31:1, 1970.
5. Biglieri, E. G., Schambelan, M., Brust, N., et al. Plasma aldosterone concentration: Further characterization of aldosterone-producing adenomas. *Circ. Res.* 34–35 (Suppl. I):I–183, 1974.
6. Bizollon, C. A., Riviere, J.-F., Franchimont, P., et al. Solid phase radioimmunoassay of plasma aldosterone. *Steroids* 23:809, 1974.
7. Brown, R. D., Swander, A., and McKenzie, J. K. Urine aldosterone radioimmunoassay: Validation of a method without chromatography. *J. Clin. Endocrinol. Metab.* 42:894, 1976.
8. Chakmakjian, Z. H., Pryor, W. W., and Abraham, G. E. A radioimmunoassay

for serum and urine aldosterone by celite column chromatography. *Anal. Lett.* 7:97, 1974.
9. Chavarri, M., Luetscher, J. A., Dowdy, A. J., et al. The effects of temperature and plasma cortisol on distribution of aldosterone between plasma and red blood cells: Influence on metabolic clearance rate and on hepatic and renal extraction of aldosterone. *J. Clin. Endocrinol. Metab.* 44:752, 1977.
10. Conn, J. W. Presidential address: (1) Painting background; (2) Primary aldosteronism, a new clinical syndrome. *J. Lab. Clin. Med.* 45:3, 1955.
11. Cope, C. L., and Loizou, S. Simplification of urinary aldosterone measurement by radioimmunoassay. *J. Clin. Pathol.* 26:628, 1973.
12. Coppage, W. S., Jr., Island, D. P., Cooner, A. E., et al. The metabolism of aldosterone in normal subjects and in patients with hepatic cirrhosis. *J. Clin. Invest.* 41:1672, 1962.
13. Crane, M. G., and Harris, J. J. Effect of aging on renin activity and aldosterone excretion. *J. Lab. Clin. Med.* 87:947, 1976.
14. Daniel, J. Y., Mion, H., and Soulas, D. Radioimmunoassay of plasma aldosterone by chromatography on Sephadex LH 20. *Clin. Chim. Acta* 55:235, 1974.
15. Deck, K. A. Eine einfache radioimmunologische Methode zur Bestimmung der Aldosteronausscheidung im Urin. *Verh. Dtsch. Ges. Inn. Med.* 78:1605, 1972.
16. Deck, K. A., Champion, P. K., Jr., and Conn, J. W. Urinary free aldosterone in healthy people and in patients with primary aldosteronism. *J. Clin. Endocrinol. Metab.* 36:756, 1973.
17. Diezi, J., Michoud, P., Aceves, J., et al. Micropuncture study of electrolyte transport across papillary collecting duct of the rat. *Am. J. Physiol.* 224:623, 1973.
18. Drewes, P. A., Demetriou, J. A., and Pileggi, V. J. Measurement of urinary aldosterone by a simplified radioimmunoassay procedure. *Clin. Biochem.* 6:88, 1973.
19. Ekins, R. P., Newman, G. B., Piyasena, R., et al. The radioimmunoassay of aldosterone in serum and urine: Theoretical and practical aspects. *J. Steroid Biochem.* 3:289, 1972.
20. Farmer, R. W., Roup, W. G., Jr., Pellizzari, E. D., et al. A rapid aldosterone radioimmunoassay. *J. Clin. Endocrinol. Metab.* 34:19, 1972.
21. Ferriss, J. B., Brown, J. J., Fraser, R., et al. Results of adrenal surgery in patients with hypertension, aldosterone excess, and low plasma renin concentration. *Br. Med. J.* 1:135, 1975.
22. Ganguly, A., Melada, G. A., Luetscher, J. A., et al. Control of plasma aldosterone in primary aldosteronism: Distinction between adenoma and hyperplasia. *J. Clin. Endocrinol. Metab.* 37:765, 1973.
23. Gomez-Sanchez, C., Kem, D. C., and Kaplan, N. M. A radioimmunoassay for plasma aldosterone by immunologic purification. *J. Clin. Endocrinol. Metab.* 36:795, 1973.
24. Haruyama, K., Nakajima, K., Fukuchi, S., et al. A simple method measuring plasma aldosterone by radioimmunoassay without extraction. *Nippon Naibunpi Gakkai Zasshi* 53:810, 1977.
25. Helber, A., and Kaufmann, W. Radioimmunologische Methode zur Aldosteronbestimmung im Urin. *Klin. Wochenschr.* 51:1164, 1973.
26. Hubl, W., Büchner, M., Stahl, F., et al. Radioimmunoassay for aldosterone in plasma without chromatography. *Endokrinologie* 66:292, 1975.
27. Ichikawa, S., Murata, K., and Shigiya, R. Application of a marker dye on Sephadex LH-20 column chromatography in radioimmunoassay of plasma aldosterone. *Endocrinol. Jpn.* 21:361, 1974.
28. Ito, T., Woo, J., Haning, R., et al. A radioimmunoassay for aldosterone in

human peripheral plasma including a comparison of alternate techniques. *J. Clin. Endocrinol. Metab.* 34:106, 1972.
29. Jowett, T. P., and Slater, J. D. H. Development of radioimmunoassays for the measurement of aldosterone in unprocessed plasma and simple plasma extracts. *Clin. Chim. Acta* 80:435, 1977.
30. Jowett, T. P., Slater, J. D. H., Piyasena, R. D., et al. Radioimmunoassay of aldosterone in plasma and urine: Validation of a novel separation technique and a rapid urine assay. *Clin. Sci. Mol. Med.* 45:607, 1973.
31. Katz, F. H., and Romfh, P. Plasma aldosterone and renin activity during the menstrual cycle. *J. Clin. Endocrinol. Metab.* 34:819, 1972.
32. Katz, F. H., Romfh, P., and Smith, J. A. Episodic secretion of aldosterone in supine man: Relationship to cortisol. *J. Clin. Endocrinol. Metab.* 35:178, 1972.
33. Kohl, K.-H., Vecsei, P., and Abdelhamid, S. Radioimmunoassays of tetrahydroaldosterone (TH-Aldo) in human urine. *Acta Endocrinol.* 87:596, 1978.
34. Kurtz, A. B., and Bartter, F. C. Radioimmunoassays for aldosterone and deoxycorticosterone in plasma and urine. *Steroids* 28:133, 1976.
35. Langan, J., Jackson, R., Adlin, E. V., et al. A simple radioimmunoassay for urinary aldosterone. *J. Clin. Endocrinol. Metab.* 38:189, 1974.
36. Lijnen, P., Amery, A., Fagard, R., et al. Direct radioimmunoassay of plasma aldosterone in normal subjects. *Clin. Chim. Acta* 84:305, 1978.
37. Lijnen, P. J., McCaa, R. E., Fagard, R. H., et al. Modified radioimmunoassay for peripheral plasma aldosterone, *F.E.B.S. Lett.* 54:84, 1975.
38. Luetscher, J. A., Jr., and Curtis, R. H. Observations on aldosterone in human urine. *Fed. Proc.* 14:746, 1955.
39. Luetscher, J. A., Jr., and Deming, Q. B. Treatment of nephrosis with cortisone. *J. Clin. Invest.* 29:1576, 1950.
40. Luetscher, J. A., Ganguly, A., Melada, G. A., et al. Preoperative differentiation of adrenal adenoma from idiopathic adrenal hyperplasia in primary aldosteronism. *Circ. Res.* 34–35 (Suppl. I):I–175, 1974.
41. Malvano, R., Gandolfi, C., Giannessi, D., et al. Radioimmunoassay of aldosterone in crude plasma extracts. *J. Nucl. Biol. Med.* 20:37, 1976.
42. Martin, B. T., and Nugent, C. A. A non-chromatographic radioimmunoassay for plasma aldosterone. *Steroids* 21:169, 1973.
43. Mattox, V. R., Mason, H. L., Albert, A., et al. Properties of a sodium-retaining principle from beef adrenal extract. *J. Am. Chem. Soc.* 75:4869, 1953.
44. Mayes, D., Furuyama, S., Kem, D. C., et al. A radioimmunoassay for plasma aldosterone. *J. Clin. Endocrinol. Metab.* 30:682, 1970.
45. McKenzie, J. K., and Clements, J. A. Simplified radioimmunoassay for serum aldosterone utilizing increased antibody specificity. *J. Clin. Endocrinol. Metab.* 38:622, 1974.
46. Nowaczynski, W., Sasaki, C., and Genest, J. Radioimmunoassay for aldosterone and normal values under various physiological conditions. *J. Steroid Biochem.* 5:123, 1974.
47. Ogihara, T., Iinuma, K., Nishi, K., et al. A non-chromatographic non-extraction radioimmunoassay for serum aldosterone. *J. Clin. Endocrinol. Metab.* 45: 726, 1977.
48. Ölgaard, K. Plasma aldosterone by radioimmunoassay determination in normal man and in patients on maintenance haemodialysis. *Scand. J. Clin. Lab. Invest.* 35:31, 1975.
49. Pakarinen, A., Koskinen, L., and Adlercreutz, H. Evaluation of radioimmunological methods for assay of plasma and urinary aldosterone. *Scand. J. Clin. Lab. Invest.* 36:331, 1976.
50. Parth, K., Zimprich, H., and Brunel, R. Determination of plasma aldosterone

in children by thin layer chromatography and radioimmunoassay. *Acta Endocrinol.* 81:330, 1976.
51. Pham-Huu-Trung, M. T., and Corvol, P. A direct determination of plasma aldosterone. *Steroids* 24:587, 1974.
52. Pratt, J. J., Boonman, R., Woldring, M. G., et al. Special problems in the radioimmunoassay of plasma aldosterone without prior extraction and purification. *Clin. Chim. Acta* 84:329, 1978.
53. Pratt, J. H., Holbrook, M. M., Dale, S. L., et al. The measurement of urinary tetrahydroaldosterone by radioimmunoassay. *J. Steroid Biochem.* 8:677, 1977.
54. Roginsky, M. S., Panetz, A. I., and Gordon, R. D. The use of amberlite XAD-2 columns for the determination of plasma aldosterone by radioimmunoassay. *Clin. Chim. Acta* 63:303, 1975.
55. Sancho, J., and Haber, E. A direct microassay for aldosterone in plasma extracts. *J. Clin. Endocrinol. Metab.* 47:391, 1978.
56. Schambelan, M., Brust, N. L., Chang, B. C. F., et al. Circadian rhythm and effect of posture on plasma aldosterone concentration in primary aldosteronism. *J. Clin. Endocrinol. Metab.* 43:115, 1976.
57. Schambelan, M., Stockigt, J. R., and Biglieri, E. G. Isolated hypoaldosteronism in adults. *N. Engl. J. Med.* 287:573, 1972.
58. Schnurr, E., and Schröder, E. Eine vereinfachte Methode zur Bestimmung der Aldosteronausscheidung. *Med. Welt.* 24:689, 1973.
59. Sealey, J. E., Bühler, F. R., Laragh, J. H., et al. Aldosterone excretion: Physiological variations in man measured by radioimmunoassay or double-isotope dilution. *Circ. Res.* 31:367, 1972.
60. Simpson, S. A., and Tait, J. F. Physico-chemical methods of detection of a previously unidentified adrenal hormone. *Mem. Soc. Endocrinol.* 2:9, 1953.
61. St. Cyr, M. J., Sancho, J. M., and Melby, J. C. Quantitation of plasma aldosterone by radioimmunoassay. *Clin. Chem.* 18:1395, 1972.
62. Stuart, J., Keane, P. M., Viol, G., et al. A rapid method for the radioimmunoassay of urinary aldosterone. *Clin. Biochem.* 6:285, 1973.
63. Underwood, R. H., and Williams, G. H. The simultaneous measurement of aldosterone, cortisol, and corticosterone in human peripheral plasma by displacement analysis. *J. Lab. Clin. Med.* 79:848, 1972.
64. Varsano-Aharon, N., and Ulick, S. A simplified radioimmunoassay of plasma aldosterone. *J. Clin. Endocrinol. Metab.* 37:372, 1973.
65. Varsano-Aharon, N., and Ulick, S. Further simplifications in the immunoassay of plasma aldosterone. *J. Clin. Endocrinol. Metab.* 39:375, 1974.
66. Vecsei, P., Penke, B., and Joumaah, A. Radioimmunoassay of free aldosterone and of its 18-oxo-glucuronide in human urine. *Experientia* 28:622, 1972.
67. Vetter, W., Vetter, H., and Siegenthaler, W. Radioimmunoassay for aldosterone without chromatography: I. Determination of urinary 18-glucuronide excretion. *Acta Endocrinol.* 74:548, 1973.
68. Vetter, W., Vetter, H., and Siegenthaler, W. Radioimmunoassay for aldosterone without chromatography: II. Determination of plasma aldosterone. *Acta Endocrinol.* 74:558, 1973.
69. Waldhäusl, W., Haydl, H., and Frischauf, H. Determination of aldosterone by Sephadex LH-20 chromatography and radioimmunoassay. *Steroids* 20:727, 1972.
70. Weinberger, M. H., Kem, D. C., Gomez-Sanchez, C., et al. The effect of dexamethasone on the control of plasma aldosterone concentration in normal recumbent man. *J. Lab. Clin. Med.* 85:957, 1975.
71. Wolfe, L. K., Gordon, R. D., Island, D. P., et al. An analysis of factors determining the circadian pattern of aldosterone excretion. *J. Clin. Endocrinol. Metab.* 26:1261, 1966.

10. Diagnostic Procedures in Hypertension

Ross M. Tucker

This chapter provides the practicing physician with clinically oriented information relating to laboratory and x-ray procedures and protocols for use in the investigation of patients with hypertension. The discussion will cover plasma renin activity measurements, blockade of the renin-angiotensin system, plasma and urine aldosterone, and catecholamines. The chapter will also review the increasing usefulness of computed tomographic and isotopic scanning procedures in the detection of adrenal tumors, along with conventional intravenous and intra-aortic radiographic contrast techniques. Finally, there is a brief description of unusual syndromes that mimic primary aldosteronism but have neither hypertension nor suppressed plasma renin activity.

Overview of the Hypertension Spectrum

Hypertension, defined as the presence of casual diastolic blood pressure of 95 mm Hg or greater, is a common disease, especially in black people. In the United States alone, there may be approximately 60 million persons with this disorder, or 15 to 20 percent of the adult population [46]. Hidden among this large number of people with hypertension are some who have a detectable cause; or secondary hypertension. In this subset are yet a smaller number with surgically correctable forms of hypertension. The three most common varieties of these correctable forms are renal artery stenosis, aldosterone-producing adenoma, and pheochromocytoma, including related neuroectodermal tumors that produce excess catecholamines [21]. The frequency of these conditions is a subject of some controversy, but a recent survey at the Mayo Clinic disclosed that each year about 26,000 patients over the age of 15 years who register there for examination have hypertension. Of this group, approximately 50 per year have surgery for relief of renovascular hypertension (0.19 percent), 11 per year have resection of a pheochromocytoma or related tumors (0.04 percent), and 3 per year have aldosterone-producing adenomas removed (0.01 percent) [75]. These frequencies are considerably lower than other previously reported estimates. At any rate, the vast majority of hypertensives have either the essential form or a secondary variety without a potential for surgical cure, including patients with polycystic and other renal parenchymal diseases. Therefore, even though most of our laboratory and x-ray testing procedures are calculated to find the surgically curable forms of hypertension, the apparent frequency of these disorders is so low that the tests are seldom positive. Some physicians might conclude that testing for secondary causes should be kept to an absolute minimum for the following reasons: (1) the surgically curable diseases causing hypertension are rare; (2) most other types of secondary hypertension have no particular potential for surgical cure, and the discovery of them might well be an academic exercise; and (3) tests for diagnosing renovascular hypertension, primary aldosterone-producing adenoma, and pheochromocytoma can be expensive and might not satisfy cost/benefit analysis requirements—a question that is not altogether philosophical in these days of third-party medical benefit schemes.

Keeping these considerations in mind, let us examine the surgically curable forms of secondary hypertension and the diagnostic procedures relating to them.

Renovascular Hypertension

Renovascular hypertension, the most common form of secondary hypertension, is caused by constricting and obstructing lesions of the renal arteries. Atheromatous plaques are the most common lesions and occur in the middle and latter decades of life with equal frequency in both sexes. Fibromuscular lesions occur with greatest frequency in women in their fourth decade [75]. In contrast to the atheromatous lesions, fibromuscular disease of the renal arteries affects the middle and distal thirds of the main vessel and frequently extends into the primary branches. Noncalcified aneurysms of intrarenal and extrarenal arteries complicate fibromuscular disease, although rupture of these aneurysms is rare.

Clinically, renovascular hypertension might be suspected when a young woman develops hypertension or when hypertension suddenly becomes more severe in an older person. In this latter group, heart failure can be the presenting symptom. In others, the dreaded hemorrhagic stroke may be the first sign of accelerating high blood pressure. Keith-Wagoner-Barker group III or group IV fundus changes in a hypertensive patient must raise the suspicion of a secondary cause.

The physical examination is helpful in guiding the physician to the diagnosis of renovascular hypertension. Pertinent findings include bruits over the carotid or femoral arteries, suggesting atherosclerotic vascular disease; there is also a characteristic, high-pitched, systolic-diastolic bruit over the abdominal aorta in the epigastrium that accompanies fibromuscular renal artery stenosis.

Patients with mild and uncomplicated hypertension who respond readily to dietary sodium and caloric restriction when indicated, with or without simple antihypertensive drug therapy, are seldom found to have significant surgically curable hypertension. Tests in this group of patients should be minimal and should include measurement of serum potassium, creatinine or urea, and hemoglobin, as well as a chest x-ray, electrocardiogram, and urinalysis. Measurement of plasma lipids, glucose, and uric acid would round out the list.

With these clinical tenets in hand, the physician's first series of laboratory and x-ray studies calculated to identify renovascular hypertension should be isotopic and radiographic ones.

Excretory Urography

Excretory urography, which is the most common screening procedure for renovascular hypertension, must include films taken within the first 2, 3, or 4 minutes after the intravenous contrast injection. Subsequent films are exposed 10, 15, 20, and sometimes 45 or 60 minutes later. When this procedure is followed, the findings suggestive of renovascular hypertension are the following:

1. Renal pole-to-pole diameter differences of 1.5 cm or greater. However, renal masses or unilateral duplication of a collecting system negates this measurement as a diagnostic parameter. Renal artery stenosis might be suspected on the side of the smaller kidney.
2. When contrast medium appears in the collecting system of one kidney on any film earlier in the series than in the other kidney, this would suggest renal artery stenosis in the kidney with the delayed appearance.
3. Delayed clearance of contrast medium on one side with persistence in the 45- or 60-minute films when the contrast medium is faded or no longer visible in the other renal pelvis would suggest renal artery stenosis on the side with the delayed clearance.
4. Irregular notching in the upper third of the ureter by periureteral arterial collaterals points to renal artery stenosis on that side.
5. Smaller calliber collecting system structures frequently occur in the kidney supplied by a stenosed artery.

Using all these urographic clues, the physician might expect to identify about 75 percent of all patients whose hypertension is caused by renal artery stenosis. The range is 53 to 83 percent in various reported series [74]; this amounts to a reasonably large number of false-negative urograms in patients who have renovascular hypertension and suggests that other screening tests might be considered when the suspicion of renal artery stenosis is high, even if the hypertensive excretory urogram is normal.

Figure 10–1 is a typical excretory urogram in a patient with unilateral left renal artery stenosis and hypertension. This film shows the appearance of contrast medium in the renal pelvis on the right at 3 minutes, while there is only a nephrogram on the left. The pole-to-pole diameters are 14 cm on the right and 10.7 cm on the left. This urogram meets two criteria for diagnosing renal artery stenosis.

Radioisotope Renography

The radioisotope renogram is also a screening procedure for detection of renovascular hypertension. Ortho-iodohippuran containing the 125 or 131 isotope of iodine as a radioactive tag is both filtered at the glomerulus and secreted by the renal tubule. Its clearance rate approximates that of the effective renal plasma flow. Detection probes placed over each renal area in the back record

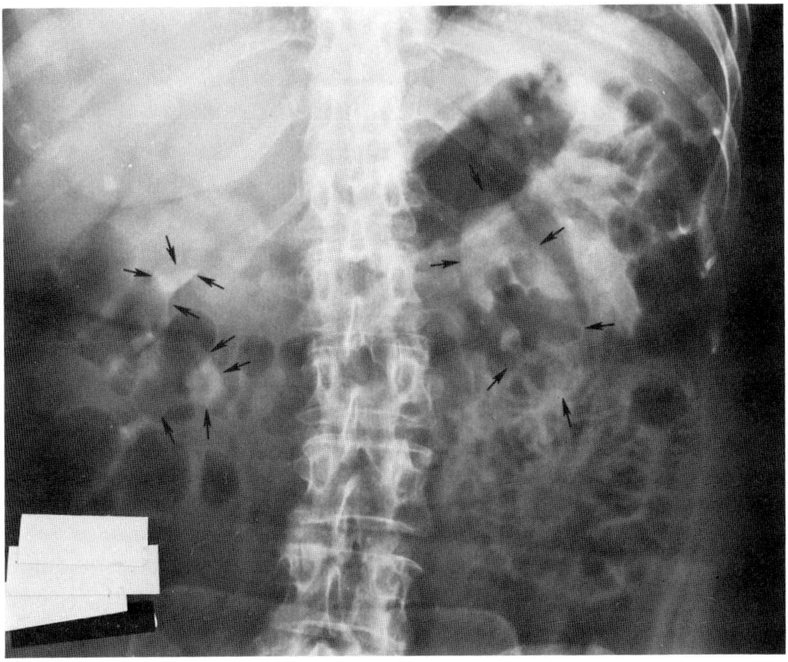

Figure 10–1
Excretory urogram. This film was exposed 3 minutes after the injection of the contrast medium. Note the obvious disparity in size, with the right kidney being larger than the left; the actual measurements were 14 cm and 10.7 cm, respectively. There is contrast medium in the calyces on the right (indicated by the arrows), whereas only a nephrogram appears on the left. These findings are highly suggestive of severe left renal artery stenosis.

radioactivity levels above background created by the radioactive ortho-iodohippuran contained within the renal parenchyma and collecting system. These activity levels are continuously plotted against time, and curves are drawn on paper accordingly. The normal curve has an early rapid rise, representing delivery of the isotope to the renal parenchyma by blood flow. This rise is terminated by a peak followed by a gradual decline, approaching the baseline asymptotically 20 to 30 minutes after the initial injection. The peak and decline occur as the isotope is cleared from the renal parenchyma and collecting system and is secreted down the ureters to the bladder.

Abnormal patterns of the peak and slope seen in renovascular hypertension include unilateral elevation of the excretion phase slope, reduced height of the early peak, or even failure to achieve a significant peak (the so-called nephrectomy pattern). One author [32] reports an abnormal radioisotope renogram with features suggesting unilateral renal artery disease in 72 percent of 180 pa-

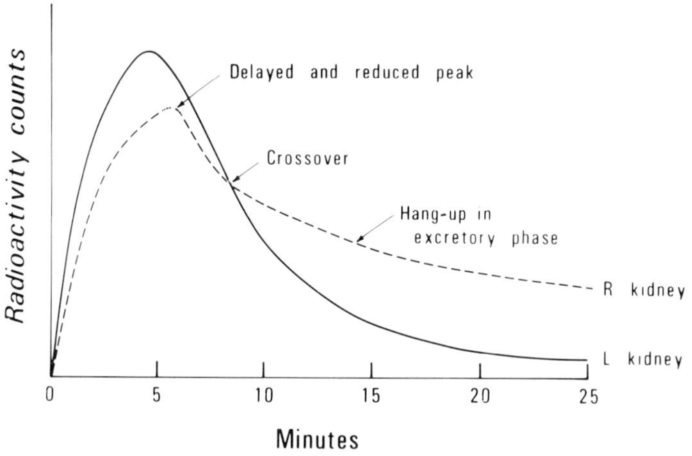

Figure 10–2
Radioisotope renogram showing the radioisotopic activity of the right kidney (*dotted line*) and the left kidney (*solid line*). There is a decrease in the height of the early peak on the right followed by a crossover pattern with delayed return of the excretory phase of the slope toward the baseline. These features suggest unilateral right renal artery stenosis.

tients who had renovascular hypertension (this amounts to a 28 percent incidence of false-negative tests).

Since the radioisotope renogram requires only tiny amounts of iodine as a tracer, few, if any, patients develop serious adverse reactions of the kind seen with excretory urographic contrast media. Moreover, some evaluation of separated renal function can be estimated from the renogram, since there is an individual probe over each kidney. On the other hand, approximately one out of four tests is falsely negative in renovascular hypertensive patients, a figure that is not particularly impressive for a screening procedure. In my own practice, the radioisotope renogram is of minor importance in the evaluation of renovascular hypertension evaluation; it is certainly not a substitute for excretory urography except in the patient who is hypersensitive to iodine. Figure 10–2 depicts a radioisotope renogram taken from a patient who had severe atheromatous right renal artery stenosis and hypertension. There is a delay in the peak of the right curve (dotted line) compared with the left (solid line). There is also a tendency for the right curve to persist higher above the baseline 10, 15, and 30 minutes after the injection; this is the "delay-and-hang-up" pattern and results in crossover at 10 minutes. These findings are all characteristic of unilateral right renal artery stenosis.

Bolus Intravenous Aortorenal Tomography

Intravenous aortorenal tomography requires a greater than usual amount of technical expertise. When it is performed properly, the abdominal aorta and main renal arteries can be visualized without the need for an arterial puncture or Seldinger catheterization of the ilioaortic system. First, an intravenous 14-gauge plastic needle is inserted into a large antecubital vein. This needle is used for the injection of a solution of 200 mg of dehydrocholate sodium (Decholin) diluted to 20 ml with normal saline as a measure of the arm-to-tongue circulation time. When this transit time measurement is completed, 80 cc of 90% sodium and meglumine diatrizoate (Hypaque-90) is injected rapidly over 3 to 5 seconds. Using the Decholin arm-to-tongue circulation time as a guide, tomographic cuts centered over the abdominal aorta at the level of the renal arteries are taken, using a stack of seven or eight films in the special cassette. These films are spaced approximately 1 cm in vertical distance above each other in the film carrier. Coupled with the arc transit of the x-ray tube above the patient, the film carrier moves horizontally below the patient. The subsequent cuts are in focus about 1 cm apart in vertical depth. After being developed, all seven films are viewed in their order of depth of focus. If the procedure is done by experienced personnel and the technical features worked out in advance, often the physician can assess the renal artery calibers quite satisfactorily, concluding that they are either normal or significantly stenosed. Occasionally, renal artery visualization is not satisfactory. Conventional intra-aortic renal arteriography is the logical next step in such a patient, as well as in the patient who has significant stenosis indicated by intravenous bolus aortorenal tomography.

Figure 10–3 depicts two films from a series of seven simultaneous aortorenal tomograms taken after a rapid intravenous injection of x-ray contrast material. The severe atheromatous stenosis of the proximal portion of the right main renal artery shows quite well as a composite picture is created from the cuts, with the planes of focus 1 cm apart in vertical distance. Only mild stenosis is present on the left.

Renal Arteriography

In the 1930s there were reported cures of hypertension involving removal of atrophic kidneys [10]. A rash of surgeries followed in hypertensive patients with unilateral small kidneys, in the hope of achieving a similar cure. None of the patients had had prior studies of renal artery caliber, and the results were dismal, with only about one-fifth of the patients receiving benefit by cure of their hypertension [6, 64, 65]. As a result, investigators began to seek more

---

Figure 10–3
(A) This radiograph is one film in a series of simultaneous tomographic cuts exposed 10 to 15 seconds after a rapid intravenous injection of contrast material. (B) This film is from the same series, with the horizontal plane of focus 1 cm anterior to that of (A). When these are viewed together, a composite picture of nearly complete atheromatous right renal artery stenosis can be seen in the proximal portion of the right main renal artery. There is mild atheromatous stenosis on the left. The renal arteries are outlined by arrows.

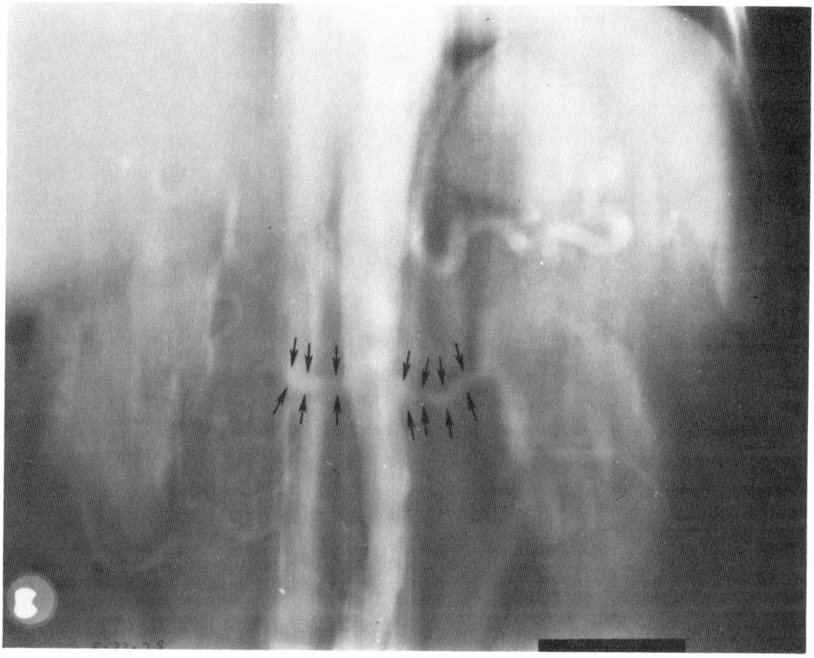

A

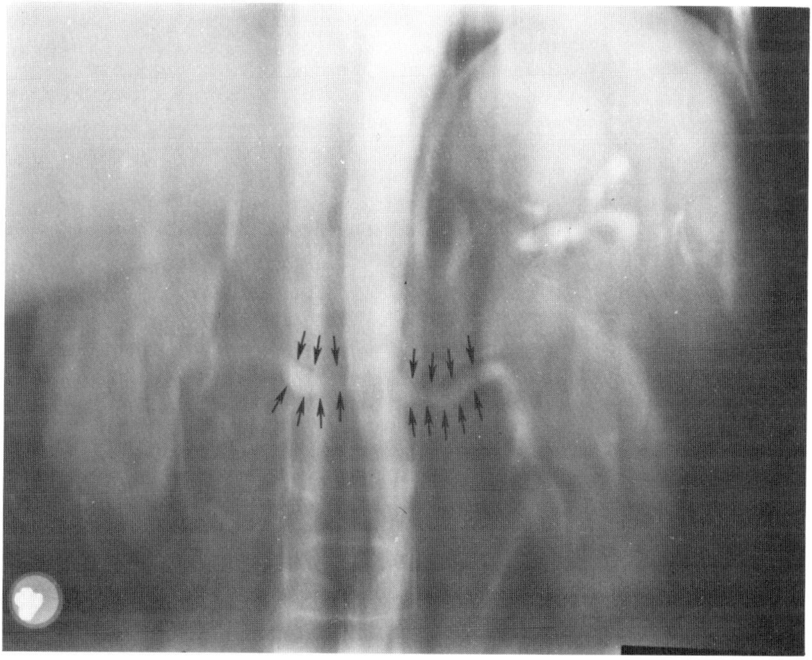

B

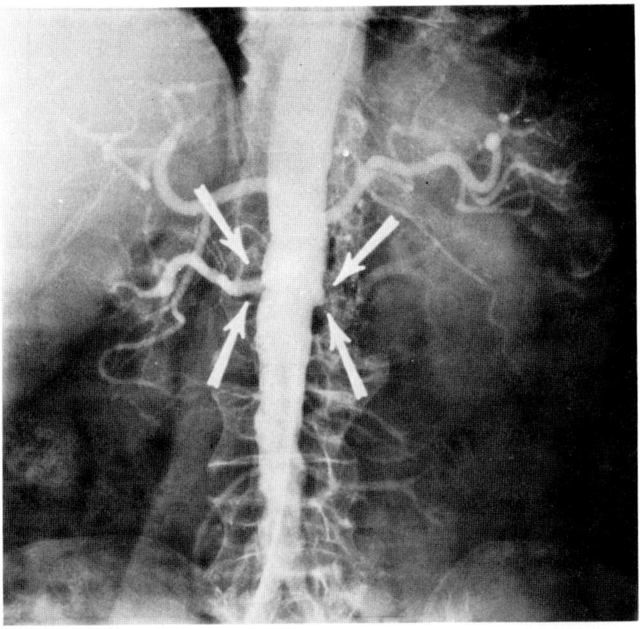

A

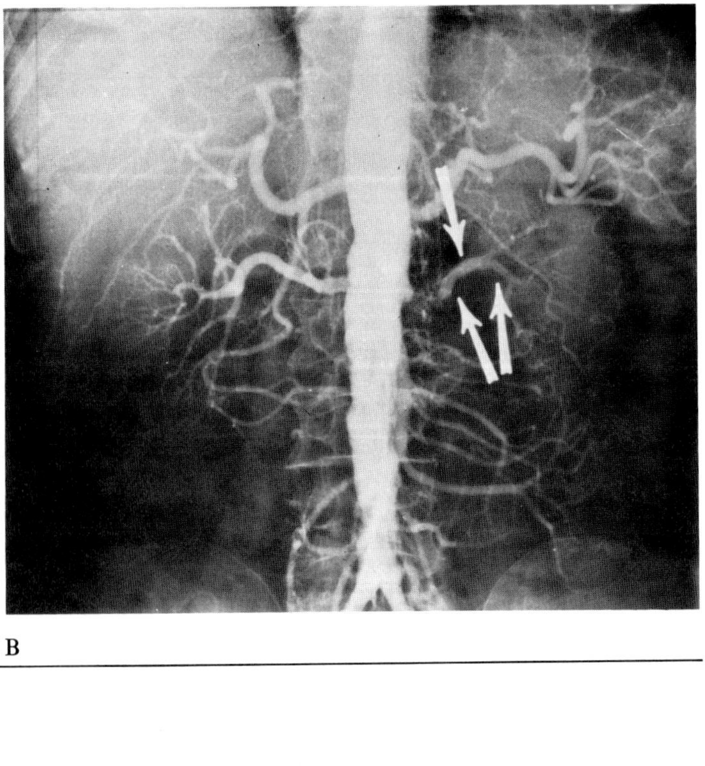

B

definitive ways of diagnosing renal ischemia than the urogram. In the 1950s renal angiography became available for diagnostic purposes in evaluating hypertension. Initially, the contrast medium was injected into the abdominal aorta by inserting the needle through the posterior lumbar approach. This method was supplanted by the transfemoral technique [58], which has the obvious advantage of allowing selective injection of contrast medium into individual visceral arteries through the manipulation of a flexible intra-aortic catheter. The selective technique reduced the confusing background vessel opacification seen with the midstream aortic injections. Unfortunately, these angiographic procedures are not without risk, as evidenced by the occurrence of iatrogenic arterial dissections [73] and renal failure [50]. The renal artery lesions that cause reduced renal blood flow can be divided into two categories, which have significant diagnostic angiographic characteristics. The atheromatous stenoses almost always begin in the aorta and extend into the proximal one-third of the main renal artery. In contrast, fibromuscular lesions almost always involve only the distal two-thirds of the main renal artery and extend into the branches, and they are seldom associated with obstructive aortic disease. Renal artery aneurysm and dissections complicate this form of renal artery stenosis [26].

Figure 10–4A is a midstream abdominal aortogram in a patient with bilateral atheromatous renal artery stenosis. It is an early film in the series and shows a moderate degree of stenosis on the right and nearly complete occlusion of the left main renal artery. Both lesions are indicated by arrows. Figure 10–4B is a subsequent film in the series from the same patient. The left renal artery can now be seen filling in a delayed fashion. The left kidney was found to be nonfunctioning by excretory urography.

Figures 10–5A and 10–5B are right and left selective renal angiograms in a patient with bilateral fibromuscular renal artery stenosis. The arrows point to the typical beaded fibromuscular disease, which is more severe on the right. As mentioned earlier, the disease affects the middle and distal two-thirds of the renal arteries and may extend into the early branches. Figure 10–5C is from the same patient as seen in Figures 10–5A and 10–5B, although it is a delayed film in the series. The arrows point to extensive collateral arteries arising from the lumbar and ureteral circulation, a common finding in severe renal artery stenosis.

Figure 10–6 is a study from another patient and was performed using the selective right renal artery catheterization technique. There is a medium-sized

---

Figure 10–4
(A) The contrast medium has been injected through a catheter lying in the lumen of the aorta. There is a severe stenosis and nearly complete obstruction of the left main renal artery. Mild atherosclerotic disease partially obstructs the right main renal artery. (B) A later film in the same series now showing delayed filling of the distal left renal artery, possibly through collaterals or merely slow flow through a 99 percent stenosis in the proximal portion of the left main renal artery.

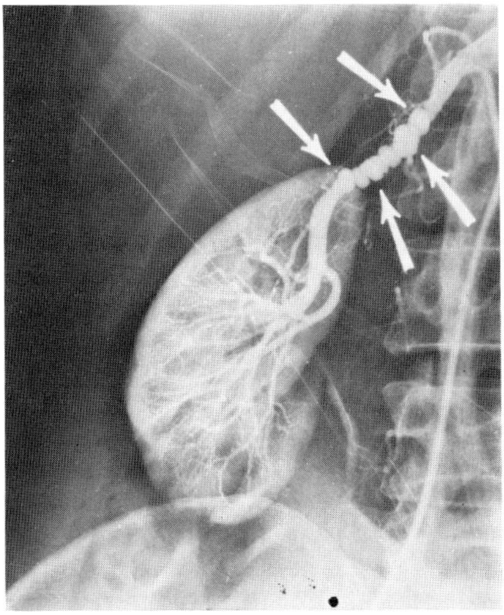

A

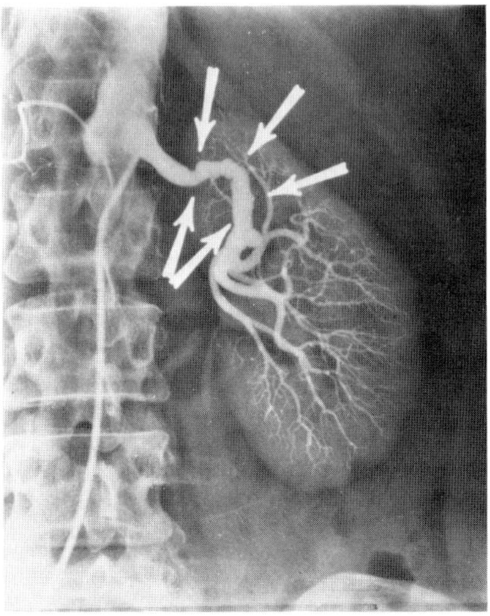

B

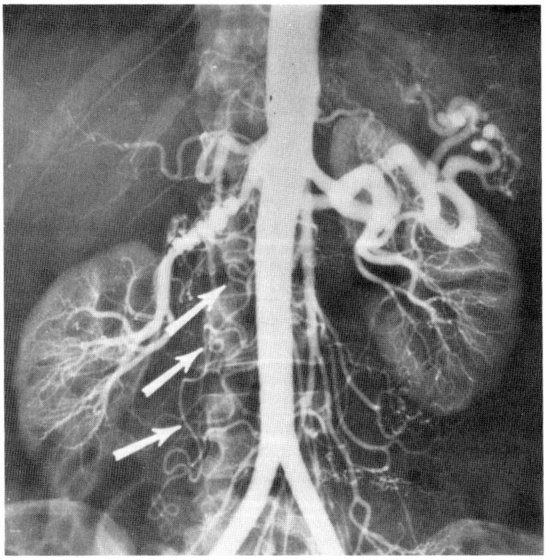

C

Figure 10–5
(A, B) The contrast medium has been injected into the right and left main renal arteries through a selective catheter. These films show the typical alternating beads and webs of fibromuscular renal artery stenosis, which begins in the middle and distal thirds of both main renal arteries and on the left appears to extend into the early branches. (C) A midstream injection from the same patient shown in Figures 10–5A and 10–5B. Note the tortuous collaterals highlighted by the arrows. Vessels such as these may be responsible for the ureteral notching seen by urography.

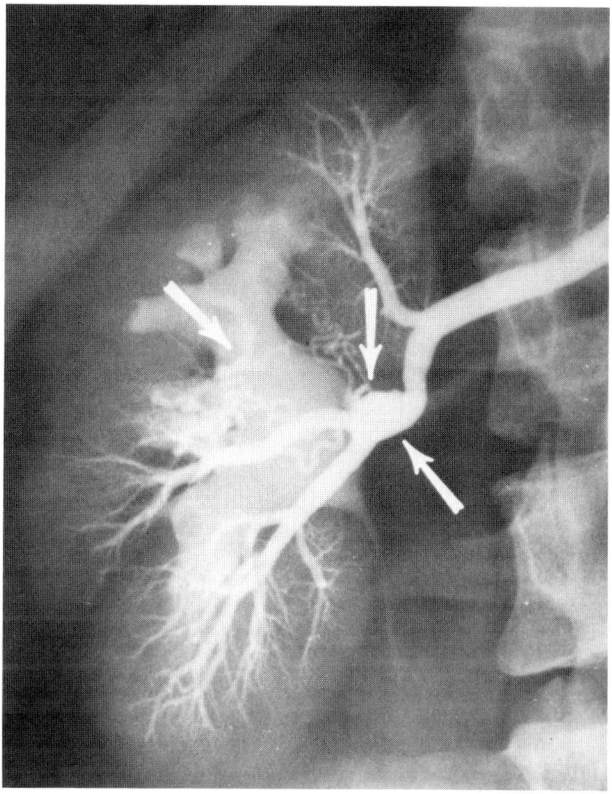

Figure 10–6
Selective right renal artery study showing a medium-sized aneurysm of the main renal artery just beyond the first branching point. There is occlusion of an intrarenal branch vessel arising from this aneurysm, with filling of the continuation of the occluded vessel by intrarenal collaterals.

noncalcified aneurysm at the second branching point. Arrows point to occlusion of the proximal portion of a branch arising from this aneurysm, with the distal continuation of the occluded vessel filling by intrarenal collaterals. This condition is probably congenital fibromuscular dysplasia, first diagnosed in this boy at age 14. Since nephrectomy would have been the only possible surgical procedure, it was elected to control his blood pressure with medication.

Much less common disorders producing stenosis of the renal arteries are the fibromuscular varieties which consist of a single discrete narrowing or a long, smooth constriction. The extrinsic compressing lesions are even less common than the atherosclerotic and fibromuscular types and may produce obstruction by tumor, fibrous bands, surgical ligatures, or crura of the diaphragm [26, 36, 63].

A number of other renal artery lesions are associated with hypertension; they include macroaneurysm without dissection [42, 45, 68], aortic dissection [59], traumatic renal artery occlusion [54, 57, 66], arteriovenous fistula [37], and embolic renal artery occlusion [16]. These conditions are interesting but rare, making them less relevant than the more common atherosclerotic or fibromuscular types.

The presence of renal artery stenosis does not necessarily imply that there is an etiologic relation between this condition and coexistent hypertension. Many such lesions are even found in normotensive patients [28, 39, 47]. However, significant hemodynamic interference is almost always caused by those lesions with greater than 75 percent stenosis on visual estimate, and seldom when stenosis is judged to be less than 25 percent [19]. Studies that characterize the lesions causing significant interruption of renal perfusion are of great importance, because those patients will most often benefit from surgical renal artery repair. There may be little improvement in hypertension as a result of repairing nonsignificant renal artery stenotic lesions. A discussion of test procedures relating to the determination of hemodynamic significance of renal artery stenotic lesions follows in the next section.

Plasma Renin Activity

Most investigators assume that the pathophysiology of blood pressure elevation associated with hemodynamically significant renal artery stenosis has at least initial relationship to increased renin release by the renal juxtaglomerular cells [7, 24, 38]. When peripheral venous plasma renin activity measurements became generally available clinically, there was an initial feeling of enthusiasm that this test could be used as a screening procedure for detection of renovascular hypertension or as a procedure for predicting blood pressure response to surgical renal artery repair or nephrectomy. Presumably, those patients with elevated plasma renin activities would have renovascular hypertension. This assumption has not enjoyed universal support from subsequent reports, however [1, 3, 12, 24, 31]. Many patients with surgically curable renovascular hypertension had normal peripheral renin activity, whereas others with essential hypertension had high values [9]. These findings make the measurement of peripheral venous renin activity of questionable value as a screening test for renovascular hypertension in populations with largely essential forms or as a predicting factor regarding the operative results for patients with angiographic evidence of renal artery stenosis.

One procedure for evaluating the peripheral venous plasma renin activity is to compare it with the 24-hour urinary excretion of sodium. This procedure must be performed in patients who have not taken diuretics for at least two weeks and who are not taking other renin-suppressing antihypertensive medications such as alpha-methyldopa (Aldomet) or propranolol (Inderal). The rationale behind this procedure is that the ambient plasma renin activity varies in an inverse way to the dietary sodium intake: the higher the dietary sodium

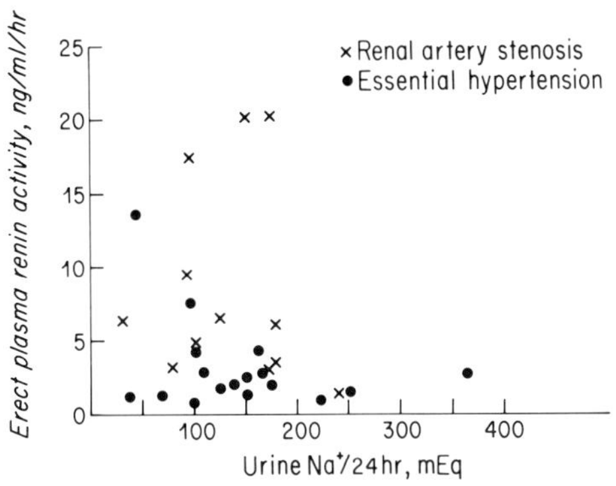

Figure 10–7
The 24-hour urine sodium excretion plotted against a normal sodium plasma renin activity measured in 28 hypertensive patients. The x's represent 11 patients with renovascular hypertension; the closed circles represent 17 with the essential form. There does not appear to be a clear delineation between the renin sodium index of those with renovascular hypertension and that of patients with the essential form.

intake, the lower the plasma renin activity, and vice versa. This renin-sodium index figure would tend to suggest the presence of renin-dependent hypertension if the data point generated by the individual patient lies above the points for normotensive persons or patients with essential hypertension. Figure 10–7 presents unpublished data from a recent series of essential and renovascular hypertensive patients. The closed circles represent patients with essential hypertension; the x's represent those with renovascular hypertension. Although many of the x's are above the points for those with essential hypertension, there is a considerable amount of overlap. We have concluded that the renin-sodium index is of value for detecting either high renin essential hypertension or renovascular hypertension but does not distinguish between the two.

Separated Ureteral Catheterization

Once renal artery stenosis has been found on the renal arteriogram, the question of whether or not this stenotic lesion is causing hypertension must be answered. As mentioned previously, there are many patients who have renal artery stenosis and normal blood pressure [28]. The converse is also true, that is, patients with essential hypertension may have renal artery narrowing that is not necessarily related to their hypertension. Finally, others with essential hypertension may develop atherosclerotic renal artery stenosis after a number of years, at which time their hypertension may become more severe.

For the purpose of relating stenosis to hypertension, a variety of functional tests have been devised, including the separated ureteral catheterization tests of Connor [13] and Stamey [67]. Although these procedures have excellent correlation with surgical results and have the advantage of providing separated measurements of renal plasma flow and glomerular filtration rate [30], they are lengthy and usually require a spinal anesthetic. In addition, there is some associated morbidity due to the postspinal headache as well as ureteral obstruction from postcatheterization edema or blood clot. The split renal function tests are no longer performed very often.

We measured the inulin clearance, urine volume, urine sodium concentration, and urine osmolality from each kidney as well as serum sodium and osmolality. The following calculations were then performed: Divide the minute urine volume from each kidney by its individual inulin clearance in milliliters per minute; subtract this result from unity and multiply it by 100. The formula for calculation of the percent renal tubular absorption of filtered water ($\% TR_{H_2O}$) utilizes the minute urine volume and the inulin clearance:

$$\text{Percent } TR_{H_2O} = \left(1 - \frac{\text{Urine volume (ml/min)}}{\text{Inulin clearance (ml/min)}}\right) \times 100$$

A kidney supplied by a significantly narrowed artery will reabsorb water more avidly than a kidney with normal circulation. We compare the values from the ipsilateral and contralateral kidneys when unilateral renal artery stenosis is present; a 1 percent or greater value for $\% TR_{H_2O}$ on the stenotic side suggests that its renal artery lesion is probably causing the hypertension.

The tubular reabsorption of filtered sodium (TR_{Na}) is calculated by dividing the inulin clearance into the sodium clearance and subtracting this result from unity. Multiplication of this result by 100 provides the $\% TR_{Na}$. A significant renal artery stenotic lesion would enhance TR_{Na} by 1 percent or greater over the nonstenotic kidney. Calculation of the percent renal tubular reabsorption of filtered sodium ($\% TR_{Na}$) utilizes the renal clearance of sodium and inulin according to the formula

$$\text{Percent } TR_{Na} = \left(1 - \frac{\text{Sodium clearance (ml/min)}}{\text{Inulin clearance (ml/min)}}\right) \times 100$$

Additional measurements indicating unilateral renal artery stenosis as a cause for hypertension would be a 15-percent or greater decrease in urine sodium concentration, a 50-percent or greater reduction in urine volume, and an increased osmolality on the stenotic side when compared with the nonstenosed kidney urine [30].

Renal Venous Renin Measurements

In the early 1960s, Boucher and colleagues devised an accurate bioassay for measuring plasma renin activity [5]. It was first used to measure peripheral venous renin activity, as mentioned earlier. Soon, Judson and Helmer were to report the measurement of renin activity in samples of blood drawn directly from the separate renal veins via a transfemoral venous catheter [34]. Strong [71], among others, suggested that the sensitivity of the test could be enhanced by preliminary acute sodium depletion with diuretic drugs and a low-sodium diet. This technique requires the patient to avoid taking diuretic and renin-suppressing drugs for approximately one month prior to the test. After this preparation, the patient ingests a 20 mEq sodium, 90 mEq potassium diet in a hospital nutrition center for three days while taking 500 mg of chlorothiazide (Diuril) twice daily. On the fourth day, renal venous and inferior vena cava renin samples are obtained. Pretreating the patient with a small dose of atropine prevents the vasovagal-induced acute blood pressure drop associated with manipulations of the inferior vena cava catheter. Using this technique, when the renal venous renin activity was increased by 50 percent in the venous effluent from the stenosed side (ratio 1.5 : 1 or greater) there was an 80 percent correlation with surgical relief of hypertension. This correlation was significantly better in patients undergoing sodium and water diuresis than in a similar group who had renal venous renin measurements under "normal sodium" circumstances.

Other techniques for inducing acute sodium depletion using drugs such as furosemide, with or without dietary sodium restriction, have not proved to be as accurate as the three-day chlorothiazide and 20 mEq sodium diet technique. Marks and co-workers [41] reviewed their own data and those from more than 400 patients reported in the literature. When the renal venous renin ratio was 1.5 : 1 or greater, there was an 88 percent possibility that there would be surgical cure or improvement by vascular repair or nephrectomy. However, there was still an overall cure or improvement rate of 80 percent when the patients were selected by arteriographic features alone. This result would suggest that increasing expertise in the interpretation of renal artery angiographic procedures may obviate the necessity for separated renal functional measurements or renal venous renin assays. Our recent data would support this hypothesis [76].

In summary, the renal venous renin ratio is an excellent test for predicting when cure or improvement of hypertension by repair of renal artery stenosis is possible. If nonlateralizing renal venous renins are found, the physician should not necessarily decide against surgical repair when the stenosis is visually severe and when hypertension is difficult to control with conventional medical programs. In such instances, the expectation for surgical cure might not be as optimistic, but it is still possible. Acute sodium depletion with the goal of about 2.5 to 3 percent of body weight loss may significantly enhance the sensitivity of this test. A ratio of 1.5 : 1 or greater in the differential renal venous activity is regarded as a positive result by most practitioners [71].

Angiotensin Blockade

In accordance with the continuing search for a diagnostic screening tool that would identify those patients having hemodynamically significant renal artery stenosis as a cause for their hypertension, investigators began to study synthetic analogues of the pressor substance, angiotensin II. They hoped to find a formulation that could attach to the vascular smooth muscle receptors commonly occupied by angiotensin II but would not trigger the adenyl cyclase system sufficiently to provoke vascular smooth muscle contraction [55, 56]. The production of these analogues was vastly implemented by the solid-phase peptide synthesis technique of Merrifield reported in 1963 [44]. One of the first useful angiotensin II analogues had only two amino acid alterations in the eight amino acid sequence of the natural hormone [35]. In this compound isoleucine was substituted for valine in the fifth position, and alanine replaced phenylalanine in the eighth or C terminal position. This analogue would competitively inhibit the vascular smooth muscle contraction response to angiotensin II. Another analogue, with sarcosine replacing aspartate in the first or N terminal position and alanine in place of phenylalanine in the eighth position, was reported by Pals [49]. This compound, 1-sarcosine, 8-alanine, angiotensin II (P-113, saralasin), was found to have similar but more effective blocking activity than the other peptide analogues of angiotensin II. It has a short half-life, approximately 5 to 10 minutes, and some true agonist as well as antagonist properties of angiotensin II. Another analogue with roughly similar properties, but which was longer acting, used sarcosine for substitution in the first position and isoleucine in the eighth position [72]. The amino acid sequence of natural angiotensin II and both of the analogues are depicted as follows. The first peptide is natural angiotensin II, with aspartine in the first and phenylalanine in the eighth position. Just below this is saralasin, in which sarcosine is substituted for aspartine in the first position and alanine for phenylalanine in the eighth position. Below this is the amino acid sequence of yet another analogue, in which sarcosine is once again substituted for aspartine in the first position but isoleucine occupies the eighth position. This analogue has properties similar to saralasin but is much longer acting.

Angiotensin II
Aspartine^{1}-arginine-valine-tyrosine-isoleucine-histidine-proline-*phenylalanine*^{8}

Sar^{1}, *ala*^{8}-*Angiotensin II (P-113, Saralasin)*
Sarcosine^{1}-arginine-valine-tyrosine-isoleucine-histidine-*alanine*^{8}

Sar^{1}, *1le*^{8}-*Angiotensin II*
Sarcosine^{1}-arginine-valine-tyrosine-isoleucine-histidine-proline-*isoleucine*^{8}

Both analogues will reverse the in vitro vascular smooth muscle contraction produced by angiotensin II but not by norepinephrine [48, 72]. The analogues will normalize blood pressure in animals made acutely hypertensive either by unilateral renal ischemia (with the contralateral ureter ligated) or by angiotensin II infusions.

In 1973 the first studies in humans were reported, using the sarcosine-1, alanine-8, peptide analogue of angiotensin II (saralasin) [8, 11, 40, 53, 69, 70]. Patients with renovascular hypertension or high-renin essential hypertension tended to have significant reductions in blood pressure during the infusion of saralasin. Sodium depletion prior to the study is necessary to allow the depressor effect to occur. Most investigators concluded that the blood pressure reduction caused by blockade of angiotensin II was strong proof for the existence of renin-dependent hypertension.

One protocol used in testing for angiotensin II-dependent hypertension with saralasin includes the avoidance of all antihypertensive drugs for one week and no diuretics for as least two weeks prior to the test. Guanethidine may be used in the interval for maintenance of blood pressure control. At 7:00 P.M. on the evening before the test, the patient ingests 80 mg of furosemide (Lasix) and weighs himself. The next morning he again weighs himself under similar conditions and records the difference as a percent weight change; usually this loss is between 2 and 4 percent. After approximately 30 minutes in the supine resting position, during which time basal blood pressures are measured every 2 minutes, the patient receives 18 mg of saralasin solution injected into the flashball of an intravenous tubing carrying a 5% dextrose and water solution over a 30-minute period. There is usually a transient elevation in blood pressure during the first 2 or 3 minutes of the infusion. The degree of blood pressure alteration produced by saralasin is calculated by taking the four lowest sequential diastolic blood pressures occurring during the infusion and calculating the mean. This value is then compared with the mean of the last four diastolic blood pressures measured just prior to the institution of the infusion. The formula used for calculation of the percent change of diastolic blood pressure in response to saralasin (%ΔDBP) follows. A positive (depressor) response is an 8 percent or greater reduction in diastolic blood pressure.

$$\text{Percent } \Delta\text{DBP} = \frac{\text{Postinfusion diastolic} - \text{preinfusion diastolic}}{\text{Preinfusion diastolic}}$$

A cooperative study group has investigated the effectiveness of saralasin in identifying patients with renovascular hypertension [29]. They found that when the ambient peripheral venous plasma renin activity was greater than 13 ng/ml/hour and there was greater than 80 percent stenosis of a renal artery noted on the angiogram, 36 of 38 patients (95 percent) had a depressor response to the saralasin infusion. There were 87 patients diagnosed by the investigators as having severe renovascular hypertension by renal angiography alone; only 55 of these patients had a depressor response (63 percent). Of the 150 patients diagnosed as having essential hypertension, 22 had a depressor response (14.6 percent). In a general way, the saralasin response was more often positive (depressor) in those patients having high renin and neutral, or true pressor, than in those with normal or low renin activity. More than 342 patients with blood pressures over 150/100 were included in this study.

Figure 10–8 shows a depressor saralasin response in a patient with severe unilateral renal artery stenosis. During the infusion of saralasin, there was a significant drop in systolic and diastolic blood pressure followed by a return

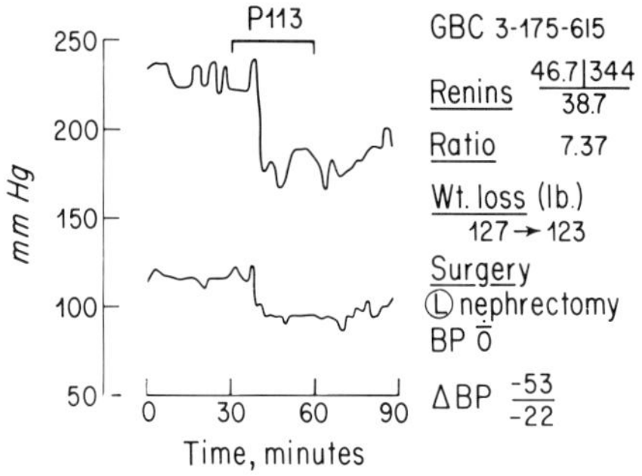

Figure 10–8
Saralasin infusion test. This patient received 18 mg of saralasin using the slow infusion technique over a 30-minute period. There is a transient increase in the systolic and diastolic blood pressure just after the initiation of the infusion, followed by a significant and sustained reduction in both parameters during the rest of the study. On termination of the infusion, the systolic and diastolic blood pressure began to return toward preinfusion values. There was a 22 mm Hg diastolic blood pressure reduction produced by the infusion (−18%). The patient subsequently underwent left nephrectomy for severe left renal artery stenosis with left renal atrophy and was normotensive after the operation without medication.

toward the preinfusion level at the termination of the infusion. This patient subsequently underwent a nephrectomy and six months after the operation had normal blood pressure without any antihypertensive drug therapy.

The saralasin infusion test does have a significantly high percentage of false-negative results in patients with renovascular hypertension (about 37 percent) to make its value as a screening procedure limited. However, performing the infusion with the patient in the seated rather than the supine position may enhance the sensitivity of this test. Studies are in progress at the present time to test this hypothesis.

Surgical Therapy for Renovascular Hypertension

Once the physician has angiographic and functional data suggesting significant renal artery stenosis, he must decide whether to suggest surgical intervention or whether to continue with medical antihypertensive therapy. The following factors should be considered: the pain, danger, and expense of a major operation and the possibility of loss of functioning renal tissue, and on the other hand, the chance that hypertension may be completely or partially relieved with fewer drugs and fewer side effects [14].

If each patient is selected for a renal angiogram only if he is a candidate for surgery, the decision-making process is easier. When a significant renal artery stenotic lesion is found, preexisting medical problems, especially atherosclerotic events such as myocardial infarction and stroke, prejudice the patient's chances of having a good surgical result [20, 43, 60] and of surviving the procedure. In one cooperative study of renovascular hypertension in which nearly 600 operative procedures were reported, 34 patients died (6.8 percent) [20]. Four-fifths of the deaths were in the group of patients with atherosclerotic renal artery stenosis, but this group comprised only three-fifths of the total patients undergoing operation. Stated in another way, the mortality rate was 9.3 percent for the atherosclerotic group and only 3.4 percent for those with fibromuscular disease. An especially worrisome combination was angina pectoris and reduced GFR (defined as a serum creatinine concentration equal to or greater than 1.4 mg/dl) in the same patient.

The risk of losing renal mass is likewise significant when the patient has surgical therapy; this may be the case when nephrectomy is elected rather than renal artery repair. Nephrectomy is sometimes necessary when complete renal infarction has occurred or when the renal pole-to-pole diameter is less than 9 cm in the kidney with the narrowed renal artery. The gross incidence of nephrectomy varies from series to series but ranges from 16 percent [43] to as high as 35 percent [20]. Two-thirds of the nephrectomies were performed as an initial approach to unilateral disease, and one-third as an accompanying procedure to contralateral arterial repair. Less frequently, nephrectomy is a secondary operation when the initial graft has failed. The incidence of nephrectomy in patients with fibromuscular renal artery disease is somewhat lower than in patients with atherosclerotic stenoses [17].

Several surgical procedures have been devised for the repair or relief of renal artery narrowing. The technical aspects are not within the scope of this chapter and may be sought elsewhere if the reader is interested [51]. The results of these procedures are quite pertinent regarding the rate of cure or significant improvement. Success rates vary from series to series, as does the definition of the categories "cured" and "improved." Taking each author's results as stated, the number of patients cured of renovascular hypertension by surgery varies from 45 to 68 percent [17, 18, 32, 43]. When the "improved" category is added to those cured, the rate increases to 66 to 93 percent. Most of the available data suggest that patients under the age of 40 with fibromuscular disease are more likely to benefit from surgical repair of the renal artery lesion than their older counterparts with atherosclerotic renal artery lesions [51]. Counterbalancing the operative mortality rates, the risk of nephrectomy, and the significant incidence of improvement or failure rather than cure is the apparent incidence of reduced survival in those patients with renovascular hypertension who were treated medically rather than surgically. In one series of patients followed from seven to fourteen years [32], those with surgical correction of renal artery stenosis had an 84 percent survival rate as compared to only 60 percent for those treated medically. Therein lies the dilemma: Surgical intervention has its problems, but nonsurgical treatment may adversely prejudice the patient's survival. There is no simple solution, and all too often the physician must make decisions when there is really no ideal answer.

Pheochromocytoma

Catecholamine-producing tumors of neuroectodermal embryological origin may arise in the adrenal medulla (typical pheochromocytoma), the carotid body (chemodectoma), the thoracolumbar sympathetic chain (ganglioneuroma), the region of the abdominal aorta just below the inferior mesenteric artery (organ of Zuckerkandl), or in various other regions in the chest or abdomen near the branches of the aorta (paragangliomas) [52]. These tumors may occur in association with von Recklinghausen's neurofibromatosis or Lindau-von Hippel disease (congenital retinal and cerebellar angiomas; cysts of pancreas, kidney, and other viscera) and Sipple's syndrome (bilateral adrenal pheochromocytoma, parathyroid adenoma, and medullary thyroid carcinoma with amyloid). Each year about 10 or 12 of these tumors are surgically removed at the Mayo Clinic from more than 26,000 patients with hypertension (0.05 percent). Most are benign (87 percent), some bilateral adrenal (4.8 percent), and a few located in extra-adrenal sites (10 percent) [52, 75].

Clinical clues to the presence of a catecholamine-secreting pheochromocytoma or other neuroectodermal tumor include episodic hypertension (42 percent) and some type of "spell" in more than half of the patients [62]. These spells are frequently characterized by the "four P's": pain in the head, palpitations, pallor, and perspiration. The attacks may be brief or prolonged. Bizarre behavior on the part of the patient may lead to psychiatric evaluation. One of our recent patients had a fever as her only symptom, which was cured by the resection of a chemodectoma. She was never found to be hypertensive preoperatively (unreported case). Cardiac arrhythmia or intracerebral hemorrhage during the acute release of catecholamines may lead to sudden death in these patients.

Diagnosis of a pheochromocytoma, paraganglioma, or ganglioneuroma that secretes excess catecholamines is made primarily by finding increased concentrations of epinephrine or norepinephrine, or both, in the plasma or increased amounts of these substances and their metabolites in the urine [61]. In the patient with episodic release of catecholamines, plasma and urine samples are most diagnostic during and just following the attacks. These values are elevated almost constantly in patients with sustained hypertension and pheochromocytoma.

Commonly measured metabolites of catecholamines in the urine are total metanephrines [metanephrines (MN) plus normetanephrines (NMN)], vanillylmandelic acid (VMA), and homovanillic acid (HVA). The chemical structure of these catecholamines and metabolites are shown in Figure 10–9. Dopamine, a precursor of norepinephrine, epinephrine, and homovanillic acid, is sometimes produced in excess quantities by the neuroblastomas of children and can be converted directly into homovanillic acid [23].

Substances that interfere with the analysis of metanephrines and produce a falsely low or normal result in patients with pheochromocytoma are x-ray con-

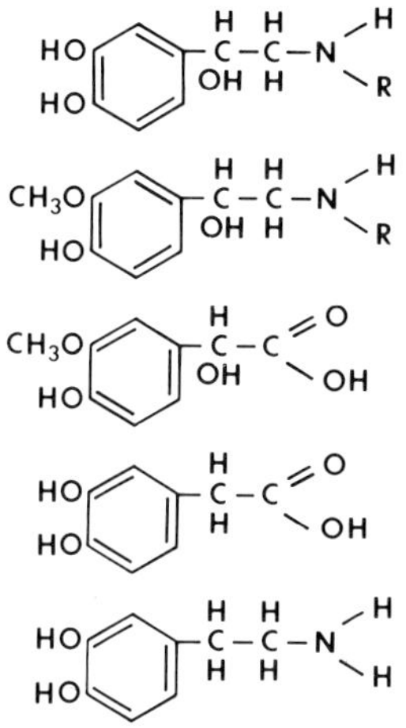

Norepinephrine R = H (NE)
Epinephrine R = CH_3 (E)

Normetanephrine R = H (NMN)
Metanephrine R = CH_3 (MN)

Vanillylmandelic acid (VMA)

Homovanillic acid (HVA)

Dopamine (precursor of NE, E and HVA)

Figure 10–9
Chemical configuration of catecholamines and metabolites.

trast media of the meglumine diatrizoate type used for excretory urograms and renal angiography. The 24-hour urine collection for metanephrines should be done before any of these procedures, or more than five days afterward. Sympathomimetic amines, monoamine oxidase inhibitors, and various nasal decongestants will raise the metanephrine excretion falsely. Alpha-methyldopa (Aldomet) will produce an abnormal spectral curve for the metanephrines, although in the non-pheochromocytoma patient the total will often be within normal limits. In this instance, the test need not be repeated unless the total metanephrine value is greater than the upper limit of normal. There was only a 4 percent incidence of false-negative urinary metanephrine excretion tests in patients with pheochromocytomas in one large series [52].

In pheochromocytoma patients, VMA analysis in a 24-hour urine collection has about a 29 percent incidence of false negatives. The level of VMA can be falsely raised by a wide variety of foods and drugs, including aspirin, monoamine oxidase inhibitors, nasal decongestants, and bronchodilators. The 24-hour HVA has a far greater incidence of false negatives than the metanephrines or VMA, but this measurement may be of value in patients whose tumors are producing excessive dopamine and metabolizing it directly to HVA within the tumor [23].

Fractionation of urinary catecholamines into norepinephrine and epinephrine may be useful because pheochromocytomas in adrenal medullary sites tend to produce excessive epinephrine, whereas those in extra-adrenal sites sel-

Table 10–1. Normal Ranges for 24-Hour Urinary Excretion of Catecholamines and Their Metabolites

Substance	Normal Range
Metanephrines	< 1.3 mg/24 hr
VMA	< 5.0 mg/24 hr
HVA	< 8.0 mg/24 hr
Catecholamines	< 250 μg/24 hr
Norepinephrine	15–80 μg/24 hr
Epinephrine	< 20 μg/24 hr
Dopamine	65–400 μg/24 hr

dom do and tend to produce norepinephrine. A surgeon might be guided in his search for the tumor by this information.

Normal values for plasma catecholamines and 24-hour urine metanephrines, VMA, HVA, epinephrine, norepinephrine, and dopamine are given in Table 10–1.

Pharmacological Tests for Pheochromocytoma

Provocative tests for pheochromocytoma are indicated in patients with spells or unsustained hypertension who have already had normal measurements of the 24-hour urinary metanephrines or VMA, or both. The rationale behind this group of pharmacological tests is the ability of certain drugs to provoke the sudden release of stored catecholamines from sympathetic nerve terminals in patients with excess production (i.e., pheochromocytoma). Drugs that provoke this response are histamine, 15 to 25 μg [60]; tyramine, 1 mg [15]; and glucagon, 1 mg [61]. The last two agents seldom produce any abnormal sensations in the patient without pheochromocytoma and are preferred by some. However, histamine has stood the test of time and seems to have the best record of diagnostic reliability, even though it produces flushing, headaches, and occasional bronchospasm.

Provocative tests for pheochromocytoma are performed with the following protocol: With the patient at rest in a quiet room and blood pressure stable for 15 to 30 minutes, immerse one of the patient's hands in ice and water slush for 60 seconds (the usual limit of tolerance) and measure the blood pressure at 30-second intervals during and 2 or 3 minutes after the immersion (this procedure is used in the histamine test only to provide a guide for evaluating the nonspecific blood pressure elevating effect of discomfort). When the blood pressure is again stable, inject rapidly 15 or 25 μg of histamine, 1 mg of glucagon, or 1 mg of tyramine intravenously. Measure the blood pressure every minute for the next 10 minutes. Draw blood samples for catecholamines at 2, 5, and 10 minutes after the injection. It may be necessary to use the antidote phentolamine (Regitine). If it is needed, inject 5 mg of phentolamine and repeat the injection as often as necessary to maintain the blood pressure at acceptable levels. This drug is an alpha-adrenergic blocker and will reverse an acute catecholamine-induced hypertensive crisis; it must always be available during any provocative pheochromocytoma test. A positive test consists of a systolic blood pressure rise of 15 percent or greater above the basal cold pressor elevation, and a significant rise in plasma catecholamines above the basal value.

The provocative test should be reserved for the patient who is normotensive but is suspected of harboring a pheochromocytoma or related catecholamine-producing tumor because of spells, documented hypertensive episodes in the past, or membership in a family with multiple endocrine neoplasia of type II with pheochromocytomas, hyperparathyroidism, and thyrocalcitonin-producing medullary thyroid cancers.

The Regitine test has little place in the diagnosis of pheochromocytoma today. The rationale behind this test was that hypertension caused by excessive alpha-adrenergic stimulation could be temporarily reversed by an intravenous injection of alpha-adrenergic blocking drugs such as Regitine. The test has been replaced by the 24-hour urine measurements of substances such as MN, NMN, or VMA.

Bolus Nephrotomography and Computed Tomographic Scanning

Large-dose intravenous x-ray contrast studies with tomographic cuts centered over the renal and suprarenal areas will often detect the adrenal, perirenal, and organ of Zuckerkandl pheochromocytoma or paraganglioma down to 2 or 3 cm in size. However, this technique does have risk of provoking the sudden release of catecholamines associated with hypertensive crisis. Ideally, the patient should be taking an adequate dose of oral alpha-adrenergic blocking drug such as phenoxybenzamine (Dibenzyline), 10 mg given twice daily for a day or two prior to the test, to prevent this crisis effect. Figure 10–10 shows a bolus nephrotomogram that identified a large paraganglioma located just below the lower pole of the left kidney (organ of Zuckerkandl). The tumor is outlined by arrows. The other anatomical structures are not in the same horizontal plane as the tumor and thus are out of focus. This tumor was not identified by the computed tomographic scan technique (described below) because the search with the latter method was limited to the suprarenal areas. The overall accuracy rate for the identification of adrenal tumors by bolus nephrotomography is listed as 67 percent in one large series [52].

Computed tomographic (CT) x-ray scanning supplies an additional technique for locating the elusive catecholamine-producing neuroectodermal tumors. Although most of these tumors are located in the conventional suprarenal areas, Remine and his colleagues [52] note that a significant number of the tumors are situated elsewhere throughout the abdomen. Of 138 tumors resected at the Mayo Clinic between 1926 and 1970, 14 were extra-adrenal. The most common extra-adrenal site was in the organ of Zuckerkandl. CT scanning of the abdomen became a frequently used diagnostic tool for the detection of pheo-

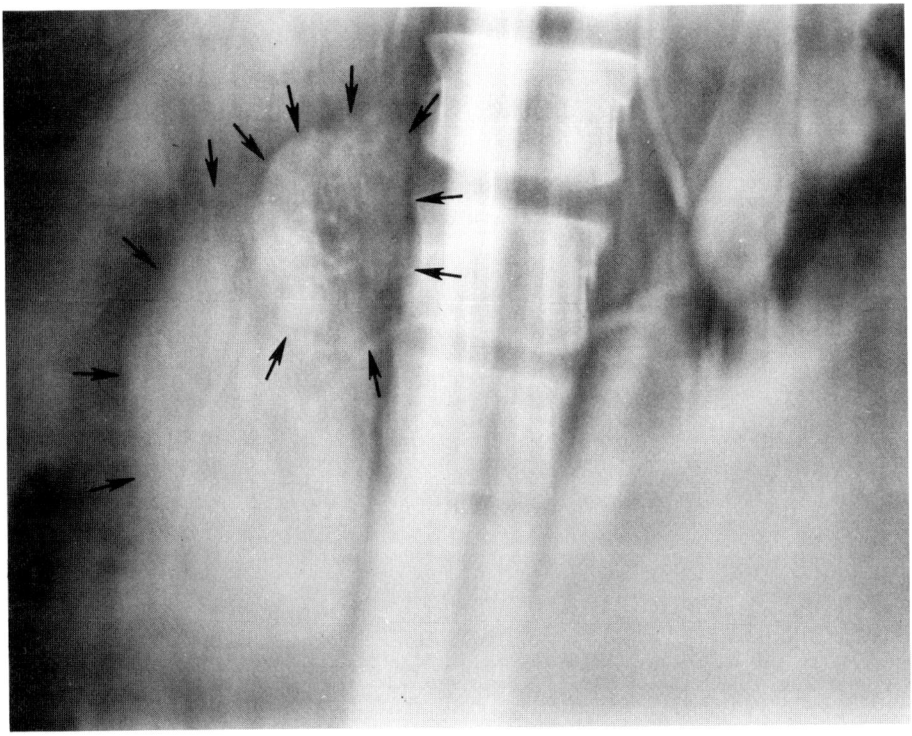

Figure 10–10
Intravenous bolus nephrotomogram in patient with hypertension and elevated catecholamine excretion in the urine. There is a vascular mass overlying the medial aspect of the lower pole of the left kidney in the region of the organ of Zuckerkandl. The other structures are not in the plane of focus in this tomogram. The tumor is outlined by arrows.

chromocytomas and paragangliomas in the latter part of 1976. In 1977, ten patients had pheochromocytomas removed at the Mayo Clinic. Eight patients had tumors located within the adrenal medulla. Seven of the eight underwent CT scanning of the abdomen, and in all seven the tumor was accurately identified and located. Intravenous bolus or routine urographic contrast studies were performed in five of the eight patients with adrenal pheochromocytomas, and in all five the tumor was likewise identified correctly.

Figure 10–11 shows an example of CT identification of a right adrenal pheochromocytoma. The patient's right-hand side is to the left of the page.

With increasing experience, we can now accurately locate nearly all catecholamine-secreting abdominal and thoracic masses with bolus nephrotomography or abdominal and chest CT scanning techniques, or both. This development is a welcome boon to the surgeon, tending to minimize blind searches throughout

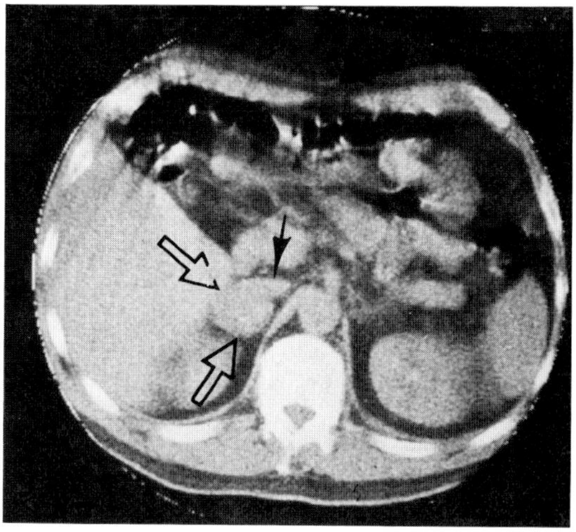

Figure 10–11
Functioning right adrenal pheochromocytoma, 3.2 cm in diameter. The tumor (*open black arrows*) is located anterior to the upper pole of the right kidney and is intimately associated with the posterior aspect of the elliptical inferior vena cava (*small black arrow*).

the abdominal recesses in search of these tumors. In the past, a negative surgical exploration usually prompted selective arteriography and venography, frequently combined with a series of plasma catecholamine assays from various locations throughout the inferior vena cava [27].

Primary Aldosteronism

The diagnosis of small adrenal cortical tumors is complicated by their size (ranging from 1.0 to 2.4 cm in the nine tumors removed at the Mayo Clinic in 1977) as well as by the variety of conditions that mimic the hypokalemia, hyperaldosteronemia, and hyperaldosteronuria associated with hypertension and suppressed plasma renin activity seen in the aldosterone-producing adenoma patient. The most common such confusing condition is bilateral diffuse or nodular adrenal hyperplasia. The aforementioned biochemical abnormalities also associated with the solitary aldosterone-producing adenoma (APA) tend to be less severe in bilateral adrenal hyperplasia. In patients with bilateral hyperplasia subtotal adrenalectomy, complete on one side and 50 percent on the other, will often correct these abnormalities. Unfortunately, many of them remain hypertensive after such surgery. Therefore, we are reluctant to suggest surgical intervention in these patients unless there is definite evidence to suggest the presence of a single APA. The laboratory and x-ray diagnostic procedures described in the following paragraphs are designed to characterize the presence of hyperaldosteronism and to locate the solitary APA tumor, if one is present. If a tumor is not located, we have little enthusiasm for blind surgical adrenal exploration and would prefer medical therapy instead, using aldosterone-blocking diuretics such as spironolactone (Aldactone). The dose is from 100 to 400 mg per day, which may require a large number of tablets since the generally available size is 25 mg per tablet.

In the hypertensive patient with hypokalemia, diuretic therapy should be discontinued completely and control of blood pressure should be maintained for the next several weeks with individually prescribed doses of a noninterfering antihypertensive drug such as guanethidine (Ismelin). The dose may vary from 25 to over 200 mg, given once daily. Therapy should be individually tailored to each patient, with the goal being identified as a standing systolic blood pressure just below 130 mm Hg. This drug is known to cause orthostatic and exercise hypotension as well as diarrhea and retrograde ejaculation; diarrhea can be controlled with diphenoxylate and atropine (Lomotil).

At the end of the two- or three-week guanethidine preparation period, the serum potassium concentration should be measured on two successive days. If this value is still less than 3.2 mEq/L, one should proceed with the measurement of peripheral venous plasma aldosterone and renin activity as well as the 24-hour urinary aldosterone excretion. Our normal ranges for plasma aldosterone concentration are 1 to 21 ng/dl, for peripheral venous renin activity 0.0 to 3.7 ng/ml/hour (erect, normal sodium diet), and for urine aldosterone excretion 2 to 16 μg/24 hours. In the same 24-hour urine specimen, the excretion of sodium should be measured to estimate dietary intake and that of potassium to document renal potassium wasting in the presence of hypokalemia. Measurements of 17-keto- and ketogenic steroids in the urine will detect the rare 17- and 21-hydroxylase deficiency found in congenital forms of mineralocorticoid excess.

At this point, it is best to defer further testing until all results are available for review. These tests are rather expensive and should not be ordered unless the indications for them are quite solid. If the plasma and urine aldosterone values exceed the normal range and the plasma renin activity is less than 1 ng/ml/hour, the physician is justified in pursuing the diagnosis of APA with further tests.

Our current practice would then suggest the measurement of the plasma aldosterone, corticosteroids, and renin activity on a blood sample drawn from the patient just prior to his arising from bed in the morning. This may require an overnight stay in the hospital (or a very accommodating venipuncture technician who will travel to the patient's home to draw the blood sample at this critical time). The patient then gets out of bed and remains ambulatory for 4 hours. The measurements are repeated at this time, generally at about 11:00 A.M. The rationale behind this test procedure is that patients with APA usually, but not always, have a reduction in the plasma aldosterone concentration after 4 hours of erect posture, or at least the values remain unchanged. In contrast, the patient with bilateral adrenal cortical hyperplasia with aldosteronism will increase the plasma aldosterone concentration after 4 hours of erect posture [4]. This information is of obvious use in helping the physician decide whether to explore the patient's adrenal areas surgically in search of the solitary tumor or to recommend medical therapy only.

Iodomethylcholesterol Adrenal Scanning

While the results of the plasma aldosterone and renin activities before and after erect posture are being analyzed, the I_{131} iodomethylcholesterol adrenal scan may be performed. This test requires the suppression of normal adrenal cortical function by dexamethasone for about three days prior to the injection of this material. The dose of dexamethasone is 0.5 mg twice daily for three days. On the third day the patient takes orally 10 to 15 drops of Lugol's iodine solution mixed in juice, which will suppress thyroid uptake of the iodine-containing isotope to be given the next day. On the fourth day, 2 mCi of I_{131} iodomethylcholesterol is injected intravenously, and adrenal scanning follows 24 and 48 hours later. Using this technique, we identified solitary APA tumors in eight of nine patients found to have this condition at surgery in 1977 (unpublished data). The rationale behind this technique is that a normal adrenal gland takes up very little of the iodomethylcholesterol isotope when ACTH is suppressed by dexamethasone. Any uptake of isotope under these conditions is suggestive of adrenal cortical hyperplasia (bilateral uptake) or a solitary tumor (unilateral uptake). An example of a solitary APA identified by isotope scanning is seen in Figure 10–12.

Computed Tomographic Adrenal Scanning

The technique of CT adrenal scanning began to enjoy increasing use for location of suprarenal adrenal cortical masses in the fall of 1976. In 1977, six of nine patients with APA tumors had CT scanning of the adrenal gland at the Mayo Clinic. The technique correctly located the presence of the tumor in each of the six patients. As mentioned above, the range in size of these tumors at the greatest diameter was from 1.0 to 2.4 cm (unpublished data). Figure 10–13 shows an example of a left adrenal APA seen by CT scan; note the slim normal right adrenal gland.

Data Analysis

At this point, the physician may have expended large amounts of diagnostic time (and money) in order to find a very rare tumor. If an APA is present, the amount of aldosterone in the urine should be elevated; the plasma renin activity should be low and should not increase significantly when the patient walks about for 4 hours; and finally, the elevated plasma aldosterone level should remain unchanged or decreased after 4 hours of erect posture. With bilateral adrenal cortical hyperplasia and hyperaldosteronism, the plasma aldosterone level should increase after 4 hours of erect posture.

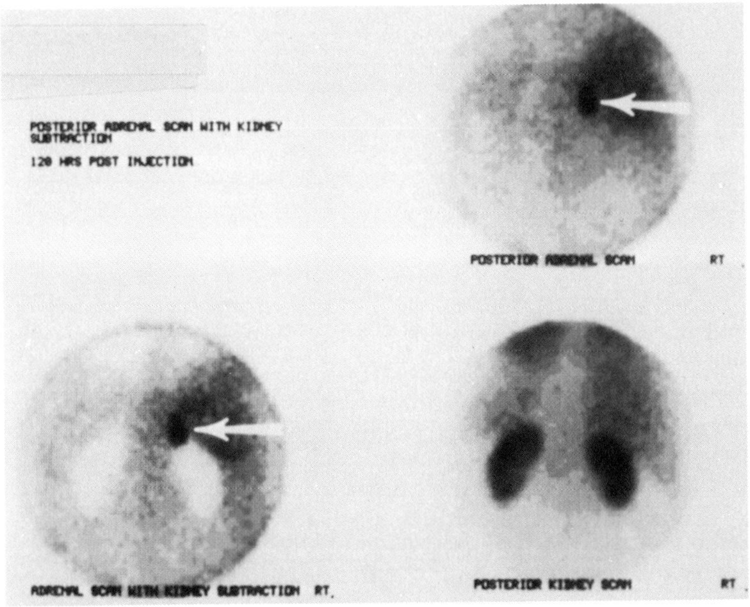

Figure 10–12
I_{131} iodomethylcholesterol adrenal scan. The top right-hand gamma camera scan is performed with the patient face down, and therefore his right is to the right of the page. The white arrow points to an area of radioisotope uptake in the region of the right adrenal gland. The right lower panel shows both kidneys having taken up an isotope of technetium. The lower left-hand scan shows residual radioactivity in the area of the right adrenal gland, with the kidney radioactivity having been subtracted electronically. This picture is consistent with a solitary functioning right adrenal adenoma.

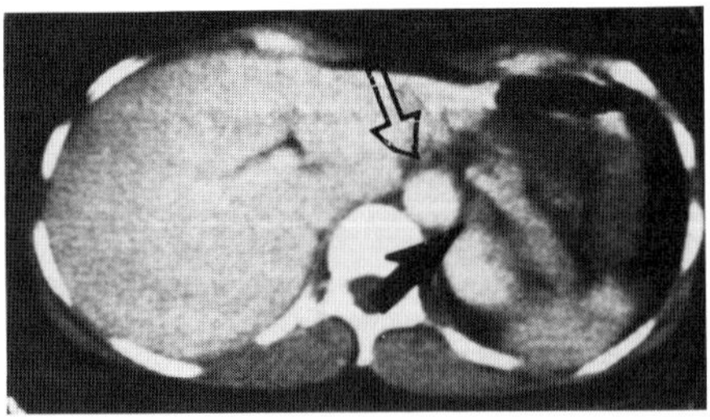

Figure 10–13
Left adrenal APA, 1.7 cm in diameter. This small tumor (*large black arrow*) is located in the triangle formed by the left lateral margin of the aorta (*open black arrow*), the posterior surface of the body of the pancreas, and the anterior surface of the upper pole of the left kidney.

If a discrete tumor is seen on the I_{131} iodomethylcholesterol adrenal scan or the CT adrenal scan and the biochemical and hormonal studies suggest that an APA is present, a surgeon should be called in. In addition, adequate doses of spironolactone and potassium chloride supplement should be prescribed to lower the blood pressure and increase the serum potassium levels to normal. If the data suggest bilateral adrenal cortical hyperplasia, a surgeon is not needed.

Since these tests are so expensive and the results difficult to analyze, the patient should be referred to a hypertension diagnostic center if the physician is not familiar with the techniques. One should proceed with the tests only if the patient's condition warrants and if he will accept surgery when a tumor is diagnosed. Finally, spironolactone medical therapy seems a better alternative to surgically induced adrenal cortical insufficiency.

Pseudohyperaldosteronism

A word is in order here about the perplexing set of conditions that produce abnormalities in many laboratory tests that mimic hyperaldosteronism if analyzed superficially. The common finding is hypokalemia, which may or may not be associated with significant blood pressure elevation. Surreptitious use of diuretics can confuse the diagnostician unless he suspects this and has access to a screening procedure that detects diuretics in the urine. Licorice glutting may also mimic hyperaldosteronism; however, these patients have a normal or low urinary aldosterone excretion and low plasma aldosterone concentration. They are hypertensive because the licorice contains a mineralocorticoid that is not detected by the urine or plasma assays for aldosterone. Similar abnormalities might occur in a patient taking fludrocortisone acetate (Florinef), a synthetic mineralocorticoid that is not detected by either plasma or urine assays for aldosterone.

Another patient in this category is the one who habitually vomits. This unusual habit results in a hydrochloric acid loss and can produce a severe degree of hypochloremic alkalosis. Hypokalemia occurs not as a result of gastric losses of potassium but as a result of potassium shifts from the extracellular to the intracellular fluid. Extracellular volume decreases from self-emesis does stimulate renal renin release, increase angiotensin II generation, and subsequent secondary hyperaldosteronism. These patients are normotensive or hypotensive, and for reasons that are not clear, they waste potassium in the urine when renal function appears normal and the serum potassium is quite low. The diagnostic clue in this situation is the lack of hypertension and the severe degree of hypokalemia and alkalosis in a patient without mental or growth retardation. Bartter's syndrome, a disorder that does include mental retardation and short stature, will be discussed later in this chapter. The differentiation between these two conditions can be quite difficult, if not impossible; this is especially true if the patient will not confide in the physician that he or she is regularly self-regurgitating. One test suggested by Dr. John Gill of the National Institutes of Health for differentiating the two conditions is based on the observation that patients with Bartter's syndrome tend to waste chloride in the urine, whereas the regurgitators ("barfers") do the opposite [22]. Renal chloride wasting, or lack of it, can be estimated by a standard inulin, chloride, and free water clearance test. The calculation for this renal chloride wasting factor is given in the following equation.

$$\text{Renal distal tubular chloride wasting factor (RWF)} = \frac{\text{Free water clearance}}{\text{Chloride clearance} + \text{free water clearance}}$$

This formula factors the free water clearance by dividing it by the chloride clearance plus the free water clearance. If the renal distal tubular chloride wasting factor is less than 0.6, the patient has chloride wasting and most likely has Bartter's syndrome. If the factor is above 0.95, he is not a renal chloride waster and is probably regurgitating gastric contents.

Another way to calculate the presence of chloride wasting is to measure the renal tubular reabsorption of chloride, as shown in the following equation.

$$\text{Percent tubular reabsorption chloride } (\%TR_{Cl}) = \left(1 - \frac{\text{Chloride clearance}}{\text{Inulin clearance}}\right) \times 100$$

When the chloride clearance is divided by the inulin clearance and subtracted from unity and the result multiplied by 100, the percentage of renal tubular reabsorption of filtered chloride is estimated. If the percentage of renal tubular reabsorption of chloride is greater than 99 percent, the patient has appropriate renal conservation of chloride and has been regurgitating. However, if the tubular reabsorption of chloride is less than 99 percent, Bartter's syndrome becomes a possibility in the patient with chronic hypochloremic-hypokalemic alkalosis and normotension. It appears that autoemesis is a much more common cause for this condition than is Bartter's syndrome. The proper identification of these patients has been quite difficult in the past, some regurgitators have been classified as having Bartter's syndrome and subjected to vigorous, but inappropriate, therapy.

Finally, patients who abuse laxatives may develop a significant degree of hypokalemia and biochemical evidence of hyperaldosteronism. Laboratory diagnosis may help to identify these normotensive and hypokalemic patients as suffering from a self-induced condition. First, they will be found not to have hypochloremic alkalosis because the diarrhea secretions being lost contain significant amounts of potassium as the bicarbonate rather than chloride. Second, phenolphthalein is one of the most common laxatives to be abused. Alkalinization of a plasma sample from the patient may reveal the typical purple color of phenolphthalein in its alkaline form. A 24-hour urine specimen will contain small amounts of sodium (less than 20 mEq) due to severe extracellular volume depletion secondary to stool losses.

Surreptitious autoemesis patients and those who abuse laxatives and diuretics often have severe psychoneuroses, which may make corrective therapy nearly impossible even when the conditions are correctly diagnosed.

Summary

Hypertension is a very common disorder. In the overwhelming majority of patients, minimal amounts of laboratory testing will suffice. A small number, however, will benefit from further studies. These evaluations may allow the physician to identify patients who have significant and operable renal artery stenoses, pheochromocytomas and paragangliomas, and aldosterone-producing adenomas. This chapter discussed the use of relevant laboratory and x-ray tests and their interpretation. Some of the opinions expressed are my own, based on experience in dealing with these conditions; other authors might well suggest other approaches. However, these differences merely reflect a complex and technologically advancing field of medicine.

References

1. Amsterdam, E., Couch, M. P., Harrison, J. H., et al. Renal vein renin activity in the prognosis of surgery for renovascular hypertension. *Am. J. Med.* 47:860, 1969.
2. Bartter, F. C. Bartter's syndrome. *Urol. Clin. North Am.* 4:253, 1977.
3. Bath, N. M., Gunnells, J. C., Jr., and Robinson, R. R. Plasma renin activity in renovascular hypertension. *Am. J. Med.* 45:481, 1968.
4. Biglieri, E. A., Schambelan, M., Brust, N., et al. Plasma aldosterone concentration: Further characterization of aldosterone producing adenomas. *Circ. Res.* 34(Suppl. 1):183, 1974.
5. Boucher, R., Veyrat, R., DeChamplain, J., et al. New procedures for measurement of human plasma angiotensin and renin activity levels. *Can. Med. Assoc. J.* 90:194, 1964.
6. Braasch, W. F. The surgical kidney as an etiological factor in hypertension. *Can. Med. Assoc. J.* 46:9, 1942.
7. Braun-Menendez, E., Fasciolo, J. C., Leloir, L. F., et al. *Renal Hypertension.* Springfield, Ill.: Thomas, 1946.
8. Brunner, H. R., Gavras, H., Laragh, J. H., et al. Angiotensin-II blockade in man by sar^{1}-ala^{8}-angiotensin II for understanding and treatment of high blood pressure. *Lancet* 2:1045, 1973.
9. Brunner, H. R., Laragh, J. H., Baer, L., et al. Essential hypertension: Renin and aldosterone, heart attack and stroke. *N. Engl. J. Med.* 286:441, 1972.
10. Butler, A. M. Chronic pyelonephritis and arterial hypertension. *J. Clin. Invest.* 16:889, 1937.
11. Case, D. B., Wallace, J. M., Keim, H. J., et al. Usefulness and limitations of saralasin, a partial competitive agonist of angiotensin II, for evaluating the renin and sodium factors in hypertensive patients. *Am. J. Med.* 60:825, 1976.
12. Cohen, E. L., Rovner, D. R., and Conn, J. W. Postural augmentation of plasma renin activity: Importance in diagnosis of renovascular hypertension. *J. A. M. A.* 197:973, 1966.
13. Connor, T. B., Thomas, W. C., Jr., Haddock, L., et al. Unilateral renal disease as cause of hypertension: Its detection by ureteral catheterization studies. *Ann. Intern. Med.* 52:544, 1960.

14. Editorial. Renovascular hypertension and the role of surgery. *J. P. M. A.* 25(2) 27, 1975.
15. Engelman, K., and Sjoerdsma, A. A new test for pheochromocytoma: Pressor responsiveness to tyramine. *J. A. M. A.* 189:81, 1964.
16. Ford, K. T., Teplick, S. K., and Clark, R. E. Renal artery embolism causing neonatal hypertension: A complication of umbilical artery catheterization. *Radiology* 113:169, 1974.
17. Foster, J. H., and Dean, R. H. Results of surgical treatment of renovascular hypertension. *J. Cardiovasc. Surg. (Torino)* Spec. Issue:169, 1975.
18. Foster, J. H., Maxwell, M. H., Franklin, S. S., et al. Renovascular occlusive disease: Results of operative treatment. The cooperative study of renovascular hypertension. *J. A. M. A.* 231:1043, 1975.
19. Fournier, A., Romeder, J. M., Salmon, D., et al. Predictive criteria of surgical curability of renovascular hypertension. *Acta Med. Scand.* 189:391, 1971.
20. Franklin, S. S., Young, J. D., Jr., Maxwell, M. H., et al. Operative morbidity and mortality in renovascular disease, cooperative study of renovascular hypertension. *J. A. M. A.* 231:1148, 1975.
21. Gifford, R. W., Jr. Evaluation of the hypertensive patient with emphasis on detecting curable causes. *Milbank Mem. Fund Q.* 47 (Part 2, No. 3): 170, 1969.
22. Gill, J. R., Jr., and Bartter, F. C. Evidence for a prostaglandin independent defect in chloride reabsorption in the loop of Henle as a proximal cause of Bartter's syndrome. *Am. J. Med.* 65:766, 1978.
23. Gitlow, S. E., Bertani, L. M., Rausen, A., et al. Diagnosis of neuroblastoma by qualitative and quantitative determination of catecholamine metabolites in the urine. *Cancer* 25:1377, 1970.
24. Gulati, O. M., Carretero, A., Oza, N. D., et al. Role of renin in the pathogenesis of renal hypertension. *Circ. Res.* 36, 37 (Suppl. I):1–187, 1975.
25. Gunnells, J. C., Jr., McGuffin, W. L., Johnsrude, F., et al. Peripheral and renal venous plasma renin activity in hypertension. *Ann. Intern. Med.* 71:555, 1969.
26. Harrison, E. G., and McCormack, L. J. Pathologic classification of renal arterial disease in renovascular hypertension. *Mayo Clin. Proc.* 46:161, 1971.
27. Harrison, T. S., and Freier, O. T. Pitfalls in the technique and interpretation of regional venous sampling for localizing pheochromocytoma. *Surg. Clin. North Am.* 54:339, 1974.
28. Holley, K. E., Hunt, J. C., Brown, A. L., et al. Renal artery stenosis: A clinical-pathologic study in normotensive and hypertensive patients. *Am. J. Med.* 37:14, 1964.
29. Horne, M. L., Keenan, R. E., Conklin, V. M., et al. Angiotensin II profiling with Saralasin: Summary of the Eaton collaborative study. *Kidney Int.* 15, (Suppl.) 9:5–115, 1979.
30. Hunt, J. C., Maher, F. T., and Greene, L. F. Functional characteristics of the separate kidneys in hypertensive man. *Am. J. Cardiol.* 17:493, 1966.
31. Hunt, J. C., Sheps, S. G., Harrison, E. G., Jr., et al. Renal and renovascular hypertension: A reasoned approach to diagnosis and management. *Arch. Intern. Med.* 133:988, 1974.
32. Hunt, J. C., and Strong, C. G. Renovascular Hypertension: Mechanism and Treatment. In J. H. Laragh (Ed.), *Hypertension Manual.* New York: Dun-Donnelley, 1974. P. 509.
33. Hussain, R. A., Gifford, R. W., Stewart, B. H., et al. Differential renal venous renin activity in diagnosis of renovascular hypertension: Review of 29 cases. *Am. J. Cardiol.* 32:707, 1973.
34. Judson, W. E., and Helmer, O. M. Diagnostic and prognostic values of renin

activity in renal venous plasma in renovascular hypertension. *Hypertension* 13: 79, 1965.
35. Khairallah, P. A., Toth, A., and Bumpus, F. M. Analogs of angiotensin II: II. Mechanism of receptor interaction. *J. Med. Chem.* 13:181, 1970.
36. Kincaid, O. W., and Davis, G. O. Renal arteriography in hypertension: Symposium on hypertension associated with renal artery disease. *Proc. Staff Meet. Mayo Clin.* 36:689, 1961.
37. Kirkpatrick, J. R. Traumatic arteriovenous fistula of the kidney: An unusual case of hypertensive encephalopathy. *J. Trauma* 15:363, 1975.
38. Laragh, J. H. Curable renal hypertension—renin, marker or cause? *J. A. M. A.* 218:733, 1971.
39. Lisa, J. R., Eckstein, D., and Solomon, C. Relationship between arterial sclerosis of the renal artery and hypertension: Analysis of 100 necropsies. *Am. J. Med. Sci.* 205:701, 1943.
40. Marks, L. S., Maxwell, M. H., and Kaufman, J. J. Saralasin bolus test, rapid screening for renin-mediated hypertension. *Lancet* 2:784, 1975.
41. Marks, L. S., Maxwell, M. H., Varady, P. B., et al. Renovascular hypertension: Does the renal vein renin ratio predict operative results? *J. Urol.* 115:365, 1976.
42. McCarron, J. P., Marshall, V. F., and Whitsell, J. C., II. Indications for surgery on renal artery aneurysm. *J. Urol.* 114:177, 1975.
43. McCombs, P. R., Berkowitz, H. D., and Roberts, B. Operative management of renovascular hypertension. *Ann. Surg.* 182:762, 1975.
44. Merrifield, R. B. Solid phase peptide synthesis: I. The synthesis of a tetrapeptide. *J. Am. Chem. Soc.* 85:2149, 1965.
45. Montero, G. H. G., and Bagley, M. Renovascular hypertension secondary to renal arterial aneurysm. *J. Urol.* 6:647, 1975.
46. National Health Survey: Blood pressure of adults by race and area, United States, 1960–1962. Washington, D.C.: National Center for Health Statistics, U.S. Department of Health, Education, and Welfare, Series 11, No. 5, 1964.
47. Oppenheimer, B. S., Klemperer, P., and Moschkowitz, L. Evidence for the Goldblatt mechanism of hypertension in human pathology. *Proc. Assoc. Am. Physicians* 54:69, 1939.
48. Pals, D. T., and Fulton, R. W. Mechanism of the antihypertensive effect of I-sar-8-ala-angiotensin II during the acute phase of experimental renal hypertension. *Arch. Int. Pharmacodyn. Ther.* 204:20, 1973.
49. Pals, D. T., Masucci, F. D., Sipos, F., et al. A specific competitive antagonist of the vascular action of angiotensin II. *Circ. Res.* 29:664, 1971.
50. Port, S. K., Wagoner, R. D., and Fulton, R. E. Acute renal failure after angiography. *Am. J. Roentgenol.* 121:544, 1974.
51. Poutasse, A. F. Surgical treatment of renal hypertension. *Am. J. Surg.* 107:97, 1964.
52. Remine, W. H., Chong, G. C., vanHeerden, J. A., et al. Current management of pheochromocytoma. *Ann. Surg.* 170(No. 5):740, May 1974.
53. Ribeiro, A. B., and Krakoff, L. A. Angiotensin blockade in coarctation of the aorta. *N. Engl. J. Med.* 295:148, 1976.
54. Richie, J. P., Bennett, C. M., and Brosman, S. A. Traumatic renal artery thrombosis with acute malignant hypertension and hyperreninemia. *Urology* 6:481, 1975.
55. Rittel, W., Iselin, B., Kappler, H., et al. Synthese eines hockwirksamen hypertensin II-amids (L-asparaginyl-L-arginyl-L-valyl-L-tyrosyl-L-isoleucyl-L-histidyl-L-prolyl-L-phenylalanin). *Helv. Chim. Acta* 40:614, 1957.
56. Schwarz, H., Bumpus, F. M., and Page, I. H. Synthesis of a biologically active

octapeptide similar to natural isoleucine angiotonin octapeptide. *J. Am. Chem. Soc.* 79:5697, 1957.
57. Sechis, M. N., Plessas, S. N., and Skalekas, G. D. Post-traumatic renovascular hypertension. *Surgery* 76:666, 1974.
58. Seldinger, S. I. Catheter placement of the needle in percutaneous arteriography, a new technique. *Acta Radiol.* 39:368, 1953.
59. Sethi, G. K., Scott, S. M., and Takaro, T. Renovascular hypertension and acute aortic dissection in a patient with renal transplant. *Am. Surg.* 42:160, 1976.
60. Shapiro, A. P., McDonald, R. H., and Scheib, E. Renal artery stenosis and hypertension: II. Current criteria for surgery. *Am. J. Cardiol.* 37:1065, 1976.
61. Sheps, S. G., and Maher, F. T. Histamine and glucagon tests in diagnosis of pheochromocytoma. *J. A. M. A.* 205:895, 1968.
62. Sjoerdsma, A., Engelman, K., Waldman, T. A., et al. Pheochromocytoma: Current concepts of diagnosis and treatment. *Ann. Intern. Med.* 65:1302, 1966.
63. Silver, D., and Clements, J. D. Renovascular hypertension from renal artery compression by congenital bands. *Ann. Surg.* 183:161, 1976.
64. Smith, H. W. Hypertension and urologic disease. *Am. J. Med.* 4:724, 1948.
65. Smith, H. W. Unilateral nephrectomy in hypertensive disease. *J. Urol.* 76:685, 1956.
66. Stables, D. P., Fouche, R. S., VanNiekerk, J. P. D., et al. Traumatic renal artery occlusion: 21 cases. *J. Urol.* 115:229, 1976.
67. Stamey, T. A., Nudelman, I. J., Good, P. H., et al. Functional characteristics of renovascular hypertension. *Medicine* 40:347, 1961.
68. Stanley, J. C., Rhodes, E. L., Gewertz, B. L., et al. Renal artery aneurysm: Significance of macroaneurysm exclusive of dissections and fibrodysplastic mural dilations. *J. Cardiovasc. Surg.* 17:85, 1976.
69. Streeten, D. H. P., Anderson, G. H., Jr., and Dalakos, T. G. Angiotensin blockade: Its clinical significance. *Am. J. Med.* 60:817, 1976.
70. Streeten, D. H. P., Anderson, G. H., Freiberg, J. M., et al. Use of an angiotensin II antagonist (Saralasin) in the recognition of "angiotensinogenic" hypertension. *N. Engl. J. Med.* 292:657, 1975.
71. Strong, C. G., Hunt, J. C., Sheps, S. G. Renal venous renin activity, enhancement of sensitivity of lateralization by sodium depletion. *Am. J. Cardiol.* 27:602, 1971.
72. Sweet, C. S., Ferrario, C. M., Khosla, M. C., et al. Antagonism of peripheral and central effects of angiotensin II by (I-sarcosine, 8-isoleucine) angiotensin II. *J. Pharmacol. Exp. Ther.* 185:35, 1973.
73. Talmer, L. B., McLaughlin, A. P., and Bookstein, J. J. Renal artery dissection: A complication of catheter arteriography. *Radiology* 117:291, 1975.
74. Tucker, R. M. Renal Arterial Hypertension. In G. M. Onesti and A. N. Best (Eds.), *Hypertension: Mechanisms, Diagnosis and Treatment.* Philadelphia: Davis, 1978.
75. Tucker, R. M., and La Barthe, D. R. Incidence of surgically treated secondary hypertension at the Mayo Clinic. *Proc. Mayo Clin.* 52:549, 1977.
76. Tucker, R. M., Strong, C. G., Brennan, L. A., et al. Renovascular hypertension: Relationship of surgical curability to renin-angiotensin activity. *Mayo Clin. Proc.* 53(No. 6):373, June 1978.

11. The Laboratory Evaluation of Urolithiasis

Lynwood H. Smith, Peter G. Werness, and John T. McCall

The formation of a stone within the urinary tract is a common complication of many different metabolic disorders [17, 29, 115, 126]. Therefore, the laboratory evaluation of patients with urinary stones must be planned, whenever possible, to define the primary metabolic disorder that is responsible for the stone formation. Once the disorder has been defined, effective treatment for preventing stone formation is often available [29, 117, 125, 126]. The laboratory evaluation of patients with urolithiasis begins by identifying the potential causes, which in turn aids in the selection of appropriate laboratory studies. An etiological classification of the multiple disorders that may be complicated by the formation of stones within the urinary tract is presented in the following outline.

- I. Renal tubular syndromes
  - A. Cystinuria
  - B. Renal tubular acidosis
    - 1. Type I—distal tubular defect
    - 2. Carbonic anhydrase inhibitors
- II. Enzyme disorders
  - A. Xanthinuria
  - B. Primary hyperoxaluria
    - 1. Type I—glycolic aciduria
    - 2. Type II—L-glyceric aciduria
- III. Hypercalcemic states
  - A. Primary hyperparathyroidism
  - B. Immobilization
  - C. Milk-alkali syndrome
  - D. Sarcoidosis
  - E. Hypervitaminosis D
  - F. Cushing's syndrome
  - G. Hyperthyroidism
  - H. Neoplastic disorders
  - I. Others
- IV. Uric acid lithiasis
  - A. Gout
  - B. Idiopathic uric acid lithiasis

This investigation was supported in part by Research Grant AM–20605 from the National Institutes of Health, Public Health Service.

C. Myeloproliferative disorders
D. Low urine output states
V. Urolithiasis associated with gastrointestinal disorders
A. Enteric hyperoxaluria
B. Uric acid lithiasis
VI. Idiopathic calcium urolithiasis
A. With hypercalciuria
1. Absorptive hypercalciuria
a. Type I
b. Type II
2. Renal hypercalciuria
B. Without hypercalciuria
1. Inhibitor deficiency
2. Increased oxalate excretion
3. Incomplete renal tubular disorders of acid-base balance
4. Hyperuricosuria
C. "Normocalcemic" hyperparathyroidism
VII. Secondary urolithiasis
A. Infected urolithiasis
B. Obstructive urolithiasis
C. Medullary sponge kidney
D. Urinary diversion

These various metabolic disorders are not discussed in this chapter. The reader is referred to detailed reviews of the causes of urolithiasis [17, 29, 115, 117, 126].

Stone Analysis

Urinary stones are always composed of at least two major parts: the crystals and the matrix skeleton. Current methods that are used clinically for the analysis of stones identify only the crystalline component. Most stones formed in the urinary tract of patients who live in the western hemisphere contain calcium salts as the principal crystalloid. Except in a few situations, which include cystinuria and xanthinuria, the predominant crystal type present in stones is not diagnostic of the underlying metabolic disorder. Extensive experience reported in the literature reveals that many types of crystals are found in stones formed within the urinary tract [44, 82, 96]. Urinary calculi often contain more than one type of crystal, perhaps reflecting the changing physical-chemical state of the urine that bathes and feeds the stone. The types of crystals found in urolithiasis are summarized in the following list.

1. Calcium salts
   a. Calcium oxalate monohydrate—whewellite

   b. Calcium oxalate dihydrate—weddellite
   c. Hydroxyapatite
   d. Carbonate apatite
   e. Calcium hydrogen phosphate dihydrate—brushite (rare)
   f. Tricalcium phosphate—whitlockite (rare)
   g. Octocalcium phosphate (rare)
2. Magnesium salts
   a. Magnesium ammonium phosphate hexahydrate—struvite
   b. Magnesium phosphate octahydrate (rare)
3. Uric acid urates
   a. Uric acid
   b. Sodium acid urate (rare)
   c. Ammonium acid urate (rare)
4. Other crystal types
   a. Cystine (rare)
   b. Xanthine (rare)

Ideally, analysis of a stone from the urinary tract should provide a quantitative chemical analysis of the components of the crystalloid and at the same time should identify the specific crystal types or habits present in the stone. Appropriate sampling is critical for accurate analysis. Many stones are layered with varying crystal habits or have a nidus of crystalline composition that is different from the main body of the stone. The use of a dissecting microscope when selecting representative sites for sampling is extremely helpful.

A number of currently available methods can provide adequate analysis of urinary stones: quantitative chemical analysis [46, 76], petrographic microscopy [97, 133], x-ray diffraction [1, 59, 82, 94, 97], and infrared spectroscopy [8, 9, 94, 128]. Other methods, including scanning and transmission electron microscopy and energy-dispersive x-ray analysis, have been used as research tools in the examination of stones.

In patients with urinary calculi, the presence of struvite ("infection stone"), cystine (cystinuria), xanthine (xanthinuria), and uric acid may be important in diagnosis and treatment. The various crystal habits of calcium oxalate and calcium phosphate may be present in calculi formed as a complication of different metabolic disorders, and in these conditions, the diagnosis and treatment depend on other data in the history and laboratory evaluation.

Crystalluria

Because urine is supersaturated in terms of the crystalline phase that forms and grows into stones within the urinary tract, crystals of this same phase would be expected to be present in the voided urine. Thus it is logical to assume that examination of freshly voided urine from patients forming calculi might be useful in the diagnosis. Moreover, the lessening or disappearance of the crystalluria should help in determining the effectiveness of specific therapy. In rare disorders such as cystinuria, when the presence of cystine crystals is diagnostic of the underlying metabolic disorder, the cause of the stone formation can be determined by microscopic examination of urine.

Unfortunately, crystals of calcium salts and uric acid occur from time to time in normal subjects, and the presence of these crystals in freshly voided urine is not diagnostic. Dyer and Nordin [31] could not find a consistent relationship between crystalluria and stone formation. Robertson and colleagues [105, 109, 110] found that patients who were recurrent stone-formers had evidence of increased crystal aggregation and growth and that these patients differed from normal subjects and patients whose stone formation was inactive. They also observed a significant decrease in crystal size and aggregation when effective therapy was used in patients with recurrent urolithiasis [106]. Using different methods to observe crystalluria, Smith has noted similar findings in a group of patients with primary hyperoxaluria [116].

Ideally, freshly voided urine should be examined immediately for the presence of crystals. With time, the nature of the crystalluria can be affected by changes in temperature and pH. Even centrifugation may affect crystal aggregation and alter the state of the crystals that were present in the voided urine. Two methods have been used to reduce the artifacts that may appear after the urine is voided. Robertson and colleagues [105, 106, 109, 110] have used the Coulter Counter to examine freshly voided urine. This method allows quantitation as well as a measure of crystal size and aggregation, but crystal identification must be made microscopically with this method. Van den Berg and co-workers [129] have separated crystals from urine at the time of voiding by vacuum filtration using a 0.2-μm Nuclepore filter (Nuclepore Corp., Pleasanton, Calif.). Once the crystals are filtered from the urine, they are stable and can be observed by using various techniques, including light microscopy, petrographic microscopy, scanning electron microscopy (Figs. 11–1 and 11–2), energy-dispersive x-ray analysis, and x-ray diffraction. Accurate assessment of crystal habit, growth, and aggregation can be made, but quantitative crystal counts are tedious. We have found that study of crystalluria has been most helpful in assessing the effect of specific types of therapy (Fig. 11–3).

Urine pH

The pH of the freshly voided urine provides important clues to the possible cause of the formation of calculi in patients with renal tubular acidosis and infected urolithiasis. The patient is asked to void at 6:00 A.M. after an overnight fast. While the patient is still fasting, the next voiding is collected for measurement of pH. If the pH is 5.5 or less, renal tubular acidosis can be ruled out. If the pH is more than 5.5, an ammonium chloride loading test is necessary [29, 81, 115]. If urine pH with fasting is greater than 6.5, infection with a bacteria that produces urease may be present. The pH should be measured immediately

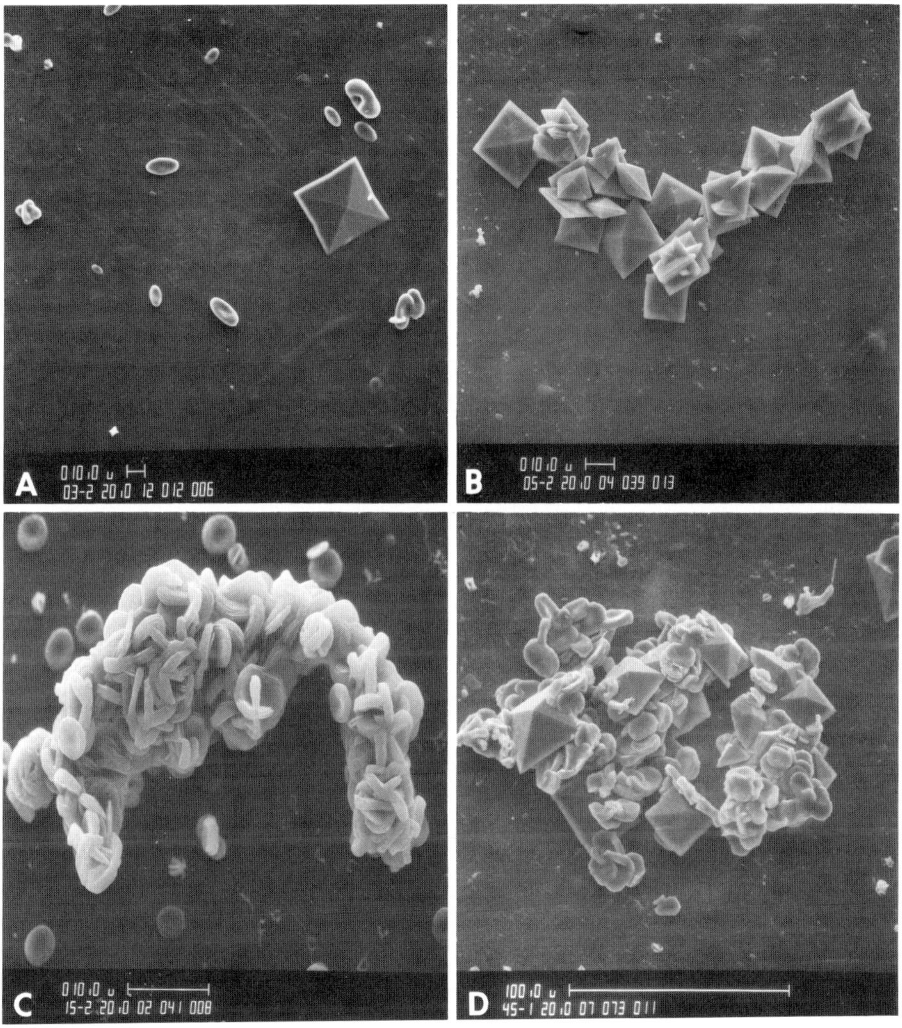

Figure 11–1
Examples of crystalluria. (A) Large calcium oxalate dihydrate (weddellite) crystal with smaller calcium oxalate monohydrate (whewellite) crystals. (B) Weddellite crystals. (C) Whewellite crystals. (D) Whewellite and weddellite crystals. (The scale of each photograph is indicated by the horizontal line at the bottom. The number to the left of the line is its length in microns.)

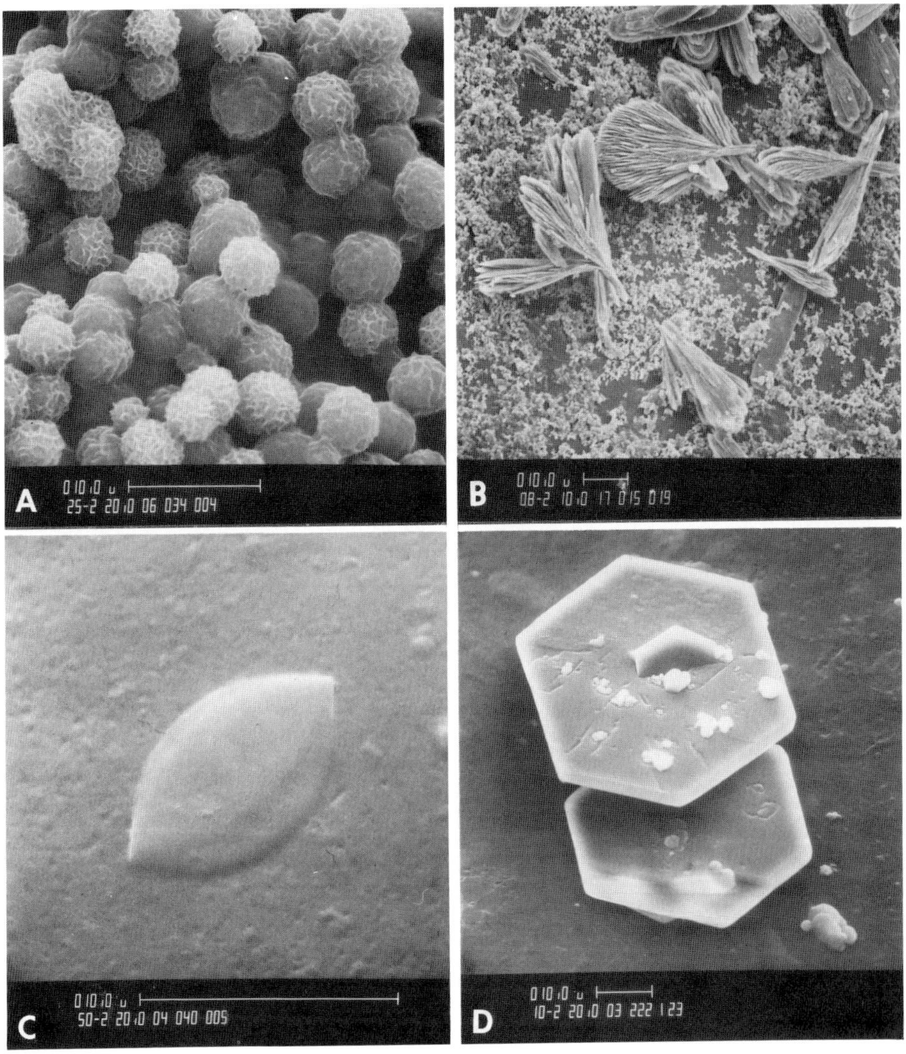

Figure 11–2
Examples of crystalluria. (A) Hydroxyapatite crystals. (B) Large calcium hydrogen phosphate dihydrate (brushite) crystals with small hydroxyapatite crystals in background. (C) Uric acid crystal. (D) Cystine crystals with small hydroxyapatite crystals on surface.

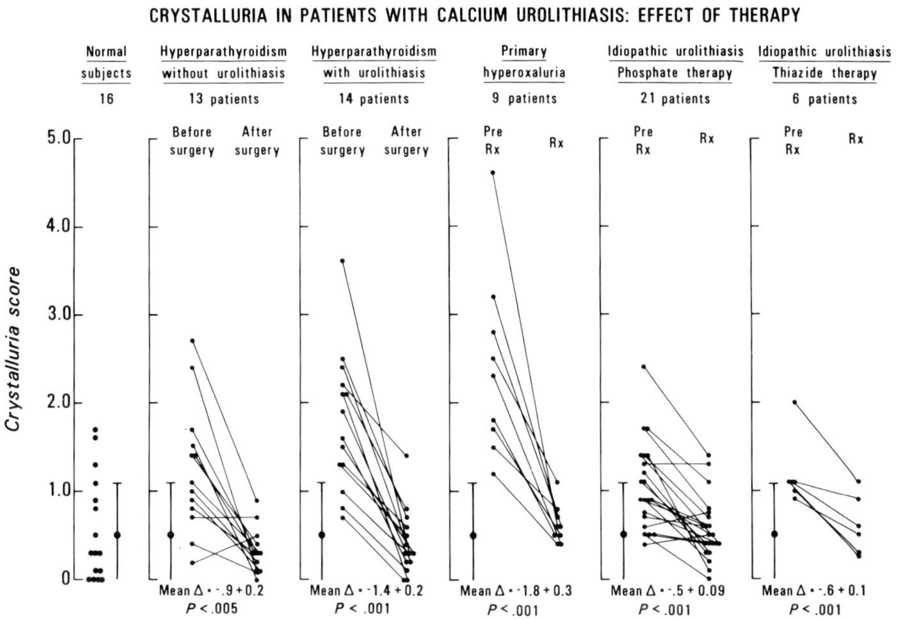

Figure 11–3
Effect of specific forms of treatment on crystalluria. "Crystalluria score" is obtained by adding the grade (0 through 5) of the quantity of crystals with each voiding during a 48-hour period and dividing by the number of voidings during the period; crystal size and aggregation are not considered. The left column shows results in normal subjects, with the mean ± SD represented by the vertical bar. Patient data are displayed as results before and after or with treatment for each patient. Individual patient results are connected by a line. The mean change with treatment and the statistical significance (*P* value) are given at the bottom of each column.

after voiding because it may change with time. Urine pH cannot be measured in the presence of bacteriuria because bacterial metabolism may alter the results.

Blood Chemistry Studies

Determinations of a number of serum parameters are useful in the evaluation of patients with urolithiasis: creatinine, blood urea nitrogen or blood urea [60, 71, 72, 87, 134], calcium [25, 57, 127], phosphorus [37, 40], uric acid [23, 26, 66], serum protein electrophoresis [27, 85], and alkaline phosphatase [18, 77]. When clinically indicated, immunoreactive parathyroid hormone [4, 11, 95, 102], cyclic adenosine monophosphate [22, 39, 83, 122, 123], ionized calcium [51, 64, 96, 103], plasma chloride [114], serum sodium and potassium concentration [10], and blood acid-base balance [24, 113] are evaluated as well. Other specific tests can also be added if clinically indicated. Serum levels of creatinine, blood urea nitrogen, or urea provide a measure of renal function. Although most patients with urolithiasis have normal or near-normal renal function, it is important to know if the function of the kidneys has decreased significantly. When the glomerular filtration rate (GFR) is reduced, the serum determinations may be altered and the excretion rates of urinary solute will be decreased.

The accurate measurement of serum calcium concentration is critical to the workup. Most of the causes of hypercalcemia complicated by urolithiasis are potentially correctable disorders; perhaps the one exception is the hypercalcemia associated with malignancy, in which stone formation is rare. Diagnosis of these disorders often begins with the documentation of hypercalcemia. Major confusion has occurred in clinical laboratories concerning the accepted normal range for the serum calcium level in healthy subjects. Commonly, a range from 9 to 11 mg/dl is used; however, careful studies in normal volunteers have placed the upper limit between 10.1 and 10.5 mg/dl [15, 16, 56, 136]. Purnell and co-workers [99] noted that 31 percent of the patients with surgically proved hyperparathyroidism had a mean preoperative serum calcium level of less than 11 mg/dl. Yendt and Gagne [136] have reported similar experience. This determination of the normal range of serum calcium is especially significant in patients with primary hyperparathyroidism and urolithiasis because they tend to have lesser elevations of serum calcium level and to have milder disease [69]. The level of serum albumin influences the calcium concentration. Because approximately 40 percent of the total serum calcium is protein-bound (primarily by albumin), low or high levels of albumin affect the protein-bound fraction of serum calcium and cause alterations in total serum calcium [104]. Levels of ionized calcium were disproportionately high in some patients with borderline hypercalcemia and urolithiasis who were subsequently found to have a parathyroid adenoma [70, 136]. Values for alkaline phosphatase, plasma chloride, and immunoreactive parathyroid hormone all provide additional information that may help in determining the cause of the hypercalcemia [3, 55, 98, 99, 132].

The level of serum phosphorus is typically low in primary hyperparathyroidism, but it may also be low in idiopathic calcium urolithiasis and renal tubular acidosis. Blood acid-base balance and levels of plasma chloride and serum sodium and potassium are often abnormal in renal tubular acidosis when a hyperchloremic acidosis is present [81].

Urine Chemistry Studies

The chemical constituents of urine should be considered in the evaluation of patients with urolithiasis. The important solutes are calcium [127], phosphorus [37, 40, 57], oxalate [45, 47, 86], uric acid [26, 66], magnesium [2], cystine [63, 120, 121], and xanthine [53]. Chemically defined inhibitors such as magnesium [2], citrate [80, 84], and pyrophosphate [62] may be important to the problem, as is the level of cyclic adenosine monophosphate (cAMP) in specific disorders [22, 39, 83, 122, 123].

Dietary intake, intestinal absorption, vitamin D metabolism, and parathyroid function may alter the urinary excretion of many of these constituents [13, 28, 30, 43, 54, 61, 65, 67, 73, 91, 92, 100, 101, 137]. Each of these factors should be considered in the interpretation of urinary chemistry results. The initial evaluation of the urine of patients with urolithiasis is best performed with the patient maintaining his usual diet and fluid intake. This setting is the one in which the patient is forming stones, and it also requires no period of adaptation to a dietary change. A recent report by Pak and colleagues [90] compared a random diet (patients taking their usual diets) with an inpatient control diet in terms of the urinary constituents; they found no consistent advantage with the inpatient diet for the initial evaluation. After the initial evaluation, specific dietary maneuvers such as fasting, low-calcium diet, high-calcium diet, and calcium loading can be carried out if indicated. These procedures will be discussed in a subsequent section. Evaluation of urine collected while the patients are taking their usual diets requires the help of a dietitian in estimating the composition of the diet, including carbohydrate, fat, protein, calcium, magnesium, phosphorus, oxalate, and purines.

Specific relationships between urinary excretion and dietary intake are important. The effect of diet on the urinary excretion of calcium has been studied extensively. Intake of calcium [48, 68, 133], carbohydrate [61], protein [65], sodium [75, 79], and phosphorus [75] can influence the excretion rate of calcium. Vitamin D, as the active metabolite $1{,}25(OH)_2D_3$, and parathyroid hormone, perhaps through $1{,}25(OH)_2D_3$, increase calcium absorption from the gut [30]. Steatorrhea decreases calcium absorption by binding calcium to fatty acids.

In health, the urinary excretion of phosphates is related to dietary intake. Parathyroid hormone decreases the tubular reabsorption of phosphate and can alter the urinary excretion markedly. Under normal conditions, dietary oxalate accounts for only 10 to 15 percent of the oxalate excreted in the urine. With a diet greatly restricted in calcium intake, the absorption of oxalate from the diet will increase, resulting in an increased urinary excretion of oxalate [73]. This relationship is exaggerated in patients with enteric hyperoxaluria, in whom intestinal absorption of oxalate is already increased [32]. The urinary excretion of uric acid is strongly influenced by the intake of purine [137]. Citrate excretion increases with an excess of parathyroid hormone and decreases with metabolic acidosis [41, 119]. Pyrophosphate excretion is proportional to phosphate intake [111, 112].

During the initial evaluation of patients with urolithiasis, 24-hour urine collections are desirable because of diurnal variations and dietary effects on the chemical constituents [19]. If time is taken with the patient to explain the method, purpose, and importance of the urine collection, adequate 24-hour collections can be obtained. Because patients who have had urinary calculi are

Table 11–1. Normal Ranges or Upper Limit of Urinary Constituents

Substance	Normal Range or Upper Limit	References
Calcium (mg/24 hr) *	< 250 to < 400	48, 58, 131
Phosphorus (mg/24 hr) *	< 1500	48
Oxalate (mg/24 hr)	15 to 50	45, 47
Uric acid (mg/24 hr) *	< 800 to < 850	6, 42
Magnesium (mg/24 hr) *	75 to 225	34, 130
Cystine (mg/24 hr)	< 30	124
Xanthine (mg/24 hr)	< 5.1 to < 8.6	135
Citrate (mg/24 hr)	300 to 900	33, 38
Pyrophosphate (mg/24 hr) *	1.0 to 3.8	62
Cyclic AMP (μmol/24 hr)	2.6 to 6.24	21

* Major dietary effect.

often on a high fluid intake (up to 4 liters or more), they must be given containers for the collection that will hold the entire 24-hour urine volume. Measurement of the urinary excretion of creatinine in the 24-hour collection provides an estimate of the completeness of the collection. Of even greater help is a careful interview with the patient after the collection, with a review of the procedure followed to ensure that no urine was lost during the collection. Collections of 24-hour urine specimens from hospitalized patients are much less desirable because diet, ambulation, intake, and medications may alter the results. Additives such as toluene that prevent bacterial growth without interfering with analyses are important in the measurement of uric acid, cystine, xanthine, and citrate [52]. Measurement of calcium, phosphorus, magnesium, pyrophosphate, oxalate, and creatinine can be performed on collections without additives. If calcium and oxalate are to be measured, concentrated hydrochloric acid should be added to reduce the pH to 2.0 or less, thus ensuring that all of the calcium and oxalate are in solution. Whenever possible, 24-hour urine collections should be refrigerated between voidings during the collection. Because many of the ranges or upper limits of the urinary constituents for normal subjects are influenced by dietary intake, absolute ranges can be stated only when defined diets are used with subjects in a steady state (Table 11–1). The values given, therefore, only provide a guide; more absolute values are provided in the references.

The results of urine studies in the evaluation of patients with urolithiasis can best be utilized by matching specific diseases with specific determinations (Table 11–2). Although each disease has a usual pattern, potential variables such as diet, intestinal absorption, and hormonal effects may alter the pattern. Cystinuria and xanthinuria are not included in the table because the results of the listed tests are normal in these conditions unless the patient has another unrelated metabolic disorder. The secondary causes of urolithiasis are also ex-

Table 11–2. Urine Chemistry Abnormalities in Patients with Urolithiasis *

Disease	Calcium	Phosphorus	Oxalate	Uric Acid	Magnesium	Citrate	Pyrophosphate
Renal tubular acidosis	↑ or N	↑ or N	N	N	N	↓↓↓	N
Primary hyperoxaluria	↓ or N	N	↑↑↑	N	N	N or ↓	N
Hypercalcemic states							
Primary hyperparathyroidism	↑↑	↑ or N	N	N	N	↑ or N	N
Others	↑↑↑	N	N	N	N	N	N
Uric acid lithiasis							
Gout	N	N	N	N or ↑	N	N	N
Idiopathic	N	N	N	N or ↑	N	N	N
Myeloproliferative disease	N	N	N	↑↑↑	N	N	N
Enteric hyperoxaluria	↓↓ to ↑	N	↑↑	N	↓↓ to N	↓↓ to N	N
Idiopathic calcium urolithiasis							
With hypercalciuria							
Absorptive	↑ or ↑↑	N or ↓	N or ↑	N or ↑	N or ↓	N or ↓	N or ↓
Renal leak	↑↑	N	N or ↑	N or ↑	N or ↓	N or ↓	N or ↓
Without hypercalciuria							
Inhibitor deficiency	N	N or ↓	N	N	↓ or N	↓ or N	↓ or N
Increased oxalate	N	N	↑	N	N	N	N
Incomplete renal tubular acidosis	N	N	N	N	N	↓ or ↓↓	N
Hyperuricosuria	N	N	N	↑↑	N	N	N

* N = normal; ↑ = mild increase; ↑↑ = moderate increase; and ↑↑↑ = large increase; same designations for decreases.

cluded because they may be associated with any of the primary metabolic diseases complicated by urinary calculi.

Overlap of abnormalities, particularly in idiopathic calcium urolithiasis, is common. For instance, a patient with one of the types of hypercalciuria may have hyperuricosuria, inhibitor deficiencies, or increased urinary excretion of oxalate, thus making classification of the patient's disorder more difficult. Until more is known about the various causes of metabolic disorders, grouping the patients is less important than defining the abnormalities found in the urine, which can be corrected by specific therapy if the metabolic activity of the stone formation warrants therapy [115].

Special Diagnostic Studies

As knowledge regarding urolithiasis and its many causes has increased, specific diagnostic studies have been developed to define better the underlying metabolic and physical-chemical disorders. Although some of these studies are currently in a developmental stage or are not practical for routine clinical evaluation, review of the background and experience with these procedures is worthwhile because they are likely to be the basis for improved clinical testing in the future.

Cystinuria

Patients with cystinuria can be classified into three major types, based on the urinary excretion of cystine and lysine in heterozygotes and the response to oral cystine loading in homozygotes [124]. This classification has been used primarily in genetic studies; the disease does not differ clinically among any of the types.

Renal Tubular Acidosis

Patients with calcium urolithiasis in whom an adequate decrease in urine pH is not obtained after an overnight fast should be given an ammonium chloride load in the evening (100 mg of NH_4Cl per kilogram is given as a solution containing 100 mg of NH_4Cl per milliliter). The patient should void at 6:00 A.M. and again at 8:00 A.M., and plasma and urinary pH and bicarbonate should be measured at the time of the second voiding. If the plasma bicarbonate concentration is 20 mEq/L without increased bicarbonate loss in the urine but the urinary pH has not decreased below 5.5, the diagnosis of type I renal tubular acidosis is confirmed and the use of ammonium chloride is discontinued. If the plasma bicarbonate does not reach this level, a second load of ammonium chloride is given, with continued monitoring of plasma and urine. If the patient is acidotic (plasma bicarbonate less than 20 mEq/L), this maneuver is unnecessary and could present a hazard to the patient.

Urolithiasis Associated with Hypercalciuria

The category of urolithiasis associated with hypercalciuria includes patients with hypercalcemia and several other disorders grouped under the diagnosis of "idiopathic hypercalciuria." A continuing problem in the evaluation of patients who have calcium urolithiasis with associated hypercalciuria is the definition of the underlying metabolic cause. In particular, patients with primary hyperparathyroidism with borderline or intermittent hypercalcemia may be very difficult to differentiate from patients with the various syndromes of idiopathic calcium urolithiasis. Nevertheless, the distinction is important because appropriate therapy is different for each of the disorders.

Beginning 10 years ago, a series of diagnostic studies have been under development which, it is hoped, will lead to accurate differentiation of these varied metabolic disorders. In 1968, Peacock and colleagues [93] reported the effect of calcium loading and deprivation on serum and urine calcium values in nine male patients with idiopathic calcium urolithiasis and in nine healthy males. The subjects were instructed to fast for approximately 20 hours, being given only distilled water (285 ml/hour) during the last 10 hours of the fast. Urine and serum calcium and creatinine levels were measured every 2 hours during the last 10 hours of the fast, at which time the urine calcium level decreased to normal. On another day, the subjects were given a calcium load (100 mg/kg) as calcium citrate, with serum and urine calcium and creatinine levels being measured. The patients who were stone-formers had an exaggerated hypercalcemia and hypercalciuria response when compared with controls. The authors concluded that these observations indicated that the hypercalciuria of idiopathic hypercalciuria was due to increased intestinal absorption of calcium.

In 1975, Pak and associates [91] modified these procedures and added the measurement of urinary cyclic AMP, with the hope of providing some assessment of parathyroid function. For seven days before testing, subjects were given a low calcium diet (approximately 400 mg per day). Fasting was started at 9:00 P.M., with 300 ml of distilled water taken at 9:00 P.M. and midnight. At 7:00 A.M. on the following morning, while still fasting, the patient drank 600 ml of distilled water, and urine was collected during the 2 hours from 7:00 to 9:00 A.M. for the measurement of calcium, creatinine, and cyclic AMP. At 9:00 A.M., venous blood was drawn for serum calcium determination, and an oral load of 1 gm of calcium was then given as a mixture of synthetic diet and calcium gluconogalactogluconate in a total volume of 300 ml. At 11:00 A.M., 300 ml of distilled water was drunk. Urine was collected during the 4 hours from 9:00 A.M. to 1:00 P.M. for the determination of calcium, creatinine, and cyclic AMP. Subject groups included normal controls and patients with hyperparathyroidism and idiopathic calcium urolithiasis. These maneuvers made it possible to differentiate three groups of patients with idiopathic calcium urolithiasis (absorptive hypercalciuria, renal hypercalciuria, and normocalciuria) from patients with primary hyperparathyroidism. A subsequent report by these workers

Table 11–3. Expected Results with Pak Test *

Metabolic Disorder	Serum		Urine Ca	Fasting Urine Ca	Urine Ca after Ca Load	Urinary Cyclic AMP	
	Ca	P				Control	After Ca Load
Absorptive hypercalciuria							
Type I	N	N	↑	N	↑	N	N
Type II	N	N	N	N	↑	N	N
Renal hypercalciuria	N	N	↑ or N	↑	↑ or N	↑	N
Normocalciuria	N	N	N	N	N	N	N
Primary hyperparathyroidism	↑	↓ or N	↑ or N	↑	↑	↑	↑

* N = normal; ↑ = increase; ↓ = decrease.
Source: C. Y. C. Pak, R. Kaplan, H. Bone, et al. A simple test for the diagnosis of absorptive, resorptive and renal hypercalciurias. *N. Engl. J. Med.* 292:497, 1975.

[90] further separated patients with absorptive hypercalciuria into two groups. In patients with type I, hypercalciuria was present with a high or a low calcium intake; in patients with type II, hypercalciuria was present only with a high calcium intake. Some abnormalities were observed in these patients (Table 11–3).

More recently, Broadus and colleagues [20] further modified these procedures, with the hope of improving the differential diagnosis between primary hyperparathyroidism with mild or intermittent hypercalcemia and the syndrome of idiopathic hypercalciuria. Patients were prepared for this test, which was called the "oral calcium tolerance test," by seven to ten days of a low calcium intake (about 400 mg per day). After an overnight fast, a control collection of blood and urine was made for determinations of basal serum calcium level, fasting calcium excretion, and basal parathyroid function as assessed by nephrogenous cAMP. An oral calcium load (1000 mg) was given, and the calciuric, calcemic, and parathyroid responses were assessed. The calciuric response is an index of calcium absorption; the calcemic response is an index of calcium tolerance; and the parathyroid response is an index of parathyroid suppressibility (Table 11–4). To date this procedure has had only limited use, but the results are encouraging. The major addition to diagnostic evaluation provided by this test is the way in which cAMP data are used to evaluate parathyroid function. The use of nephrogenous cAMP expressed as a function of glomerular filtration (nanomoles per deciliter of glomerular filtration) provides excellent correlation with parathyroid function while avoiding many of the pitfalls of using the urinary excretion of cAMP [21].

Special mention should be made of the measurement of parathyroid hormone. Theoretically, an assay that could provide accurate information about the level of immunoreactive parathyroid hormone would be extremely helpful in the differentiation of patients with hyperparathyroidism. Initial results with a clinical assay developed by Arnaud and colleagues [3, 4, 99] were very encouraging. They found an inverse correlation between serum calcium level and parathyroid hormone activity in normal subjects; in patients with surgically proved primary hyperparathyroidism, the hormonal activity was elevated and there was a positive correlation between serum calcium level and hormone activity. Unfortunately, in the patients under consideration, the serum calcium and hormonal levels are often borderline or intermittently elevated, with variations between assays from different laboratories. At least part of the problem may be caused by the heterogeneity of circulating forms of human parathyroid hormone [5, 12]. It is hoped that with improved methods for measuring parathyroid hormone, the measurement of this hormone will be an additional tool for the differential diagnosis of these patients.

In addition to these special studies, the measurement or calculation of activity products, states of saturation, and the inhibitor activity for crystal growth and aggregation in the calcium oxalate and calcium phosphate crystal systems have been used as research tools [7, 14, 20, 35, 36, 49, 50, 74, 78, 88, 89, 105, 107,

Table 11–4. Expected Results with Calcium Tolerance Test

Measurement	Absorptive Hypercalciuria	Renal Hypercalciuria	Primary Hyperparathyroidism
Calcium excretion (mg/dl GF)	↑ (Fasting excretion normal value)	↑ (Fasting excretion above normal value)	↑ (Fasting excretion may or may not be above normal value)
Serum calcium (mg/dl)	↑ (20% hypercalcemic)	Slight ↑ or no change	↑ (All hypercalcemic)
Nephrogenous cyclic AMP (nmol/dl GF)	↓ (Mean decrease > 50%) greater than normal subject	↓ Same as normal subject	↓ Much less than normal subject

Source: A. E. Broadus, M. Dominguez, and F. C. Bartter. Pathophysiological studies in idiopathic hypercalciuria: Use of an oral calcium tolerance test to characterize distinctive hypercalciuric subgroups. *J. Clin. Endocrinol. Metab.* 47:751, 1978.

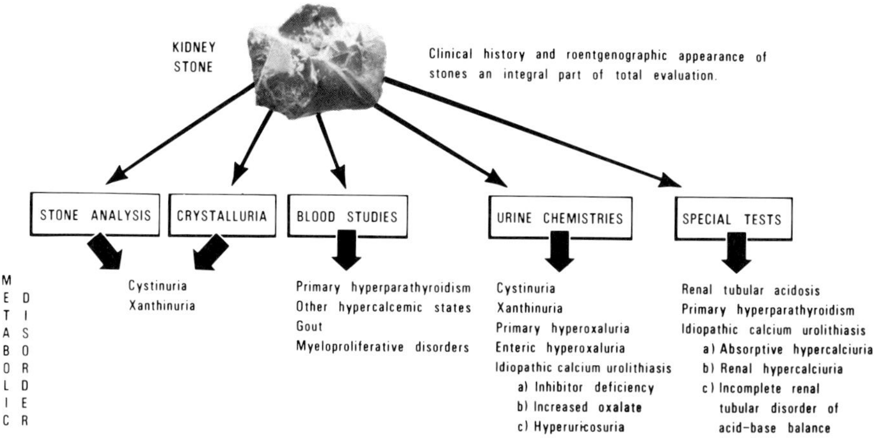

Figure 11–4
Flow diagram showing the diagnostic use of laboratory studies.

108, 118]. To date, these procedures are complex and are not applicable to the routine laboratory evaluation of patients with urolithiasis.

Conclusion

A flow diagram can be developed that applies the various diagnostic studies to the metabolic abnormalities associated with urolithiasis (Fig. 11–4). The flow diagram includes the clinical history, the roentgenographic appearance of the stones, and the results of various laboratory studies in making an accurate diagnosis, which is important for effective treatment. Because our understanding of the causes of the formation of calculi in the urinary tract is increasing rapidly, it is likely that our diagnostic approaches will change and improve.

References

1. Alexander, L., and Klug, H. P. Basic aspects of x-ray absorption in quantitative diffraction analysis of powder mixtures. *Anal. Chem.* 20:886, 1948.
2. *Analytical Methods for Atomic Absorption Spectrophotometry.* Norwalk, Conn.: Perkin-Elmer Corporation, 1968.
3. Arnaud, C. D., Littledike, E. T., Tsao, H. S., et al. Calcium homeostasis, parathyroid hormone and calcitonin in health and disease. *Excerpta Medica International Congress Series* No. 238, 1970. Pp. 360–372.
4. Arnaud, C. D., Tsao, H. S., and Littledike, T. Radioimmunoassay of human parathyroid hormone in serum. *J. Clin. Invest.* 50:21, 1971.
5. Arnaud, C. D., Wilson, D. M., and Smith, L. H. Primary Hyperparathyroidism, Renal Lithiasis and the Measurement of Parathyroid Hormone in Serum

by Radioimmunoassay. In L. Cifuentes Delatte, A. Rapado, and A. Hodgkinson (Eds.), *Urinary Calculi: Recent Advances in Aetiology, Stone Structure and Treatment*. Basel: Karger, 1973. Pp. 346–353.

6. Atsmon, A., de Vries, A., and Frank, M. *Uric Acid Lithiasis*. Amsterdam: Elsevier, 1963.
7. Barker, L. M., McPhillips, J. J., Lawrence, G. D., et al. Studies on mechanisms of calcification: I. Properties of urinary derivatives which inhibit cartilage calcification. II. Electron microscopic observations of the effect of inhibitors on crystal formation. *Johns Hopkins Med. J.* 127:2, 1970.
8. Beischer, D. E. Analysis of renal calculi by infrared spectroscopy. *J. Urol.* 73:653, 1955.
9. Bellanato, J., Cifuentes Delatte, L., Hidalgo, A., et al. Application of Infrared Spectroscopy to the Study of Renal Stones. In L. Cifuentes Delatte, A. Rapado, and A. Hodgkinson (Eds.), *Urinary Calculi: Recent Advances in Aetiology, Stone Structure and Treatment*. Basel: Karger, 1973. Pp. 237–246.
10. Berman, E. Biochemical applications of flame emission and atomic absorption spectroscopy. *Appl. Spectrosc.* 29:1, 1975.
11. Berson, S. A., and Yalow, R. S. Parathyroid hormone in plasma in adenomatous hyperparathyroidism, uremia, and bronchogenic carcinoma. *Science* 154: 907, 1966.
12. Berson, S. A., and Yalow, R. S. Immunochemical heterogeneity of parathyroid hormone in plasma. *J. Clin. Endocrinol. Metab.* 28:1037, 1968.
13. Bien, E. J., Yü, T. F., Benedict, J. D., et al. The relation of dietary nitrogen consumption to the rate of uric acid synthesis in normal and gouty man. *J. Clin. Invest.* 32:778, 1953.
14. Bisaz, S., Felix, R., Neuman, W. F., et al. Quantitative determination of inhibitors of calcium phosphate precipitation in whole urine. *Mineral Electrolyte Metab.* 1:74, 1978.
15. Boonstra, C. E., and Jackson, C. E. The clinical value of routine serum calcium analysis. *Ann. Intern. Med.* 57:963, 1962.
16. Boonstra, C. E., and Jackson, C. E. Serum calcium survey for hyperparathyroidism: Results in 50,000 clinic patients. *Am. J. Clin. Pathol.* 55:523, 1971.
17. Bordier, P., Ryckewart, A., Gueris, J., et al. On the pathogenesis of so-called idiopathic hypercalciuria. *Am. J. Med.* 63:398, 1977.
18. Bowers, G. N., Jr., and McComb, R. B. A continuous spectrophotometric method for measuring the activity of serum alkaline phosphatase. *Clin. Chem.* 12:70, 1966.
19. Briscoe, A. M., and Ragan, C. Diurnal variations in calcium and magnesium excretion in man. *Metabolism* 15:1002, 1966.
20. Broadus, A. E., Dominguez, M., and Bartter, F. C. Pathophysiological studies in idiopathic hypercalciuria: Use of an oral calcium tolerance test to characterize distinctive hypercalciuric subgroups. *J. Clin. Endocrinol. Metab.* 47: 751, 1978.
21. Broadus, A. E., Mahaffey, J. E., Bartter, F. C., et al. Nephrogenous cyclic adenosine monophosphate as a parathyroid function test. *J. Clin. Invest.* 60:771, 1977.
22. Brown, B. L., Albano, J. D. M., Ekins, R. P., et al. A simple and sensitive saturation assay method for the measurement of adenosine 3′:5′-cyclic monophosphate. *Biochem. J.* 121:561, 1971.
23. Brown, R. A., and Freier, E. F. Evaluation of an improved automated carbonate procedure for serum urate. *Clin. Biochem.* 1:154, 1967.
24. Burnett, R. W., and Noonan, D. C. Calculations and correction factors used in determination of blood pH and blood gases. *Clin. Chem.* 20:1499, 1974.

25. Cali, J. P., Moore, L., Mandel, J., et al. Standard Reference Materials: A Referee Method for the Determination of Calcium in Serum. U.S. Department of Commerce, National Bureau of Standards, Special Publication 260, 1972. P. 30.
26. Caraway, W. T. Uric acid. *Standard Methods Clin. Chem.* 4:239, 1963.
27. Chin, H. P. *Cellulose Acetate Electrophoresis: Techniques and Applications.* Ann Arbor, Mich.: Ann Arbor-Humphrey Science Publishers, 1970.
28. Coburn, J. W., Hartenbower, D. L., and Norman, A. W. Metabolism and action of the hormone vitamin D: Its relation to diseases of calcium homeostasis. *West. J. Med.* 121:22, 1974.
29. Coe, F. L. *Nephrolithiasis: Pathogenesis and Treatment.* Chicago: Year Book, 1978.
30. DeLuca, H. F. Recent advances in our understanding of the vitamin D endocrine system. *J. Lab. Clin. Med.* 87:7, 1976.
31. Dyer, R., and Nordin, B. E. C. Urinary crystals and their relation to stone formation (letter to the editor). *Nature* 215:751, 1967.
32. Earnest, D. L., Johnson, G., Williams, H. E., et al. Hyperoxaluria in patients with ileal resection: An abnormality in dietary oxalate absorption. *Gastroenterology* 66:1114, 1974.
33. Elliot, J. S., and Ribeiro, M. E. The urinary excretion of citric, hippuric, and lactic acid in normal adults and in patients with calcium oxalate urinary calculus disease. *Invest. Urol.* 10:102, 1972.
34. Evans, R. A., Sutton, R. A. L., Forbes, M. A., et al. Urinary excretion of calcium and magnesium in patients with calcium-containing renal stones. *Lancet* 2:958, 1967.
35. Finlayson, B. Renal lithiasis in review. *Urol. Clin. North Am.* 1:181, 1974.
36. Finlayson, B., and Miller, G. H., Jr. Urine ion equilibria: A numerical approach demonstrated by application to antistone therapy. *Invest. Urol.* 6:428, 1969.
37. Fiske, C. H., and Subbarow, Y. The colorimetric determination of phosphorus. *J. Biol. Chem.* 66:375, 1925.
38. Gamble, W., Orten, J. M., and Smith, A. H. Citric acid cycle in certain alterations of acid-base balance in human subjects. *J. Appl. Physiol.* 16:593, 1961.
39. Gilman, A. G. A protein binding assay for adenosine 3′:5′-cyclic monophosphate. *Proc. Natl. Acad. Sci. U.S.A.* 67:305, 1970.
40. Goldenberg, H., and Fernandez, A. Simplified method for the estimation of inorganic phosphorus in body fluids. *Clin. Chem.* 12:871, 1966.
41. Grollman, A. P., Harrison, H. C., and Harrison, H. E. The renal excretion of citrate. *J. Clin. Invest.* 40:1290, 1961.
42. Gutman, A. B., and Yü, T.-F. Uric acid nephrolithiasis. *Am. J. Med.* 45:756, 1968.
43. Harrison, H. E., and Harrison, H. C. The interaction of vitamin D and parathyroid hormone on calcium phosphorus and magnesium homeostasis in the rat. *Metabolism* 13:952, 1964.
44. Herring, L. C. Observations on the analysis of ten thousand urinary calculi. *J. Urol.* 88:545, 1962.
45. Hodgkinson, A. Determination of oxalic acid in biological material. *Clin. Chem.* 16:547, 1970.
46. Hodgkinson, A. A combined qualitative and quantitative procedure for the chemical analysis of urinary calculi. *J. Clin. Pathol.* 24:147, 1971.
47. Hodgkinson, A. *Oxalic Acid in Biology and Medicine.* London: Academic Press, 1977.

48. Hodgkinson, A., and Pyrah, L. N. The urinary excretion of calcium and inorganic phosphate in 344 patients with calcium stone of renal origin. *Br. J. Surg.* 46:10, 1958.
49. Howard, J. E. Studies on urinary stone formation: A saga of clinical investigation. *Johns Hopkins Med. J.* 139:239, 1976.
50. Howard, J. E., and Thomas, W. C., Jr. Some observations on rachitic rat cartilage of probable significance in the etiology of renal calculi. *Trans. Am. Clin. Climatol. Assoc.* 70:94, 1958.
51. Husdan, H., Leung, M., Oreopoulos, D., et al. Measurement of serum and plasma ionic calcium with the "Space-Stat 20 Ionized Calcium Analyzer." *Clin. Chem.* 23:1775, 1977.
52. Hutner, S. H., and Bjerknes, C. A. Volatile preservatives for culture media. *Proc. Soc. Exp. Biol. Med.* 67:393, 1948.
53. Jørgensen, S., and Poulsen, H. E. Enzymic determination of hypoxanthine and xanthine in human plasma and urine. *Acta Pharmacol. Toxicol.* (*Kbh.*) 11:223, 1955.
54. Kaplan, R. A., Haussler, M. R., Deftos, L. J., et al. The role of 1α, 25-dihydroxy vitamin D in the mediation of intestinal hyperabsorption of calcium in primary hyperparathyroidism and absorptive hypercalciuria. *J. Clin. Invest.* 59:756, 1977.
55. Keating, F. R., Jr. The clinical problem of primary hyperparathyroidism. *Med. Clin. North Am.* 54:511, 1970.
56. Keating, F. R., Jr., Jones, J. D., Elveback, L. R., et al. The relation of age and sex to distribution of values in healthy adults of serum calcium, inorganic phosphorus, magnesium, alkaline phosphatase, total proteins, albumin and blood urea. *J. Lab. Clin. Med.* 73:825, 1969.
57. Kessler, G., and Wolfman, M. An automated procedure for the simultaneous determination of calcium and phosphorus. *Clin. Chem.* 10:686, 1964.
58. Knapp, E. L. Factors influencing the urinary excretion of calcium: I. In normal persons. *J. Clin. Invest.* 26:182, 1947.
59. Lagergren, C. Biophysical investigations of urinary calculi: An x-ray crystallographic and microradiographic study. *Acta Radiol.* [*Suppl.*] (*Stockh.*) 133:1, 1956.
60. Larsen, K. Creatinine assay by a reaction-kinetic principle. *Clin. Chim. Acta* 41:209, 1972.
61. Lemann, J., Jr., Piering, W. F., and Lennon, E. J. Possible role of carbohydrate-induced calciuria in calcium oxalate kidney-stone formation. *N. Engl. J. Med.* 280:232, 1969.
62. Lewis, A. M., Thomas, W. C., Jr., and Tomita, A. Pyrophosphate and the mineralizing potential of urine. *Clin. Sci.* 30:389, 1966.
63. Lewis, H. B. Cystinuria: A review of some recent investigations. *Yale J. Biol. Med.* 4:437, 1932.
64. Li, T.-K., and Piechocki, J. T. Determination of serum ionic calcium with an ion-selective electrode: Evaluation of methodology and normal values. *Clin. Chem.* 17:411, 1971.
65. Licata, A. A., Bou, E., and Bartter, F. C. The effects of dietary protein on urinary calcium in nephrolithiasis (abstract). *Am. J. Clin. Nutr.* 30:622, 1977.
66. Liddle, L., Seegmiller, J. E., and Laster, L. The enzymatic spectrophotometric method for determination of uric acid. *J. Lab. Clin. Med.* 54:903, 1959.
67. Lindemann, R. D., Adler, S., Yiengst, M. J., et al. Influence of various nutrients on urinary divalent cation excretion. *J. Lab. Clin. Med.* 70:236, 1967.
68. Litin, R. B., Diessner, G. R., and Keating, F. R., Jr. Urinary excretion of calcium in patients with renal lithiasis. *J. Urol.* 86:17, 1961.

69. Lloyd, H. M. Primary hyperparathyroidism: An analysis of the role of the parathyroid tumor. *Medicine (Baltimore)* 47:53, 1968.
70. Low, J. C., Schaaf, M., Earll, J. M., et al. Ionic calcium determination in primary hyperparathyroidism. *J.A.M.A.* 223:152, 1973.
71. Marsh, W. H., Fingerhut, B., and Kirsch, E. Determination of urea nitrogen with the diacetyl method and an automatic dialyzing apparatus. *Am. J. Clin. Pathol.* 28:681, 1957.
72. Marsh, W. H., Fingerhut, B., and Miller, H. Automated and manual direct methods for the determination of blood urea. *Clin. Chem.* 11:624, 1965.
73. Marshall, R. W., Cochran, M., and Hodgkinson, A. Relationships between calcium and oxalic acid intake in the diet and their excretion in the urine of normal and renal-stone-forming subjects. *Clin. Sci.* 43:91, 1972.
74. Marshall, R. W., and Robertson, W. G. Nomograms for the estimation of the saturation of urine with calcium oxalate, calcium phosphate, magnesium ammonium phosphate, uric acid, sodium acid urate, ammonium acid urate and cystine. *Clin. Chim. Acta* 72:253, 1976.
75. Massry, S. G., Friedler, R. M., and Coburn, J. W. Excretion of phosphate and calcium: Physiology of their renal handling and relation to clinical medicine. *Arch. Intern. Med.* 131:828, 1973.
76. McCall, J. T., and Smith, L. H. Chemical Analysis of Calculi From the Urinary Tract. In F. W. Sunderman and F. W. Sunderman, Jr. (Eds.), *Laboratory Diagnosis of Kidney Diseases*. St. Louis: Green, 1970. Pp. 309–312.
77. McComb, R. B., and Bowers, G. N., Jr. Study of optimum buffer conditions for measuring alkaline phosphatase activity in human serum. *Clin. Chem.* 18:97, 1972.
78. Meyer, J. L., and Smith, L. H. Growth of calcium oxalate crystals: II. Inhibition by natural urinary crystal growth inhibitors. *Invest. Urol.* 13:36, 1975.
79. Modlin, M. The interrelation of urinary calcium and sodium in normal adults. *Invest. Urol.* 4:180, 1966.
80. Moellering, H., and Gruber, W. Determination of citrate with citrate lyase. *Anal. Biochem.* 17:369, 1966.
81. Morris, R. C., Jr. Renal tubular acidosis: Mechanisms, classification and implications. *N. Engl. J. Med.* 281:1405, 1969.
82. Morriss, R. H., and Beeler, M. F. X-ray diffraction analysis of 464 urinary calculi. *Am. J. Clin. Pathol.* 48:413, 1967.
83. Murad, F. Clinical studies and applications of cyclic nucleotides. *Adv. Cyclic Nucleotide Res.* 3:355, 1973.
84. Natelson, S., Pincus, J. B., and Lugovoy, J. K. Microestimation of citric acid: A new colorimetric reaction for pentabromoacetone. *J. Biol. Chem.* 175:745, 1948.
85. Nerenberg, S. T. *Electrophoresis: A Practical Laboratory Manual*. Philadelphia: Davis, 1966.
86. Olthuis, F. M. F. G., Markslag, A. M. G., Elhorst, J. T. K., et al. Urinary oxalate estimation. *Clin. Chim. Acta* 75:123, 1977.
87. Owen, J. A., Iggo, B., Scandrett, F. J., et al. The determination of creatinine in plasma or serum, and in urine: A critical examination. *Biochem. J.* 58:426, 1954.
88. Pak, C. Y. C. Physicochemical basis for formation of renal stones of calcium phosphate origin: Calculation of the degree of saturation of urine with respect to brushite. *J. Clin. Invest.* 48:1914, 1969.
89. Pak, C. Y. C., and Chu, S. A simple technique for the determination of urinary state of saturation with respect to brushite. *Invest. Urol.* 11:211, 1973.
90. Pak, C. Y. C., Fetner, C., Townsend, J., et al. Evaluation of calcium urolith-

iasis in ambulatory patients: Comparison of results with those of inpatient evaluation. *Am. J. Med.* 64:979, 1978.

91. Pak, C. Y. C., Kaplan, R., Bone, H., et al. A simple test for the diagnosis of absorptive, resorptive and renal hypercalciurias. *N. Engl. J. Med.* 292:497, 1975.
92. Peacock, M., Hodgkinson, A., and Nordin, B. E. C. Importance of dietary calcium in the definition of hypercalciuria. *Br. Med. J.* 3:469, 1967.
93. Peacock, M., Knowles, F., and Nordin, B. E. C. Effect of calcium administration and deprivation on serum and urine calcium in stone-forming and control subjects. *Br. Med. J.* 2:729, 1968.
94. Pollack, S. S., and Carlson, G. L. A comparison of x-ray diffraction and infrared technics for identifying kidney stones. *Am. J. Clin. Pathol.* 52:656, 1969.
95. Potts, J. T., Jr., and Krutzik, S. R. Parathyroid Hormone Radioimmunoassay: Clinical Applications. In *Nichols Institute Radioimmunoassay Manual* (3rd ed.). San Pedro, Calif.: Nichols Institute, 1976. Pp. 1–18.
96. Prien, E. L. Crystallographic analysis of urinary calculi: A 23-year survey study. *J. Urol.* 89:917, 1963.
97. Prien, E. L., and Frondel, C. Studies in urolithiasis: I. The composition of urinary calculi. *J. Urol.* 57:949, 1947.
98. Purnell, D. C., Scholz, D. A., Smith, L. H., et al. Treatment of primary hyperparathyroidism. *Am. J. Med.* 56:800, 1974.
99. Purnell, D. C., Smith, L. H., Scholz, D. A., et al. Primary hyperparathyroidism: A prospective clinical study. *Am. J. Med.* 50:670, 1971.
100. Rasmussen, H. Ionic and hormonal control of calcium homeostasis. *Am. J. Med.* 50:567, 1971.
101. Rasmussen, H., DeLuca, H., Arnaud, C., et al. The relationship between vitamin D and parathyroid hormone. *J. Clin. Invest.* 42:1940, 1963.
102. Reiss, E., Canterbury, J. M., and Egdahl, R. H. Experience with a radioimmunoassay of parathyroid hormone in human sera. *Trans. Assoc. Am. Physicians* 81:104, 1968.
103. Robertson, W. G. Measurement of ionized calcium in biological fluids. *Clin. Chim. Acta* 24:149, 1969.
104. Robertson, W. G., and Peacock, M. New techniques for the separation and measurement of the calcium fractions of normal human serum. *Clin. Chim. Acta* 20:315, 1968.
105. Robertson, W. G., and Peacock, M. Calcium oxalate crystalluria and inhibitors of crystallization in recurrent renal stone-formers. *Clin. Sci.* 43:499, 1972.
106. Robertson, W. G., Peacock, M., Marshall, R. W., et al. The effect of ethane-1-hydroxy-1, 1-diphosphonate (EHDP) on calcium oxalate crystalluria in recurrent renal stone-formers. *Clin. Sci. Mol. Med.* 47:13, 1974.
107. Robertson, W. G., Peacock, M., Marshall, R. W., et al. Saturation-inhibition index as a measure of the risk of calcium oxalate stone formation in the urinary tract. *N. Engl. J. Med.* 294:249, 1976.
108. Robertson, W. G., Peacock, M., and Nordin, B. E. C. Activity products in stone-forming and non-stone-forming urine. *Clin. Sci.* 34:579, 1968.
109. Robertson, W. G., Peacock, M., and Nordin, B. E. C. Calcium crystalluria in recurrent renal-stone formers. *Lancet* 2:21, 1969.
110. Robertson, W. G., Peacock, M., and Nordin, B. E. C. Calcium oxalate crystalluria and urine saturation in recurrent renal stone-formers. *Clin. Sci.* 40:365, 1971.
111. Russell, R. G. G., and Hodgkinson, A. The urinary excretion of inorganic

pyrophosphate by normal subjects and patients with renal calculus. *Clin. Sci.* 31:51, 1966.
112. Russell, R. G. G., Wadstrom, L. B., Lindstedt, S., et al. The origin of inorganic pyrophosphate in urine. *Clin. Sci.* 37:419, 1969.
113. Siggaard-Anderson, O. *The Acid-Base Status of the Blood* (4th ed.). Baltimore: Williams & Wilkins, 1974.
114. Skeggs, L. T., Jr., and Hochstrasser, H. Multiple automatic sequential analysis. *Clin. Chem.* 10:918, 1964.
115. Smith, L. H. Medical evaluation of urolithiasis: Etiologic aspects and diagnostic evaluation. *Urol. Clin. North Am.* 1:241, 1974.
116. Smith, L. H. Application of Physical, Chemical, and Metabolic Factors to the Management of Urolithiasis. In H. Fleisch, W. G. Robertson, L. H. Smith, and W. Vahlensieck (Eds.), *Urolithiasis Research.* New York: Plenum, 1976. Pp. 199–211.
117. Smith, L. H. Urolithiasis. In C. W. Gottschalk and L. E. Earley (Eds.), *Strauss and Welt's Diseases of the Kidney* (3rd ed.). Boston: Little, Brown, 1979. Pp. 893–932.
118. Smith, L. H., Meyer, J. L., and McCall, J. T. Chemical Nature of Crystal Inhibitors Isolated from Human Urine. In L. Cifuentes Delatte, A. Rapado, and A. Hodgkinson (Eds.), *Urinary Calculi: Recent Advances in Aetiology, Stone Structure and Treatment.* Basel: Karger, 1973. Pp. 318–327.
119. Smith, L. H., van den Berg, C. J., Wilson, D. M., et al. Urolithiasis in primary hyperparathyroidism (abstract). *Kidney Int.* 12:461, 1977.
120. Spackman, D. H., Stein, W. H., and Moore, S. Automatic recording apparatus for use in the chromatography of amino acids. *Anal. Chem.* 30:1190, 1958.
121. Stein, W. H. A chromatographic investigation of the amino acid constituents of normal urine. *J. Biol. Chem.* 201:45, 1953.
122. Steiner, A. L., Kipnis, D. M., Utiger, R., et al. Radioimmunoassay for the measurement of adenosine 3′,5′-cyclic phosphate. *Proc. Natl. Acad. Sci. U.S.A.* 64:367, 1969.
123. Steiner, A. L., Pagliara, A. S., Chase, L. R., et al. Radioimmunoassay for cyclic nucleotides: II. Adenosine 3′,5′-monophosphate and guanosine 3′,5′-monophosphate in mammalian tissues and body fluids. *J. Biol. Chem.* 247:1114, 1972.
124. Thier, S. O., and Segal, S. Cystinuria. In J. B. Stanbury, J. B. Wyngaarden, and D. S. Fredrickson (Eds.), *The Metabolic Basis of Inherited Disease* (3rd ed.). New York: McGraw-Hill, 1972. Pp. 1504–1519.
125. Thomas, W. C., Jr. Medical aspects of renal calculous disease: Treatment and prophylaxis. *Urol. Clin. North Am.* 1:261, 1974.
126. Thomas, W. C., Jr. *Renal Calculi: A Guide to Management.* Springfield, Ill.: Thomas, 1976.
127. Trudeau, D. L., and Freier, E. F. Determination of calcium in urine and serum by atomic absorption spectrophotometry (AAS). *Clin. Chem.* 13:101, 1967.
128. Tsay, Y.-C. Application of infrared spectroscopy to analysis of urinary calculi. *J. Urol.* 86:838, 1961.
129. van den Berg, C. J., Cahill, T. M., and Smith, L. H. Crystalluria. In H. Fleisch, W. G. Robertson, L. H. Smith, and W. Vahlensieck (Eds.), *Urolithiasis Research.* New York: Plenum, 1976. Pp. 365–366.
130. Wacker, W. E. C., and Vallee, B. L. Magnesium metabolism. *N. Engl. J. Med.* 259:475, 1958.
131. Watson, L., and Dale, N. E. The urinary excretion of calcium, phosphorus

and creatinine in normal subjects and in patients with skin cancer. *Clin. Sci.* 31:77, 1966.

132. Wills, M. R., and McGowan, G. K. Plasma-chloride levels in hyperparathyroidism and other hypercalcaemic states. *Br. Med. J.* 1:1153, 1964.
133. Wood, E. A. *Crystals and Light: An Introduction to Optical Crystallography.* Princeton, N.J.: Van Nostrand, 1964.
134. Wybenga, D. R., DiGiorgio, J., and Pileggi, V. J. Manual and automated methods for urea nitrogen measurement in whole serum. *Clin. Chem.* 17:891, 1971.
135. Wyngaarden, J. B. Xanthinuria. In J. B. Stanbury, J. B. Wyngaarden, and D. S. Fredrickson (Eds.), *The Metabolic Basis of Inherited Disease* (3rd ed.). New York: McGraw-Hill, 1972. Pp. 992–1002.
136. Yendt, E. R., and Gagne, R. J. A. Detection of primary hyperparathyroidism, with special reference to its occurrence in hypercalciuric females with “normal” or borderline serum calcium. *Can. Med. Assoc. J.* 98:331, 1968.
137. Zöllner, N. Influence of Diet on Urinary Uric Acid Excretion. In H. Fleisch, W. G. Robertson, L. H. Smith, and W. Vahlensieck (Eds.), *Urolithiasis Research.* New York: Plenum, 1976. Pp. 155–163.

12. Renal Acidosis

James C. M. Chan

Historical Aspects

The first published description of acid-base disturbances in the English language medical literature occurred in 1831 [48]. In a letter to the editor of the *Lancet,* during the 1831 cholera epidemic of London, O'Shaughnessy described an excessive loss of carbonate of soda in the watery diarrhea. No differentiation between carbonate and bicarbonate was made, but such a distinction would not have been expected at the time. The next description of acid-base disturbances was in 1877, when Walter [64] gave hydrochloric acid to rabbits by stomach tube and reported a serious depletion of the carbon dioxide in the blood. In 1909, Henderson [29] described in his famous monograph the interplay between the metabolic and respiratory components, which later developed into the acid-base equation commonly known as the Henderson-Hasselbalch equation. In the same year, Sorensen [63] perfected the first electrode to measure hydrogen-ion concentration in the blood and also coined the term *pH* to represent the reverse logarithmic concentration of hydrogen ion. In 1923, Bronsted [7] and Lowry established the foundation for the modern definition of acid-base physiology by defining an acid as a substance that donates hydrogen ion and a base as a substance that accepts hydrogen ion. Also in 1923, Van Slyke [70], in collaboration with Wu in the Peking Union Medical College and McLean in the Rockefeller Institute, perfected the equipment that has since come to be known as the Van Slyke machine for measuring the partial pressure of carbon dioxide (Pco_2) in blood. This technique has many clinical implications in the early detection of diabetic ketoacidosis. In the pre-insulin period, these advances led to early treatment of acid-base disturbances and a marked improvement in the survival rates of patients in diabetic ketoacidosis and impending diabetic coma.

The Henderson-Hasselbalch equation is presented as follows:

$$pH = pK + \log \frac{HCO_3^-}{S \cdot Pco_2}$$

where HCO_3^- is the bicarbonate concentration (24.0 mEq/L), S is the solubility constant of carbonate acid (S = 0.03 at 37° C), and Pco_2 is the partial pressure of carbon dioxide in blood (Pco_2 = 40 mm Hg), and pK is the dissociation constant for both carbon dioxide and carbonic acid.

Translated to clinical usage, the pH of blood is determined by the interplay between the metabolic component and the respiratory component.

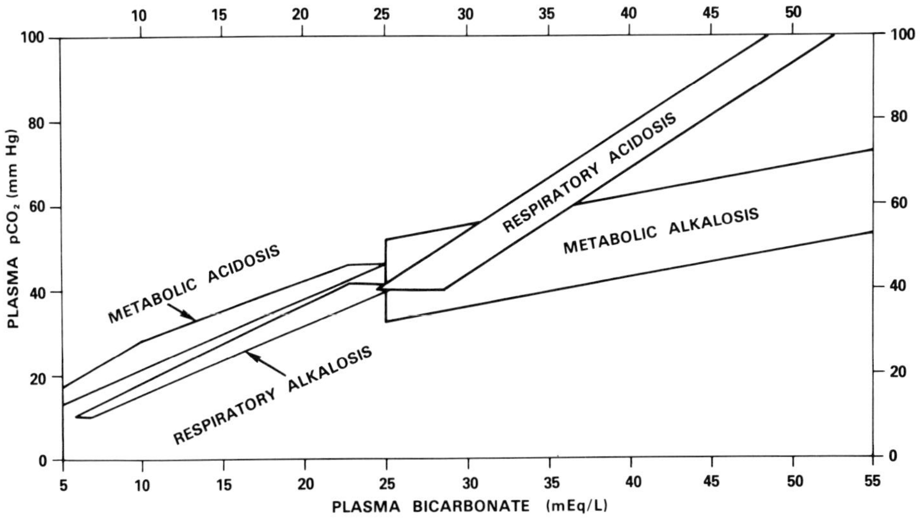

Figure 12–1
The interrelationship between plasma bicarbonate and Pco_2 in the blood, showing the 95th percentile confidence limits.

Interrelationship Between Metabolic and Respiratory Components

The interplay between the metabolic component in blood (as represented by the plasma bicarbonate in mEq/L) and the respiratory component (as represented by the plasma Pco_2 in mm Hg) is shown in Figure 12–1 [2, 49, 65]. There is a narrow confidence limit for the respiratory compensation to acid-base disturbance. The ninety-fifth percentile confidence limits for respiratory acidosis and metabolic alkalosis are wide and are less useful clinically.

For the purpose of illustration, let us discuss the condition of a child with severe metabolic acidosis secondary to diarrhea dehydration. The plasma bicarbonate has fallen to 10 mEq/L, and in the absence of any secondary process, the respiratory response (hyperventilation) will bring the Pco_2 down to 20 mm Hg, within the ninety-fifth percentile confidence limits for metabolic acidosis. However, if the plasma Pco_2 should fall above the ninety-fifth percentile confidence limits, an independent secondary process interfering with carbon dioxide exchange would have to be sought for, such as a pneumonitis. On the other hand, if the Pco_2 were to fall below the ninety-fifth percentile confidence limits, an independent secondary process stimulating the respiratory center would have to be sought for, such as salicylate intoxication. Thus any Pco_2 value falling out of the ninety-fifth percentile confidence limits for metabolic acidosis would indicate a secondary process other than a normal respiratory compensation.

Blood Buffering

The first line of defense against acid-base disturbances occurs in the blood [49]. In the plasma, the bicarbonate, inorganic phosphate, and protein serve as buffers. In the erythrocytes, hemoglobin, oxyhemoglobin, inorganic and organic phosphate, and bicarbonate contribute as buffers. At a normal blood pH of 7.40, the plasma and erythrocyte bicarbonate buffering system is responsible for 40 percent of the total buffering capacity of the blood. As metabolic acidosis develops and the blood pH falls to, for example, 7.20, more and more bicarbonate is used up, and thus determination of the total blood bicarbonate concentration is a reflection of the degree of metabolic acidosis.

In addition to the blood buffering system, the body utilizes two other systems for defense of the hydrogen ion concentration: the respiratory system, as mentioned previously, and the renal system.

The respiratory compensation to any acid-base disturbance is prompt. In contrast, the renal response to acid-base disturbance is gradual, with stepwise increments of net acid excretion to a hydrogen ion load over three or four days until maximum renal acidification occurs and the excretion of hydrogen ion reaches a plateau.

Renal Excretion of Hydrogen Ion

The proximal renal tubule reabsorbs between 4000 and 6000 mEq per day of bicarbonate and is one of the major mechanisms for regulation of acid-base equilibrium in the body [50, 51, 61]. In the distal renal tubule, two mechanisms are called into play. The first process is the formation of titratable acid, which consists primarily of the buffering of hydrogen ion with filtered phosphate. The second process is the formation of ammonium by the buffering of hydrogen ion by secreted ammonia. Ammonia is produced in the tubular cells by the action of glutaminase on glutamine. The total amount of net acid excretion varies from 1 to 2 mEq/kg/day. In health, little bicarbonate is excreted in the final urine composition; nearly all of it is reabsorbed in the proximal tubule with small amounts in the distal tubule, leaving virtually no bicarbonate in the final urine composition.

Acid-Base Variables in Normal Blood

The body keeps the blood pH within a very narrow and precise range [1, 20, 35, 52] (Table 12–1). The blood pH from the neonate to the adult varies from 7.41 to 7.39. However, the plasma P_{CO_2} and the total CO_2 are lower in the younger age group as compared to adults. It is not known why normal neonates and children under age 2 have a plasma total CO_2 of approximately 21 mEq/L. Various hypotheses have been proposed; one of these postulates that the immature renal tubule in the younger age group results in a lowered level of tubular

Table 12–1. Normal (Mean ± S.D.) Blood Acid-Base Data in Various Age Groups

	Premature Infants 2nd to 3rd Week of Life	Neonates	Children	Adults
Blood pH	7.40 + 0.08	7.40 ± 0.06	7.40 ± 0.04	7.40 ± 0.03
Plasma P_{CO_2} (mm Hg)	34.0 ± 9.0	33.5 ± 3.6	33.9 ± 3.5	39.0 ± 2.6
Plasma total CO_2 (mEq/L)	21.0 ± 2.0	21.0 ± 1.8	21.2 ± 1.4	25.2 ± 2.8

reabsorption of bicarbonate. According to the second hypothesis, the more rapid respiratory rate in infants and young children results in a low P_{CO_2}, and therefore, as a compensatory effort, the total CO_2 is low. The third hypothesis postulates that increased hydrogen ion production from the rapidly growing skeletal system in infancy and early childhood results in a lowering of the blood total CO_2.

Clinical Disorders of Hydrogen Ion Metabolism

In view of the extensive literature concerning hydrogen ion metabolic disorders, only the clinical disorders of metabolic acidosis are presented here. These disorders are listed in Table 12–2. It should be noted that a major mechanism for the development of metabolic acidosis involves one of four factors: (1) an increased production of noncarbonic, nonmetabolic, fixed acid; (2) increased extrarenal or renal loss of bicarbonate or alkaline substances; (3) dilutional reduction of bicarbonate concentration in extracellular fluid by administration of bicarbonate-free isotonic or hypertonic fluids; or (4) renal tubular acidosis secondary to a defect in the acidification mechanism.

Electrolyte Pattern

Figure 12–2 illustrates the plasma electrolyte pattern [51] in two different types of metabolic acidosis. In the normal state the cation column consists of sodium and potassium, whereas the anion column consists of bicarbonate, chloride, protein, phosphate, sulfate, and organic anions. The difference between sodium, chloride, and bicarbonate is what is conventionally known as the undetermined anion (UA). The UA fraction is usually less than 8 mEq/L.

In metabolic acidosis secondary to reduced renal parenchyma, as in uremia [58], retention of hydrogen ion results in the reduction of plasma bicarbonate. The renal failure also gives rise to the retention of anion variables, resulting in a large UA fraction (up to nearly three times that of normal). In distinct contrast is the normal UA fraction in renal tubular acidosis. In this clinical condition, the reduction of plasma bicarbonate is due to hydrogen ion retention with-

Table 12–2. Clinical Disorders of Metabolic Acidosis

Mechanism	Condition
Increased production of noncarbonic acid	*Beta-hydroxybutyric and acetoacetic acid*
	Insulin deficiency
	Starvation or fasting
	Ethanol intoxication
	Ketotic hypoglycemia with hypoalaninemia
	Lactic acid
	Muscular exercise
	Insufficient oxygenation of tissues (hypoxia)
	Phenformin therapy
	Ethanol ingestion
	Type I glycogen storage disease
	Fructose-6-diphosphate deficiency
	Leukemia
	Diabetes mellitus
	Cirrhosis
	Pancreatitis
	Incompletely identified organic acids
	Methanol intoxication
	Ethylene glycol intoxication
	Paraldehyde intoxication
	Salicylate intoxication
	Propionyl CoA carboxylase deficiency
	Methylmalonic aciduria
	Acidifying salts
	Ammonium chloride
	Arginine hydrochloride
	Lysine hydrochloride
	Hyperalimentation
	Sulfuric acid
	Methionine
	Nutramigen and high-protein milk formula
Increased extrarenal losses of bicarbonate (or combustible base) in gastrointestinal secretions	*Loss of base*
	Diarrhea
	Drainage of pancreatic, biliary, or small bowel secretions
	Ureterosigmoidostomy
	Ingestion of calcium chloride, cholestyramine, and magnesium sulfate
Dilutional reduction of bicarbonate concentration in extracellular fluid by administration of bicarbonate-free isotonic or hypertonic fluid	*"Dilutional acidosis"*
	Oliguric or salt-retaining states
	Impaired renal acidification
	Infants

Table 12–2. (Continued)

Mechanism	Condition
Renal acidosis from inappropriately reduced amount of bicarbonate delivered to extracellular fluid by the kidneys	*Diminished renal mass* Uremic acidosis Post-transplant acidosis
	Impaired renal acidification Classic type I (distal) renal tubular acidosis Type II (proximal) renal tubular acidosis Leigh's syndrome Hyperparathyroidism Polycystic kidney disease

Source: Modified from T. Sebastian et al., Metabolic Acidosis with Special Reference to the Renal Acidosis. In B. M. Brenner and F. C. Rector (Eds.), *The Kidney*. Philadelphia: Saunders, 1976. Reprinted by permission.

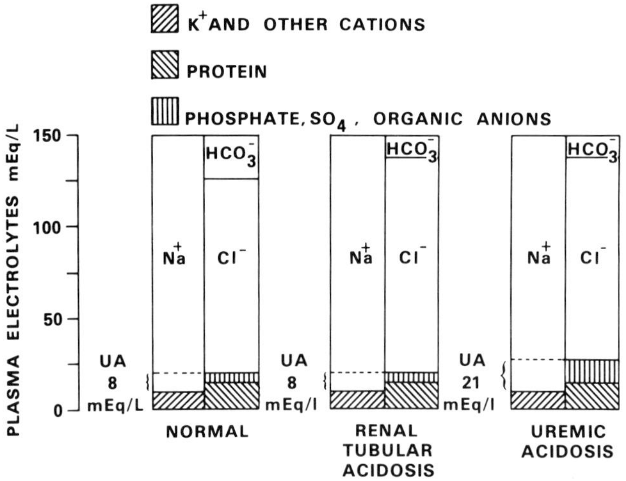

Figure 12–2
Plasma cations (sodium, Na^+; potassium, K^+) and anions (bicarbonate, HCO_3^-; chloride, Cl^-; phosphate; sulfate, SO_4; and organic anions). UA = undetermined anions.

out renal impairment; therefore, the chloride components must expand in order to meet the requirements of the law of electrical neutrality (this is the best physiological explanation for the hyperchloremia that invariably accompanies the metabolic acidosis of renal tubular acidosis).

It should be noted that a number of other clinical disorders of metabolic acidosis are also associated with a normal anion gap and thus are often accompanied by hyperchloremia. These disorders include diarrhea acidosis [1]; ureteral ileostomy [60]; sustained loss of small intestinal and pancreatic secretion (through nasal gastric suction or through drainage of fistulas) [61]; acidosis secondary to total parenteral nutrition [8, 42]; intake of acidifying salts [67]; conditions such as dilutional acidosis [40]; following the use of diuretics with carbonic anhydrase inhibitory effect [59]; or acidosis secondary to the use of cation exchange resins [61].

The disorders of metabolic acidosis associated with an increased anion gap include acute and chronic renal failure [12, 15] and ingestion of toxins [61] (e.g., ethylene glycol, paraldehyde, methyl alcohol, salicylate). Other conditions associated with an increased UA are diabetic [21], lactic [30, 46, 47, 56], and alcoholic acidosis [32]; sulfur injection [5]; inborn errors of amino acid metabolism [22]; and nonketotic hyperosmolar coma [3].

Net Acid Excretion

The excretion of hydrogen ion, net acid excretion, consists of equal parts of titratable acid and ammonium in a normal subject (Fig. 12–3). On administration of ammonium chloride [4, 19], arginine hydrochloride, or other acidifying salts, increasing amounts of net acid excretion will occur and will then reach a plateau after three or four days.

The components of the net acid excretion also show interesting changes. Primarily, the titratable acidity will increase in response to the acid load by 100 to 150 percent and will then level off when all the filtered phosphate has been used up in the buffering of hydrogen ion to form titratable acid [53]. The excretion of ammonium also increases with acid loading by 150 to 250 percent. However, since the enzyme-substrate-related mechanism of ammonium formation has been maximally utilized, it too will level off. Normally, maximum net acid excretion with appropriate ammonium chloride loading exceeds 3 mEq/kg/day. With a single challenge of 75 mEq/m^2 of ammonium chloride, the urinary pH usually falls to less than 5.5 and the net acid excretion increases to 85 ± 20 $\mu Eq/min/1.73\ m^2$ at 3 to 6 hours after such a loading dose (Fig. 12–4).

In distinct contrast, patients with end-stage kidney failure are unable to excrete appropriate amounts of net acid and indeed may excrete only one-tenth the amount of the normal controls subjected to a similar acid loading (see Fig. 12–3). The response in the uremic patients is also slower and grossly inadequate. The impairment in excretion is reflected more strongly in the failure to

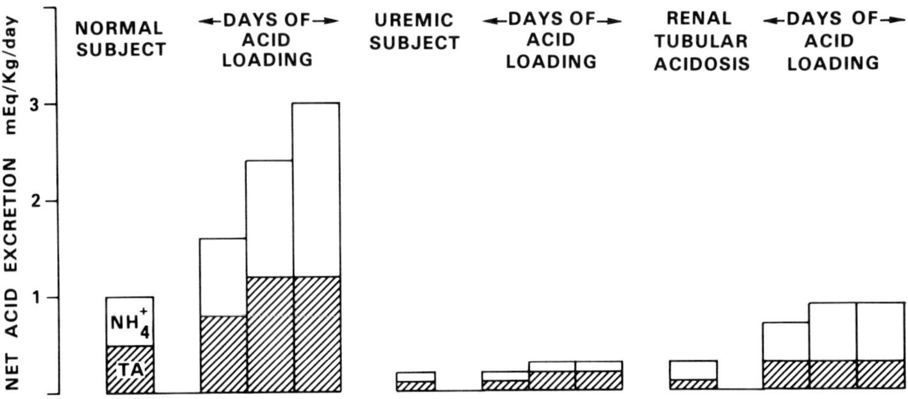

Figure 12–3
Net acid excretion, consisting of urinary titratable acidity (TA) plus ammonium (NH_4).

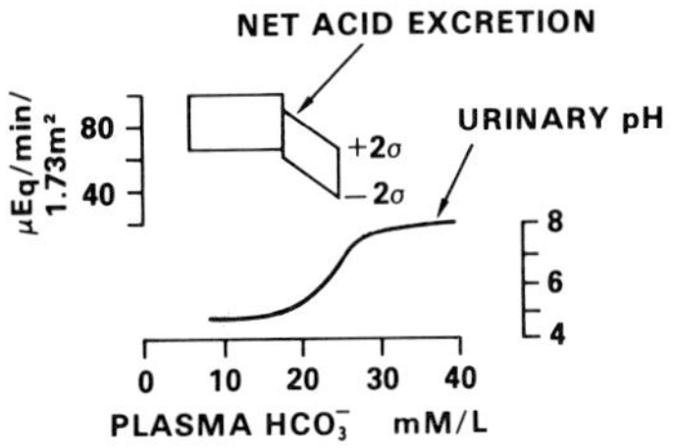

Figure 12–4
Normal renal tubular response to acute metabolic acidosis induced by an acidifying salt (ammonium chloride [NH_4Cl] at a challenge dose of 75 mEq/m^2 given orally).

form ammonium (which is dependent on the action of glutaminase on glutamine). The excretion of titratable acidity may also increase, but the total amount is far from adequate [53].

In patients with renal tubular acidosis, the total amount of net acid excretion is 0.3 mEq/kg/day, consisting of ammonium to titratable acid in the ratio of 2 : 1. With acid loading, the titratable acid increases by 100 to 200 percent and then levels off rapidly. The ammonium formation may increase by 200 to 300 percent, but it will also level off at an inadequate level (see Fig. 12–3).

Renal Tubular Acidosis

Classification

Renal tubular acidosis (RTA) can either be a primary renal disease or can be secondary to other disorders. Various classifications of this disorder have been presented. The following sections represent an attempt at a simplified version of classification.

PROXIMAL RTA. *Primary Type.* Proximal, or type II, RTA is characterized by a low renal plasma bicarbonate threshold with a consequent excessive urinary loss of bicarbonate. At normal plasma bicarbonate levels, the fractional excretion of filtered bicarbonate is over 15 percent. This excretion rate diminishes during spontaneous (or induced) metabolic acidosis, indicating an almost intact acidification mechanism in the distal tubule [13].

The fractional excretion of filtered bicarbonate is calculated as follows:

$$(U_{HCO_3^-} \times P_{cr}) \div (P_{HCO_3^-} \times U_{cr})$$

where U = urine,
P = plasma,
HCO_3^- = bicarbonate, and
cr = creatinine.

Secondary Type. Proximal RTA may be associated with other dysfunctions of the proximal tubule, such as Fanconi's syndrome, vitamin D deficiency, secondary hyperparathyroidism, the nephrotic syndrome, medullary cystic disease, heavy metal and drug intoxications, transplanted renal allografts [19], and certain systemic diseases [13].

DISTAL RTA. *Primary Type.* Distal (classic, or type I) RTA is characterized by a renal tubular inability to lower the urinary pH because of a defect in producing adequate amounts of titratable acidity and ammonium, which then leads to a systemic metabolic acidosis [13]. Renal tubular bicarbonate reabsorption is not reduced because the fractional excretion of filtered bicarbonate is less than 5 percent. Recent data tend to suggest that the metabolic acidosis may be related to an increased endogenous acid production [16].

Secondary Type. Distal RTA syndromes have been described that are secondary to pyelonephritis, medullary sponge kidney, hypergammaglobulinemic state, vitamin D deficiency or intoxication, primary hyperparathyroidism, idiopathic hypercalciuria, amphotericin B toxicity, acute tubular necrosis, kidney allografts, and probably other disorders [13, 19].

DISTAL RTA WITH BICARBONATE WASTING. A distal type of RTA with bicarbonate wasting has also been described in which the renal acidification defect is associated with an impairment of 5 to 10 percent in the fractional reabsorption of filtered bicarbonate at a normal plasma bicarbonate level. The fact that the fractional excretion of filtered bicarbonate does not change during severe acidosis differentiates this type of RTA from the hybrid type [53].

HYBRID RTA. Hybrid RTA has mixed characteristics of both type II (proximal RTA) and type I (distal RTA). It is characterized by inadequate net acid ex-

Table 12–3. Symptoms of Children with Primary RTA

Patient	Age at Diagnosis	Type of RTA	Symptoms
1	1 week	Type 1–2 hybrid (Leigh's syndrome)	Failure to thrive, lactic acidosis
2	2 weeks	Type 1–2 hybrid	UTI, dehydration, failure to thrive, severe metabolic acidosis
3	2 weeks	Distal (type I)	Dehydration, UTI, poor weight gain
4	3 weeks	Proximal (type II)	Failure to thrive, persistent metabolic acidosis
5	4 weeks	Distal (type I)	Dehydration, UTI, poor weight gain
6	4 months	Distal (type I) with HCO_3^- wasting	Enuresis, UTI
7	12 months	Type 1–2 hybrid (Leigh's syndrome)	Growth failure, nystagmus
8	18 months	Distal (type I)	Growth failure, polyuria
9	22 months	Proximal (type II)	Growth failure, polydipsia, polyuria, hyperchloremic metabolic acidosis
10	28 months	Distal (type I)	Growth failure
11	4 years	Distal (type I)	Severe hyperchloremic metabolic acidosis; end-stage renal failure from massive nephrocalcinosis and parenchymal fibrosis
12	4½ years	Proximal (type II) 7% bicarbonaturia	Growth failure

UTI = urinary tract infection.

cretion and is accompanied by bicarbonaturia that is in excess of 15 percent of the bicarbonate filtered in the presence of normal plasma bicarbonate level. Under severe metabolic acidosis, the bicarbonaturia decreases to about 3 percent.

INCOMPLETE RTA. Incomplete RTA is characterized by a normal blood pH, inappropriately high urinary pH, and impaired net acid excretion with normal or exaggerated compensatory ammonium excretion during ammonium chloride-induced metabolic acidosis.

Clinical Experience and Observations

Over the last 6 years we treated a number of children with renal tubular acidosis (Table 12–3). The presenting symptoms are growth failure, dehydration, urinary tract infection, and vomiting. The age of diagnosis varies from 1 week to 4½ years [16].

The patients with classic distal RTA were studied with ammonium chloride loading. These patients were given ammonium chloride (75 mEq/m^2) in gelatin-coated tablets. The induced metabolic acidosis is reflected in a reduction in the serum bicarbonate (Fig. 12–5). However, in the presence of severe metabolic acidosis (serum bicarbonate of 10 mM/L), in no instance was the urinary pH below 6.5. This is indicative of a distal renal tubular defect in establishing a sharp pH gradient [14]. In addition, the lower panel of Figure 12–5 shows an inadequate net acid excretion. In normal subjects with induced metabolic acidosis, the net acid excretion should exceed 65 $\mu Eq/min/1.73\ m^2$. The inability of these patients to excrete normal amounts of net acid constitutes evidence of a distal renal tubular acidification defect.

Patient C.S. was given the conventional alkaline therapy of 2 mEq/kg/day. Her growth failure is evidenced by height that is below the third percentile [16]. Patient D.G. was treated similarly and has stayed at the third percentile for height and weight. R.G. is younger than D.G. by 2 years. At the age of 2 weeks, R.G. developed symptoms similar to those of the older brother. At the insistence of the mother, a diagnostic workup was initiated, confirming the presence of distal, classic RTA. At this time, the mother became frustrated with medical advice and decided on her own to treat the younger brother with the same amount of Shohl's solution as the older brother was taking. In retrospect, therefore, R.G. was taking between 4 and 10 mEq/kg/day of alkaline solution. As a result, he is growing at the 25th percentile for height and weight, as compared to the older brother who is at the third percentile [16].

Measurement of Endogenous Acid Production

In order to delineate a possible mechanism for the increased need of the alkali solution in patients with RTA, we carried out a number of experiments to estimate the rate of acid production in patients with classic, distal RTA. The quantitation of endogenous acid production is fraught with difficulties, both conceptually and analytically, because hydrogen ion production is derived from several sources endogenously and thus is not accessible to external measurements. In 1956, Hunt [31] proposed that a major bulk of endogenous acid production could be quantitated by measuring the urinary sulfate component. He carried out experiments in humans in which he proposed that sulfur-containing amino acids such as methionine and cystine would result in urinary sulfate excretion when they were completely oxidized into hydrogen ion and sulfate. By quantitating urinary sulfate excretion, one can extrapolate the amount of hydrogen ion produced in this metabolic process. In 1961 and 1965–66 Relman and Lemann [37, 38, 55] confirmed Hunt's observation and extended it to include a second major component of endogenous acid production, namely, the incomplete oxidation of organic acids leading to dissociation into organic anion and hydrogen ion. They showed that with the excretion and quantitation of organic

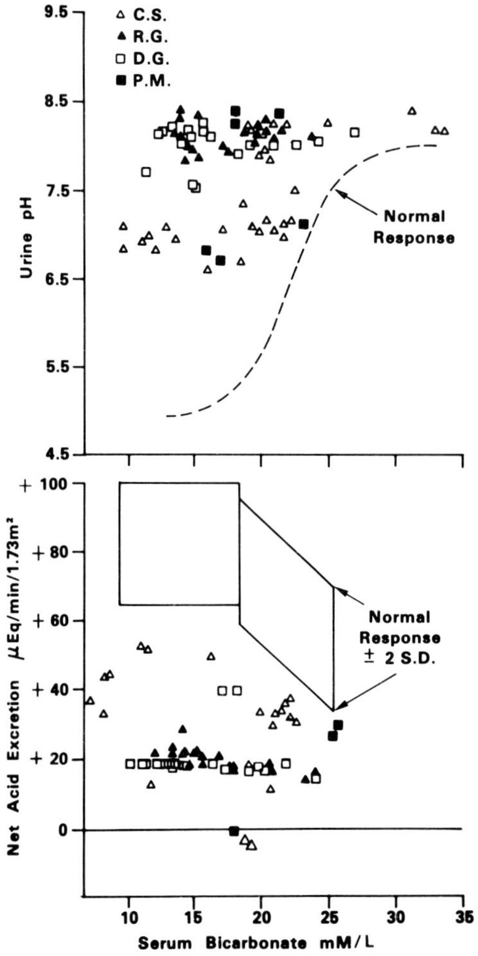

Figure 12–5
Children with distal (type I, classic) RTA demonstrating a failure of the urinary pH and net acid excretion to respond appropriately after a challenge dose of 75 mEq/m^2 of ammonium chloride. (Reprinted, by permission, from J. C. M. Chan, Acid-base, calcium, potassium and aldosterone metabolism in renal tubular acidosis. *Nephron* 23:152–158 [Karger, Basel, 1979].)

anion in the urine, one can extrapolate the amount of hydrogen ion produced in the metabolic process.

In 1969, Kilderberg and colleagues [35] applied these concepts and methodologies of Hunt and of Relman and associates [31, 37, 38] to the study of endogenous acid production in rapidly growing premature infants and found that the rapid growth of the skeletal system contributed to hydrogen ion production. These researchers utilized a stoichiometrical reaction that has been described in the literature for some time, namely, that calcium retained in the body, when combined with secondary and primary phosphate and water to form hydroxyapatite, results in the release of hydrogen ion. Since infants are fed their normal calcium intake in the form of milk formula, if one assumes that all the calcium retained goes to form hydroxyapatite, it seems reasonable that their hypothesis is correct.

In a study [35] involving premature infants who were fed their normal milk formula (Similac), it was found that the undetermined anion absorption is close to zero with a 6.7 ± 0.6 mEq/day of undetermined anion as intake and 6.6 ± 0.7 mEq/day of undetermined anion in the stool as output. (The undetermined anion of food or stool is calculated as the difference between sodium, potassium, calcium, and phosphorus minus the sum of chloride plus phosphorus, assuming that the phosphorus valence is 1.8 at a normal blood pH.) This finding can be taken as indirect additional evidence that no significant net absorption of potential base occurs through the gastrointestinal tract. It has also been shown that the net production of hydrogen ion through the complete oxidation of sulfur-amino acids, incomplete oxidation of organic acids, and hydrogen ion contributions from hydroxyapatite production varies between 1.9 and 2.6 mEq/kg/day in the short term (six days) according to studies in 4 premature infants on their normal milk formula [35]. This finding is in agreement with our study in 18 premature infants [11, 13] (gestation age 34.7 ± 2.8 weeks), where the endogenous net acid production was shown to be 1.8 ± 1.0 mEq/kg/day (Fig. 12–6).

By applying the concepts and methodologies of these investigators to the study of normal, healthy children [11, 13], one can calculate that in children with average body weights of 20.5 kg the endogenous hydrogen ion production is 1.40 mEq/kg/day, which is balanced by the hydrogen ion excretion of 1.35 mEq/kg/day and results in an acid balance of nearly zero.

With these normal children used as control subjects, the hydrogen ion production and excretion of the four children with classic, distal RTA are presented in Table 12–4. It is clear that the hydrogen ion production is twice as high in the study subjects as it is in the controls [16]. In the presence of this increased acid production and of the impaired acid excretion, there is a positive hydrogen ion balance.

A representative study of the hydrogen ion balance data [16] in one of these children is shown in Figure 12–7. On the left-hand panel of the figure are shown the acid balance data during metabolic acidosis (the total CO_2 is 15

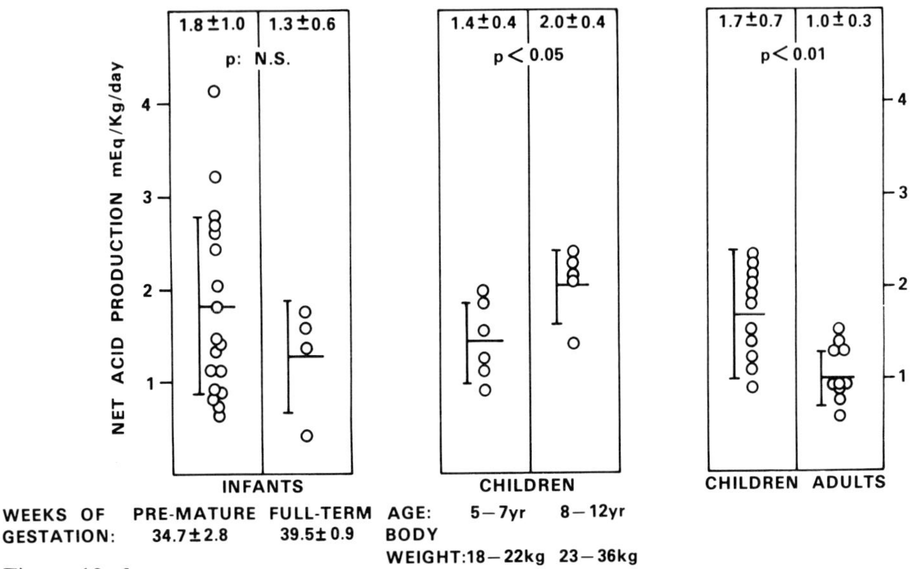

Figure 12–6
Endogenous acid production in various age groups. (Redrawn from data of J. C. M. Chan, Hydrogen ion production secondary to metabolism of sulfur-amino acids and organic acids. *Nutr. Metab.* 22:288–294 [Karger, Basel, 1978].)

mEq/L). On the lower panel of the figure are shown the acid balance data plotted according to the method of Relman: the endogenous acid production from the zero axis downward, the conventional alkaline therapy at 2 mEq/kg/day from the bottom line upward, and the net acid excretion further upward (shaded area). The distance between the zero axis and the heavy (acid balance) line represents a positive accumulation of hydrogen ion. It is obvious that in view of the increased acid production, the conventional alkali therapy is insufficient to neutralize the hydrogen ion production, resulting in positive accumulation of hydrogen ion. With progressive increments of alkali therapy, the metabolic acidosis is corrected (right-hand panel of Fig. 12–7). It is interesting to note that the acid production after correction of acidosis is equal to that of the acidotic period. The alkali therapy of 4 to 5 mEq/kg/day resulted in the retention of 72 mEq of base, which is reflected in the correction of the systemic acidosis. An interesting facet from this set of data involves the proximal tubular response to excessive alkali therapy and to the progressive increase in net base excretion, which results in a stepwise increment of alkali excretion with the acid balance pointing toward zero at the end of the study.

Mechanism of Growth Failure in Renal Tubular Acidosis

The mechanism of growth failure secondary to the metabolic acidosis of RTA has not yet been delineated. It would seem reasonable to assume that no growth

Table 12–4. Acid Balance in RTA: Patients with Classic (Type I, Distal) RTA Compared to Normal Subjects

Patient	Body Weight (kg)	Mean Daily Net Acid Production (mEq/kg)	Mean Daily Net Acid Excretion (mEq/kg)	Mean Daily Acid Balance (mEq/kg)	Serum Total CO_2 (mEq/L)		
					Initial	Final	Change
1	18.2	2.4	0.9	1.5	19	21	− 2
2	22.5	1.6	0.1	1.5	17	14	3
3	17.5	2.5	0.1	2.4	15	11	4
4	10.9	2.8	1.3	1.5	21	11	9
Mean ± S.D. 17 collections in 4 patients with RTA		2.4 ± 0.5	0.6 ± 0.6	1.5 ± 0.1	18 ± 3	14 ± 5	4 ± 5
Mean ± S.D. normal children weighing 20.5 ± 1.6 kg		1.4 ± 0.4	1.4 ± 0.5	0.1 ± 0.3	25 ± 2	25 ± 3	0.0 ± 3
P		< 0.05	< 0.05	< 0.05			

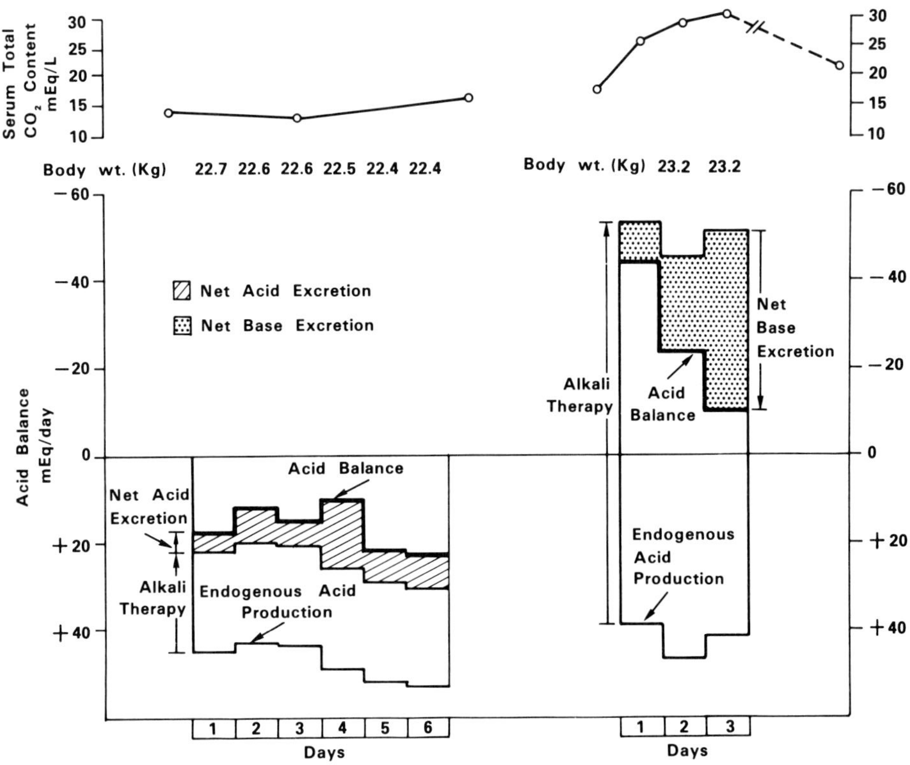

Figure 12–7
Net acid balance studies in a child with distal (classic, type I) RTA. Details in text. (Reprinted, by permission, from J. C. M. Chan, Hydrogen ion production secondary to metabolism of sulfur-amino acids and organic acids. *Nutr. Metab.* 22:288–294 [Karger, Basel, 1978].)

is possible unless the skeletal system begins to grow. To test this hypothesis [16], a representative calcium balance of one of the subjects was examined. On the left-hand panel of Figure 12–8 are shown the calcium balance data during metabolic acidosis. The intake of calcium is plotted from the zero axis downward and the stool and urinary excretion from the bottom line upward, according to the method of Albright, so that the clear area between the zero axis and the calcium balance line represents a positive accumulation of calcium. It is obvious that after correction of metabolic acidosis (right-hand panel of the figure) there is a nearly twofold increase in the calcium balance, which is secondary mainly to a 50-percent reduction in stool calcium loss. The reduction in urinary calcium excretion is also a contributing factor to the overall improvement in the calcium metabolism.

It would seem reasonable to deduce from this set of data that metabolic acidosis interferes with calcium absorption in the gastrointestinal tract.

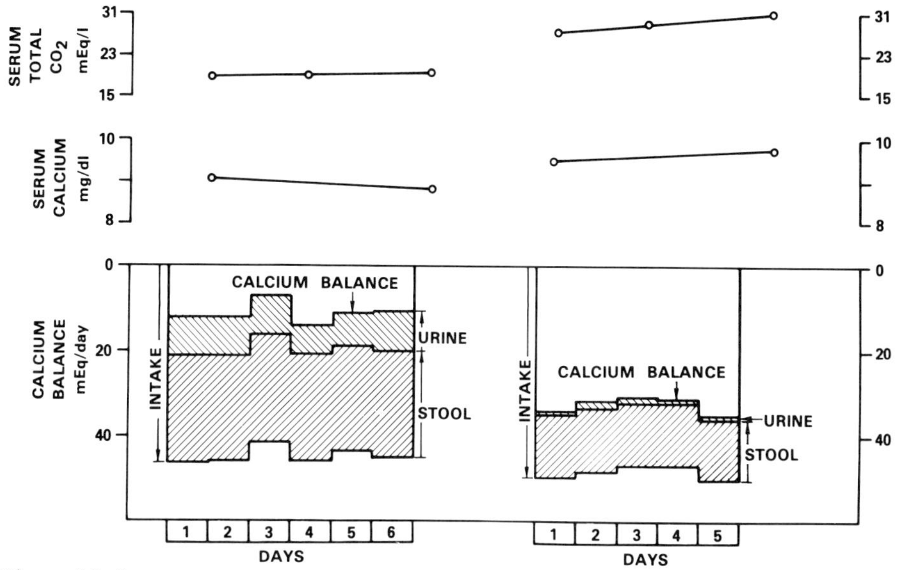

Figure 12–8
Calcium balance data in a child with distal (classic, type I) RTA (see text for details). (Reprinted, by permission, from J. C. M. Chan, Acid-base, calcium, potassium and aldosterone metabolism in renal tubular acidosis. *Nephron* 23:152 [Karger, Basel, 1979].)

Other Conditions Related to Metabolic Acidosis

Metabolic Acidosis and Infant Feeding

A number of years ago, Healy [27] drew attention to the fact that metabolic acidosis can occur in normal infants who are fed Nutramigen. The exact mechanism of this metabolic acidosis was not delineated. In order to test the hypothesis that the endogenous acid production in certain milk formulae may be higher than previously assumed, we carried out a study on a 9-week-old infant at the Children's Hospital of Los Angeles [10], who was admitted with sepsis, dehydration, elevated blood urea nitrogen, and severe metabolic acidosis (Fig. 12–9). With rehydration and bicarbonate therapy, the blood urea nitrogen returned to normal levels, and the blood total CO_2 and metabolic acidosis were corrected. However, upon institution of SMA milk formula, metabolic acidosis recurred. With the substitution of glucose water for this milk formula and without bicarbonate therapy, the metabolic acidosis was corrected. When Nutramigen was used, metabolic acidosis recurred, with blood total CO_2 falling to 15 mEq/L. With small amounts of bicarbonate therapy and "Jello-water," metabolic acidosis was corrected, with total CO_2 back up to 28 mEq/L. At this point, the child was admitted to the Clinical Research Center at the Children's Hos-

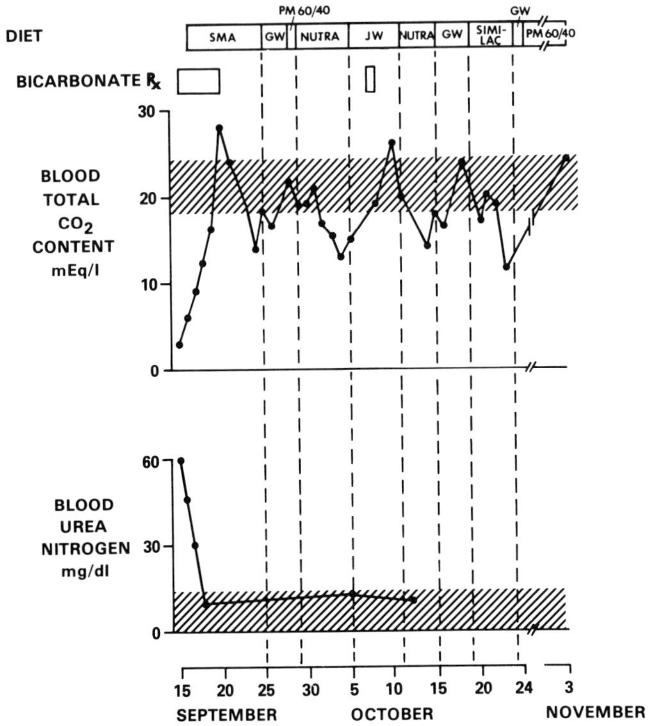

Figure 12–9
Clinical course in a 9-week-old infant with sepsis who was fed various milk formulae. Note that the recurrence of metabolic acidosis is most severe with Nutramigen and occurs to a lesser extent with SMA milk formula. GW = glucose water; PM 60/40 = milk formula; JW = Jello-water; Nutra = Nutramigen. (See text for details.) (Reprinted, by permission, from J. C. M. Chan, The effect of milk formulae on acid balance. *Nutr. Metab.* 16:140–154 [Karger, Basel, 1974].)

pital of Los Angeles, where hydrogen balance studies were performed. As shown in Figure 12–10, the acid production increased with Nutramigen as well as with Similac, resulting in positive accumulation of hydrogen ion and recurrence of metabolic acidosis. However, the acid production was markedly diminished during glucose water ingestion and was adequately dealt with by the net acid excretion.

It would seem reasonable to deduce that the increased endogenous acid production secondary to Nutramigen may have accounted for the development of the metabolic acidosis.

In a recent study by Moore and colleagues [43] on 180 healthy, full-term infants, it was demonstrated that formula (SMA)-fed infants suffer from a significant incidence (41 percent) of severe metabolic acidosis (base excess

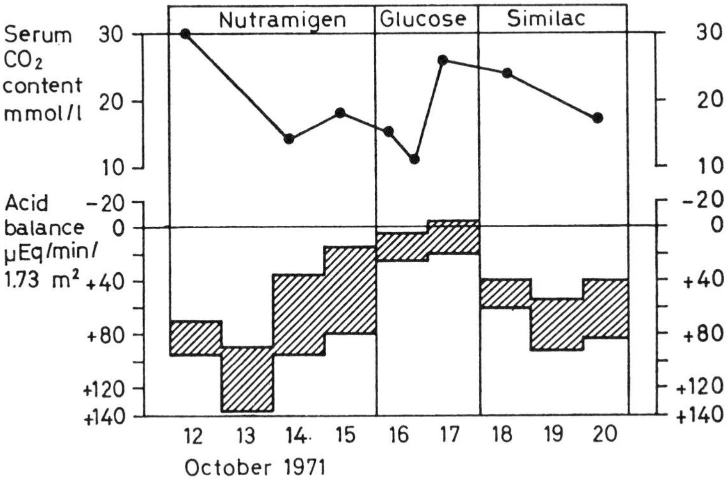

Figure 12–10
Endogenous acid production and net acid excretion in the same infant 1 month after apparently successful treatment of sepsis. The effect of various milk formulae on the net acid balance is shown. Nutramigen is associated with markedly increased endogenous acid production and recurrence of severe metabolic acidosis; these phenomena occur to a lesser extent with Similac. (See text for details.) (Reprinted, by permission, from J. C. M. Chan, The effect of milk formulae on acid balance. *Nutr. Metab.* 16:140–154 [Karger, Basel, 1974].)

exceeding 10 mM/L) as compared to the 5 percent incidence in breast-fed infants. Moore and colleagues attributed this difference to the more acidogenic pH, higher titratable acidity, and endogenous acid load from the milk formula [43]. The exact mechanism for the acidosis can be delineated only by a net acid balance study. However, the quantitation of preformed acids or bases is seriously faulted on both a theoretical and a practical basis. In fact, if one examines carefully the anion gap ($Na^+ K^- Cl^-$ 1.8P) of any milk formula, it is obvious that such a preformed base is very large and that in comparison, the preformed acid in milk formula is very small indeed. If one approaches acid-base metabolism along the lines of preformed cation or anion gap in a food substance, then milk (by virtue of a large anion gap) is very alkalogenic. This line of reasoning, advocated by some authorities, neglects the significant acid contribution from endogenous metabolism. Indeed, currently available data would indicate that milk formulae are acidogenic despite a large anion gap.

Metabolic Acidosis Secondary to Total Parenteral Nutrition

In a longitudinal study of five infants and children receiving total parenteral nutrition, it was shown that the acidosis occurs when the net acid excretion is less than the estimated acid production [17]. When the acid excretion exceeds the level of the estimated acid production, neutralization of the acid-base state is obtained.

There is a controversy concerning the etiology of the metabolic acidosis in this situation. On the one hand, data from one group of investigators [28] show that the acidogenic properties of amino acid mixtures are secondary to the cation gap, and that with hydrolysate solutions with an anion gap, metabolic acidosis is not seen [28]. If this postulation is correct, then hydrolysate solutions with the anion gap should have a tendency to produce metabolic alkalosis. In addition, the theoretical possibility exists that a mixture of the two solutions (with the cation gap being neutralized by the anion gap) should exert a neutral acid-base effect. However, metabolic alkalosis is rarely seen; instead, metabolic acidosis is seen in both types of amino acid infusions [23]. Thus it would seem more reasonable to study the endogenous acid production accompanying either one of these types of alimentation solution. Attention has been directed to the fact that the lysine hydrochloride in the synthetic amino acid solutions is strongly acidogenic and that the endogenous acid production, therefore, would be increased [18]. However, this issue is of lesser importance due to the fact that lower concentrations of the alimentation solutions are now being used because the potential acidogenic properties of amino acid solutions are becoming widely recognized.

Metabolic Acidosis in Chronic Renal Failure

The work of Goodman, Lemann, and Lennon [24] showed that there is positive accumulation of hydrogen ion in chronic renal failure at an average value of 20 to 30 mEq/day (Fig. 12–11). In view of the stable metabolic acidosis of 18 mM in the presence of this daily accumulation of hydrogen ion, it seems reasonable to assume that an additional buffering system is used, namely, that of the skeletal system [24]. This bone buffering of excess hydrogen ion may contribute to the development of osteoporosis and bone diseases in patients with chronic renal failure.

Acid-Base Disturbances in Patients on Hemodialysis

With the failure of the renal excretion of hydrogen ion, patients on a hemodialysis program usually suffer from metabolic acidosis. Due to the presence of the acetate in the dialysate solution, which freely diffuses across the dialysis membrane during the usual 4 to 5 hours of hemodialysis, it has been shown that in children, the metabolic acidosis is corrected in about half of the cases (Fig. 12–12). The clinical implications of persistent metabolic acidosis that is not corrected by the dialysis procedure are interesting and require additional studies. Recent data imply that the use of bicarbonate instead of acetate in the commercially available dialysate tends to reduce patient morbidity [25]. This finding emphasizes the importance of this somewhat neglected area of investigation.

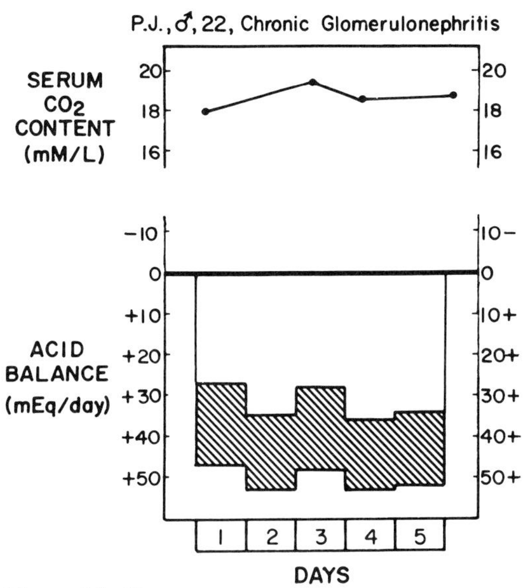

Figure 12–11
Net acid balance studies in a patient with chronic renal failure. The endogenous acid production is plotted from the zero axis downward and the net acid excretion from the bottom line upward. The net acid balance is the distance between the zero axis and the uppermost line. Note the accumulation of 20 to 30 mEq/day of acid. (Reprinted, by permission, from A. D. Goodman, J. Lemann, Jr., E. J. Lennon, et al., Production, excretion and net balance of fixed acid in patients with renal acidosis. *J. Clin. Invest.* 44:495, 1965.)

Metabolic Acidosis After Kidney Transplantation

A number of years ago, we became interested in the acid-base status of patients after kidney transplantation [19]. We were able to document that in children, the blood total CO_2 varies between a mean of 19 and 21 mM/L in cadaveric and life-related subjects (Fig. 12–13). In order to test the renal tubular acidification functions of these subjects, we carried out acid loading studies (75 mEq/m^2 of ammonium chloride administered orally). We showed that in normal subjects as well as in single-kidney subjects after donating their kidney, the urinary pH could not be brought down lower than 5.0. The minimum urinary pH stayed above 6.0 and was suggestive of an impaired ability of the distal tubule in establishing a sharp pH gradient. It has been postulated [4, 19] that this acidification defect may be related to the long period of ischemia during the transplant procedure, resulting in acute tubular necrosis and renal tubular acidosis. However, on close examination of the glomerular filtration rate, it was found that life-related and cadaveric transplant children have a glomerular filtration rate (GFR) between 80 and 100 ml/min/1.73 m^2; on fractionation of the net acid excretion by

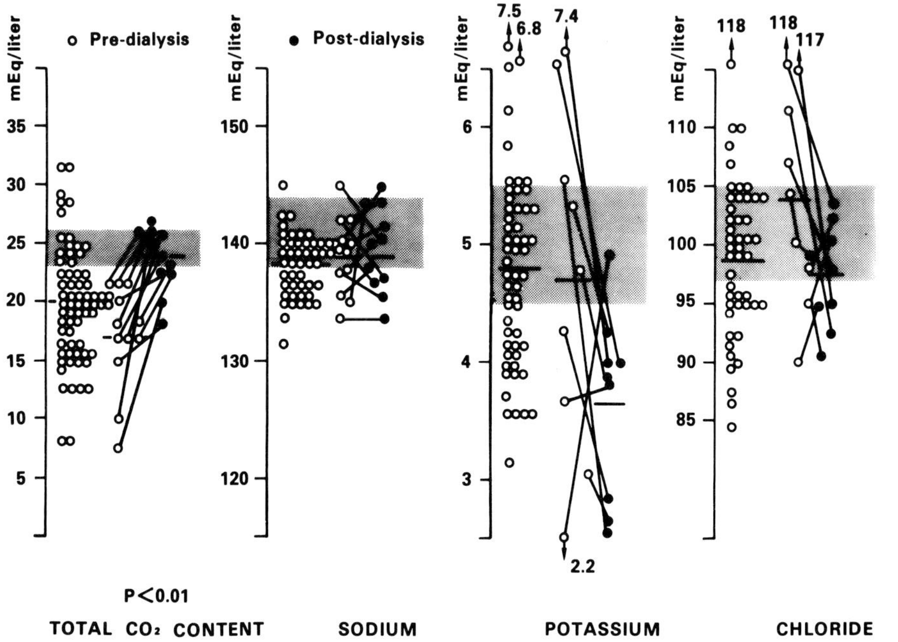

Figure 12–12
Blood acid-base data in 16 children on maintenance hemodialysis before and after a 4- to 5-hour hemodialysis procedure. Only half of the subjects have correction of the metabolic acidosis after the dialysis. (Reprinted, by permission, from J. C. M. Chan, Late complications of long-term hemodialysis in children: Clinical aspects and some measurable variables concerning parathyroid hormone, divalent ions, acid-base metabolism, anemia, nutrition, growth, and survival data. *J. Urol.* 120:578, 1978. © 1978, The Williams & Wilkins Co., Baltimore.)

GFR, the ability to excrete net acid per functioning nephron is comparable between the cadaveric-transplant subjects and the normal as well as the control (single-kidney) subjects [19]. It would seem reasonable, therefore, to assume that the metabolic acidosis occurring after transplantation may be related to the reduction in total GFR and total nephron mass. The clinical implications of the subclinical metabolic acidosis have not been determined.

Conclusions

In summary, it is important to recognize that the endogenous acid production in distal renal tubular acidotic subjects is higher than previously described and that increased amounts of alkaline therapy at dosages from 3 to 4 mEq/kg/day will be required to correct the metabolic acidosis, which will then result in sustained improvement in growth.

It should be recognized that metabolic acidosis will occur when the amount

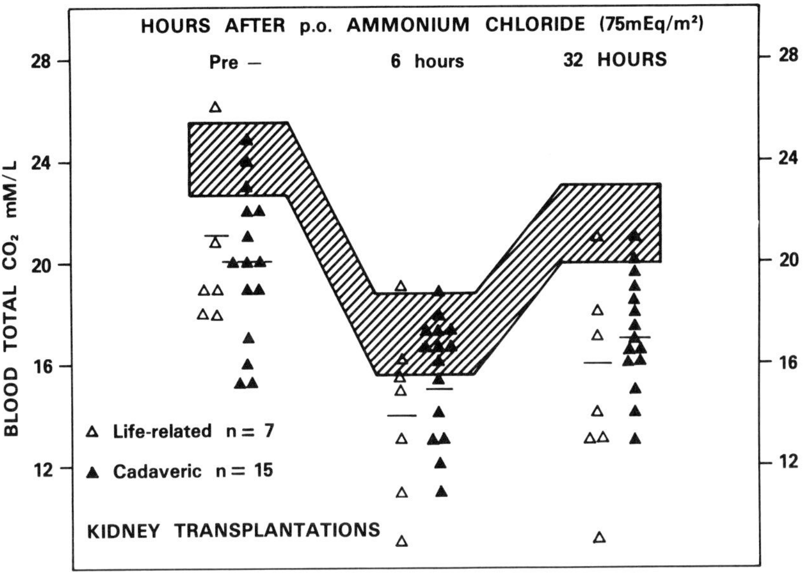

Figure 12–13
Blood acid-base data in 22 children 6 to 12 months after successful kidney transplantation. Note the metabolic acidosis in the baseline state, after ammonium chloride loading, and 6 to 32 hours afterward. Response to acid loading as reflected in the blood total CO_2 for normal single-kidney subjects is shown in the shaded areas. Note the return to normal total CO_2 in the healthy subjects with one kidney as compared to the transplanted children. (Drawn from data of J. C. M. Chan et al., The adaptation of hydrogen ion excretion associated with nephron reduction in post-transplant patients. *Pediatr. Res.* 7:712, 1973.)

of endogenous acid production exceeds the renal net acid excretory capacity. This imbalance may occur in renal failure, total parenteral nutrition, sepsis, and the ingestion of certain milk formulae in the presence of impaired renal function.

It should also be recognized that children on maintenance hemodialysis, as well as after transplantation, have asymptomatic metabolic acidosis. The clinical implication of the acidosis is yet to be determined.

Appendix 1

Renal Acidification: Testing Procedures

Light breakfast before ammonium chloride loading is permitted because of the nausea induced by the administration of ammonium chloride on an empty stomach.

At 7:30 A.M., a specimen of arterialized capillary blood is obtained for control acid-base status. During the succeeding 6 hours, fluids are administered orally at the rate of 20 ml/kg to ensure a good urine flow.

At 8:00 A.M. (zero time), ammonium chloride (a gelatin-coated rather than enteric-coated tablet) is given orally in the dosage of 75 mEq/m^2 during a 60-minute period. The bladder is emptied at 9:00 A.M.

Urine is collected at 2-hour intervals, and blood specimens for acid-base determinations are obtained at the midpoint of the urine collection period.

Aliquots of the 2-hour urine collection are utilized for determinations of net acid. Subsequently, urine is collected for a total of 6 hours after ammonium chloride administration.

For the 6 hours of the study, the patient reclines comfortably in bed and is permitted no food except free access to dextrose water.

Appendix 2

Urinary Titratable Acidity and Ammonium: Method of Determination

The quantitation of urinary titratable acidity plus ammonium minus bicarbonate, referred to as *net acid excretion,* is important in the study of renal and acid-base physiology.

The titrimetric method presented here is modified from Jorgensen [33], Kilderberg [34], and Sorensen [62] for the rapid determination of net acid excretion to the endpoints of pH 7.40, Pco_2 of 0 mm Hg, and temperature of 37° C.

Equipment

The following equipment is needed for the titrimetric method: a Radiometer pH meter (PHM 61-SG); an automatic titrator (TTT 60) with autoburette (ABU 12); a burette assembly, 2.5 ml (B 220); a titration assembly (TTA 60); and a constant temperature water bath plus thermostated jacket.

Method

A 1-ml urine sample is pipetted into thermostated vials, into which is also pipetted 1 ml of 0.100 normal HCl. This mixture is heated in a boiling water bath for 2 minutes to drive out all CO_2. After cooling for 10 minutes, the titration is carried out with 0.100 N NaOH (standardized with potassium biphthalate) to pH 7.40 at 37° C. The blank of distilled water is similarly treated. Concentration of titratable acidity (TA) is calculated as the difference in volume of NaOH required to titrate the sample and the blank, multiplied by the normality of the NaOH, times 1000; the result is the concentration of TA in millimoles per liter.

Next 1 ml of 8% formaldehyde is added, which causes the pH to drop. Without resetting the titrator, one continues the titration back to a pH of 7.40. The blank is treated in an identical fashion. The difference in the volume of NaOH used between the sample and the blank, divided by the 1-ml sample, multiplied by the normality of NaOH, times 1000 will give the net acid concentration (NAC)) in millimoles per liter. The ammonium concentration is the difference between the NAC and the TA.

The reproducibility of this method was evaluated by Chan [9] in 10 consecutive determinations of the same sample of urine. The average TA was 24.2 mM/L with S.E. of ± 0.15 mM/L; the ammonium was 38.1 mM/L with S.E. of ± 0.34 mM/L; the NAC was 62.3 mM/L with S.E. of ± 0.20. No significant change was found in urine stored at −20° C up to 30 days [9].

Appendix 3

Urinary Bicarbonate: A Titrimetric Method for Determination

The measurement of urinary bicarbonate usually relies on the Van Slyke method of 1917, which involves vacuum extraction and manometric measurements [68, 69]. This method is cumbersome and requires such meticulous care in maintenance and cleaning that the measurement of urinary bicarbonate has remained mainly a research procedure.

The titrimetric measurement of bicarbonate used in our laboratory is not new but was previously applied only to blood bicarbonate measurements. In 1965, Gyory and Edwards [26] proposed a new titrimetric method for simultaneous determination of urinary bicarbonate and titratable acidity that is comparable in accuracy to the values obtained by the Van Slyke manometric apparatus. The principle of this method lies in the observation that after the initial pH of the urine is determined, an excess of acid added to the sample will combine with urinary bicarbonate which on boiling will form carbon dioxide. The urine can be back-titrated with standard alkali to the endpoint of the original pH, thus permitting the calculation of urinary bicarbonate.

Equipment

The equipment used in this procedure is the same as that for urinary titratable acid and ammonium (see Appendix 2).

Method

After the initial pH of the urinary sample is determined in a thermostated vial at 37° C, a 1-ml sample of urine is pipetted into a titration vial containing 1 ml of 0.1 N HCl. The mixture is placed in a boiling water bath for 20 minutes to expel the CO_2. On cooling to room temperature, titration is continued to the original pH of the urine. A similarly treated blank is used as a control. The difference between the sample and the blank, multiplied by the normality of the NaOH, times 1000 will give the urinary bicarbonate in millimoles per liter.

General Comments Concerning Titrimetric Methods

The quantitative determination of urinary titratable acidity, ammonium, and bicarbonate by this automatic titrator method is convenient not only for research but also for routine use. Certain problems encountered with the Natelson microgasometer are avoided with the automatic titrator. Difficulty in obtaining consistent results is one of the major drawbacks of the microgasometer, and this problem is not encountered with the automatic titrator. In addition, the possibility of error is greater in the microgasometer because of gas leakage through the stopcock mechanism. The microgasometer is unable to measure accurately large quantities of bicarbonate (i.e., in excess of 70 mEq/L) in view of the large volume of gas formed in the reaction chamber [39]. By increasing the normality of the HCl in the titrimetric method, any quantity of urinary bicarbonate can be determined by this method.

Appendix 4

Tubular Reabsorption of Bicarbonate and the Bicarbonate Threshold

The renal tubular reabsorption of bicarbonate and the threshold at which bicarbonaturia appears (i.e., Tm bicarbonate) is important in renal physiology, especially in the diagnosis of proximal renal tubular acidosis. The simultaneous measurement of glomerular filtration rate is also a necessary component of the computations.

Equipment

The equipment used in this study includes a Foley catheter, a heparin lock, and inulin. The remainder of the equipment is similar to that used in the determination of urinary bicarbonate (see Appendix 3).

Method

In order to establish an initial state significant of metabolic acidosis (plasma bicarbonate less than 14 mEq/L), either spontaneous acidosis must be present or metabolic acidosis must be induced by an ammonium chloride loading (see Appendix 1). In a manner similar to any clearance methodology, a Foley catheter is placed in the bladder, a venous heparin lock is then set up in one limb, and infusion of inulin and bicarbonate solution is set up in the other limb.

After verifying that a state of metabolic acidosis is established, the bicarbonate-inulin perfusion is initiated. The concentration and rate of perfusion are computed to elevate the blood bicarbonate concentration by 1 mEq per hour. Significant bicarbonaturia is suggested by the urinary pH exceeding 7.5, at which point the rate of bicarbonate infusion is doubled.

The bladder is air-washed every 20 minutes and blood samples taken at the midpoint of each period. Urinary and plasma pH and bicarbonate and inulin concentrations are measured.

The tubular reabsorption of bicarbonate is calculated according to the clearance principle of

$$\frac{UV}{P} \div 100 \text{ ml GFR}$$

where U = urinary concentration of bicarbonate in milliequivalents per liter,
V = urinary flow rate in milliliters per minute,
P = plasma concentration of bicarbonate in milliequivalents per liter, and
GFR = glomerular filtration rate as estimated by inulin clearance.

The filtered urinary bicarbonate can then be calculated from the amount of renal tubular reabsorption and the quantity of urinary excretion of bicarbonate, and the titration curve is constructed accordingly.

It is necessary that a physician and a nurse be in attendance throughout the procedure because of the risks of tetany secondary to metabolic alkalosis, hypokalemia, and the possibility of fluid overload.

References

1. Albert, M. S. Acid-base disorders in pediatrics. *Pediatr. Clin. North Am.* 23(4):639, 1978.
2. Anuda, J. A. C., and Kurtzman, N. A. Metabolic acidosis and alkalosis. *Clin. Nephrol.* 7:201, 1977.
3. Bartter, F. C. Hyper-renal hypoosmolalitats Syndrome. *Fortschutte der Medizin* 82:55, 1964.
4. Better, O. S., Chaimovitz, C., Naveh, Y., et al. Syndrome of incomplete renal tubular acidosis after cadaver kidney transplantation. *Ann. Intern. Med.* 71:39, 1969.
5. Blum, J. E., and Coe, F. C. Metabolic acidosis after sulfur injection. *N. Engl. J. Med.* 297:869, 1977.
6. Booth, B. E., Tsai, H. C., and Morris, R. C., Jr. Metabolic acidosis in the vitamin D-deficient chick. *Metabolism* 26:1099, 1977.
7. Bronsted, J. N. Einige Bemerkungen uber der Begriff der Sauren und Basen. *Rec. Trav. Chem. Pays-Bas* 42:718, 1923.
8. Chan, J. C. M. The influence of synthetic amino acid and casein hydrolysate solutions on the endogenous acid production and urinary excretion of acid in total intravenous alimentation. *Pediatr. Res.* 6:789, 1972.
9. Chan, J. C. M. The rapid determination of urinary titratable acid and ammonium and evaluation of freezing as a method of preservation. *Clin. Biochem.* 5:94, 1972.
10. Chan, J. C. M. The effect of milk formulae on acid balance. *Nutr. Metab.* 16:140, 1974.
11. Chan, J. C. M. Hydrogen ion production secondary to metabolism of sulfur-amino acids and organic acids. *Nutr. Metab.* 22:288, 1978.
12. Chan, J. C. M. Peritoneal dialysis for renal failure in children: Clinical aspects and electrolyte changes as observed in 20 cases. *Clin. Pediatr.* 17:349, 1978.
13. Chan, J. C. M. Renal electrolyte and mineral disorders in children. *Curr. Probl. Pediatr.* 8:1, 1978.

14. Chan, J. C. M. Urinary sulfate excretion in children with classic renal tubular acidosis. *Nutr. Metab.* 22:257, 1978.
15. Chan, J. C. M. Late complications of long-term hemodialysis in children: Clinical aspects and some measurable variables concerning parathyroid hormone, divalent ions, acid-base metabolism, anemia, nutrition, growth, and survival data. *J. Urol.* 120:578, 1978.
16. Chan, J. C. M. Acid-base, calcium, potassium and aldosterone metabolism in renal tubular acidosis. *Nephron* 23:152, 1979.
17. Chan, J. C. M., Asch, M. J., Lin, S., et al. Hyperalimentation with amino acid and casein hydrolysate solutions: Mechanisms of acidosis. *J. A. M. A.* 220:1700, 1972.
18. Chan, J. C. M., Chaimovitz, C., and Ma, R. S. W. Acidity, osmolality, electrolyte and amino acid concentration of casein-hydrolysate and synthetic amino acid solutions. *Clin. Biochem.* 6:46, 1973.
19. Chan, J. C. M., Grushkin, C. M., Malekzadeh, M., et al. The adaption of hydrogen ion excretion associated with nephron reduction in post-transplant patients. *Pediatr. Res.* 7:712, 1973.
20. Edelman, C. M., Jr., Rodriquez-Soriano, J., Borchis, H., et al. Renal bicarbonate reabsorption and hydrogen ion excretion in normal infants. *J. Clin. Invest.* 46:1309, 1967.
21. Felig, P. Diabetic ketoacidosis. *N. Engl. J. Med.* 290:1360, 1974.
22. Finkelstein, J. D. Enzyme Defects in Sulfur Amino Acid Metabolism in Man. In D. M. Greenburg (Ed.), *Metabolism of Sulfur Compounds.* New York: Academic, 1975.
23. Fraley, D. S., Adler, S., Bruns, F., and Segal, D. Metabolic acidosis after hyperalimentation with a casein hydrolysate, occurrence in a starved patient. *Ann. Intern. Med.* 88:352, 1978.
24. Goodman, A. D., Lemann, J., Jr., Lennon, E. J., et al. Production, excretion and net balance of fixed acid in patients with renal acidosis. *J. Clin. Invest.* 44:495, 1965.
25. Graefe, V., Milutinovich, J., Follette, W. C., et al. Less dialysis—induced morbidity and vascular instability with bicarbonate in dialysate. *Ann. Intern. Med.* 88:332, 1978.
26. Gyory, A. Z., and Edwards, K. D. G. Simultaneous titrimetric determination of bicarbonate and titratable acid of urine. *Aust. J. Exp. Biol. Med. Sci.* 45:495, 1965.
27. Healy, C. E. Acidosis and failure to thrive in infants fed Nutramigen. *Pediatrics* 49:910, 1972.
28. Heird, W. C., Dell, R. B., Driscoll, J. M., Jr., et al. Metabolic acidosis resulting from intravenous alimentation mixtures containing synthetic amino acids. *N. Engl. J. Med.* 287:254, 1972.
29. Henderson, L. J. Dos Gleicheur cht zurischen Basen und Sauren in tierischen Organizmus. *Engebn. Physiol.* 8:254, 1909.
30. Hirschman, G. H., and Chan, J. C. M. Complex acid-base disorder in subacute encephalopathy (Leigh's syndrome). *Pediatrics* 61:278, 1978.
31. Hunt, J. N. The influence of dietary sulfur on the urinary out-put of acid in man. *Clin. Sci.* 15:119, 1956.
32. Jenkins, D. W., Eckel, R. E., and Craig, J. W. Alcoholic ketoacidosis. *J. A. M. A.* 217:177, 1971.
33. Jorgensen, K. Titrimetric determination of the net excretion of acid/base in urine. *Scand. J. Clin. Lab. Invest.* 9:281, 1957.
34. Kilderberg, P. *Clinical Acid-Base Physiology: Studies in Neonates, Infants and Young Children.* Baltimore: Williams & Wilkins, 1968.

35. Kilderberg, P., Engel, K., and Winters, R. W. Balance of net acid in growing infants, endogenous and transintestinal aspects. *Acta Paediatr.* (Uppsala) 58:321, 1969.
36. Lee, S. W., Russell, J., and Avioli, L. V. 25-hydroxy-cholecalciferol to 1,25-dihydroxycholecalciferol: Conversion impaired by systemic metabolic acidosis. *Science* 195:994, 1977.
37. Lemann, J., Jr., Lennon, E. J., Goodman, A. D., et al. The net balance of acid in subjects given large loads of acid and alkali. *J. Clin. Invest.* 44:507, 1965.
38. Lemann, J., Jr., Litzow, J. R., and Lennon, E. J. The effects of chronic acid loads in normal man: Further evidence for the participation of bone mineral in the defense against chronic metabolic acidosis. *J. Clin. Invest.* 45:1608, 1966.
39. Lin, S. L., and Chan, J. C. M. Urinary bicarbonate: A titrimetric method for determination. *Clin. Biochem.* 6:207, 1973.
40. Makoff, D. L., Da Silva, J. A., and Rosenbaum, B. J. Hypertonic expansion: Acid-base and electrolyte changes. *Am. J. Physiol.* 218:1201, 1970.
41. McSherry, E., and Morris, R. C., Jr. Attainment acid maintenance of normal stature with alkali therapy in infants and children with classic renal tubular acidosis. *J. Clin. Invest.* 61:509, 1978.
42. Meng, H. C., Stahlman, M. T., and Otten, A. The use of crystalline amino acid mixture for parenteral nutrition in low-birth-weight infants. *Pediatrics* 59:699, 1977.
43. Moore, A., Ansell, C., and Barrie, H. Metabolic acidosis and infant feeding. *Br. Med. J.* 1:129, 1977.
44. Natelson, S. *Microtechniques of Clinical Chemistry* (2nd ed.). Springfield, Ill.: Thomas, 1963.
45. Oh, M. S., and Carrol, H. J. Current concepts: The anion gap. *N. Engl. J. Med.* 297:814, 1977.
46. Oliver, P. B. Phenformin and lactic acidosis. *Ann. Intern. Med.* 38:548, 1969.
47. Orrigen, C. E., Eustace, J. C., and Wunsch, C. D. Natural history of lactic acidosis after grand-mal seizures: A model for the study of an anion-ion gap acidosis not associated with hyperkalemia. *N. Engl. J. Med.* 297:796, 1977.
48. O'Shaughnessy, W. R. Experiments in blood in cholera. *Lancet* 1:490, 1831.
49. Peters, J. P., and Van Slyke, D. D. *Hemoglobin and Oxygen, Carbonic Acid and Acid-Base Balance.* Baltimore: Williams & Wilkins, 1932.
50. Pitts, R. F. Renal production and excretion of ammonia. *Am. J. Med.* 36:720, 1964.
51. Pitts, R. F., and Alexander, R. S. The nature of the renal tubular mechanism for acidifying the urine. *Am. J. Physiol.* 144:239, 1945.
52. Rector, F. C., Jr. Acidification of the Urine. In J. Orloff and R. W. Berliner (Eds.), *Handbook of Physiology,* Section 8: *Renal Physiology.* Baltimore: Williams & Wilkins, 1973.
53. Relman, A. S. Renal acidosis and renal excretion of acid in health and disease. *Adv. Intern. Med.* 12:295, 1964.
54. Relman, A. S. The acidosis of renal disease. *Am. J. Med.* 44:706, 1968.
55. Relman, A. S., Lennon, E. J., and Lemann, J., Jr. Endogenous production of fixed acid and the measurements of the net balance of acid in normal subjects. *J. Clin. Invest.* 40:1621, 1961.
56. Ritz, E., and Heikland, A. Lactic acidosis. *Clin. Nephrol.* 7:231, 1977.
57. Schuartz, A. B., and Lyons, J. *Acid-Base and Electrolyte Balance, Normal Regulation and Clinical Disorders.* New York: Grune & Stratton, 1977.
58. Schwartz, W. B., Hall, P. W., IV, Hays, R. M., et al. On the mechanism of acidosis in chronic renal failure. *J. Clin. Invest.* 38:39, 1959.
59. Schwartz, W. B., Jansen, R. L., and Relman, A. S. The deposition of acid ad-

ministered to sodium-depleted subjects: The renal response and the role of whole body buffers. *J. Clin. Invest.* 33:587, 1954.
60. Schwartz, W. B., and Kassirer, J. P. Effects of Ureteral Transplantation. In M. B. Strauss and L. G. Welt (Eds.), *Diseases of the Kidney* (1st ed.). Boston: Little, Brown, 1963. P. 759.
61. Sebastian, A., McSherry, E., and Morris, R. C., Jr. Metabolic Acidosis with Special Reference to Renal Acidosis. In B. M. Brenner and F. C. Rector (Eds.), *The Kidney*. Philadelphia: Saunders, 1976.
62. Sorensen, S. P. L. Enzymstudiem: I. Über die quantitative Messung proteolytische Spaltungen. *Biochem.* 7:45, 1908.
63. Sorensen, S. P. L. Enzymstudiem: II. Über die Messung und die Bedeutung der Wasserstoffionenkon-zentration bei enzymatischen Prozessen. *Biochem. Z.* 21:301, 1909.
64. Walter, F. Untersuchungen über die Wirkung der Sauren auf der thierischen Organism. *Arch. Exp. Pathol. Pharmacol.* 7:148, 1877.
65. Weil, W. B. A unified guide to parenteral fluid therapy. *J. Pediatr.* 75:1, 1969.
66. West, C. D., and Smith, W. C. An attempt to elucidate the cause of growth retardation in renal disease. *Am. J. Dis. Child.* 91:460, 1956.
67. Wrong, O., and Davies, H. E. F. The excretion of acid in renal disease. *Q. J. Med.* 28:259, 1958.
68. Van Slyke, D. D. Studies of acidosis: II. A method for the determination of carbon dioxide and carbonates in solution. *J. Biol. Chem.* 30:347, 1917.
69. Van Slyke, D. D., and Neill, J. M. The determination of gases in blood and other solutions by vacuum extraction and manometric measurement. *J. Biol. Chem.* 61:523, 1924.
70. Van Slyke, D. D., Wu, H., and Nichea, F. C. Studies of gas and electrolyte equilibrium in the blood: V. Factors controlling the electrolyte and water distribution in the blood. *J. Biol. Chem.* 56:765, 1923.

13. Nuclear Medicine Procedures in Nephrology

James S. Robertson

Any administration of radioactive material to a patient for diagnostic, therapeutic, or research purposes could rightfully be regarded as being a nuclear medicine procedure. In nephrology, however, several such procedures are more typically conducted in laboratories bearing other designations, and it is logical to describe these procedures in contexts other than that of nuclear medicine. In particular, attention is called to the discussions of [^{125}I] iothalamate clearance, [^{131}I] Hippuran clearance, and radioimmunoassay, which are concerned with the uses of radioactive agents but which appear in other chapters of this book. Radionuclides have been used to study renal blood flow [20], the glomerular filtration rate [27, 53], and effective renal plasma flow [12]. Some other applications of radionuclides in nephrology, including animal studies, are presented in the book by Blaufox and Funck-Brentano [6]. In the present chapter attention is confined to two types of basic nuclear medicine procedures, kidney scanning and the production of renograms.

Imaging

Definition

In nuclear medicine the term *imaging* refers to any of several methods that are used for producing a mapping of the distribution of a radioactive agent. The procedure is sometimes called *scintigraphy* and the resultant mapping is called a *scintiscan,* which implies that the mapping, or picture, is obtained through the use of a scintillator for radiation detection. The procedure is also often called *scanning,* which may or may not be accurate depending on the method used.

Instrumentation

By far the most popular scintillator currently in routine use is the thallium-activated sodium iodide crystal NaI(Tl). The passage of a gamma ray through such a crystal causes it to emit flashes of light. In a typical system, the flashes of light produced in the crystal are in turn detected by a photomultiplier tube, which responds by producing an electrical pulse. These electrical pulses may be analyzed electronically to select those pulses that correspond to the gamma ray energy of interest. In the final output, the selected signals are translated by recording devices into marks on paper or spots on photographic film, or they may be displayed on a cathode ray tube (CRT).

Historically, scintiscans have been (and to a large extent still are) achieved through the use of radiation detection devices called rectilinear scanners, in which the detector moves back and forth in a boustrophedon pattern across the area of interest. The location of the output from the recording device is mechanically or electronically synchronized with the location of the detector so that there is a correspondence between the location of the source of activity and that of its representation in the display. This imaging method is correctly referred to as scanning.

Another imaging method involves the use of gamma scintillation cameras, which achieve a comparable end result, but which (at least for renal imaging) typically remain stationary. However, by extension this method is also sometimes called scanning. Modern gamma cameras have NaI(Tl) crystals that are 25 cm or greater in diameter by a few millimeters thick. The crystals are seen by an array of photomultiplier tubes mounted in concentric rings on the back side of the crystal. The light flashes produced by a given gamma ray appear more intense to the photomultiplier tubes near the site of the flashes in the crystal than to those further away. This difference provides localizing information that is used by appropriate electronic circuits to assign a location in the display to each event. Thus with a gamma camera the picture is built up throughout its entirety over a period of time as dictated by the random emission of gamma rays, rather than being constructed line by line as with the rectilinear scanner. Usually a parallel-hole collimator is used with a gamma camera, but diverging collimators may be used to enlarge the field of view, or converging or "pinhole" collimators may be used to produce magnified images.

Biological Factors

If the radioactive agent localizes in a particular organ, the shape and location of that organ may be defined in a scintigram. Clearly, however, such a result must involve more than simply anatomy. In order for the radioactivity to become localized at a site of interest it first has to be delivered to that location, usually in the circulating blood. Next, there must be an extraction that transfers the activity from the blood to the organ. The activity may remain trapped or may be eliminated from the organ by return to the blood or by an excretory process. The choice of the radioactive agent to be used thus depends in part on what mixture of anatomical and physiological information is desired. The interplay of glomerular filtration, tubular secretion, and tubular absorption processes makes the kidney a particularly interesting organ for study with radioactive tracers.

Radiopharmaceuticals

Numerous radiopharmaceuticals are available for use in renal studies. Arnold and colleagues [1] have made comparisons of 17 different agents for renal imaging in the rabbit and have reviewed the results obtained with some of these agents in humans. Partly as a result of the chemical and physical differences among these agents, they differ in the mechanisms of their uptake and excretion and thus provide different kinds of information about the kidneys.

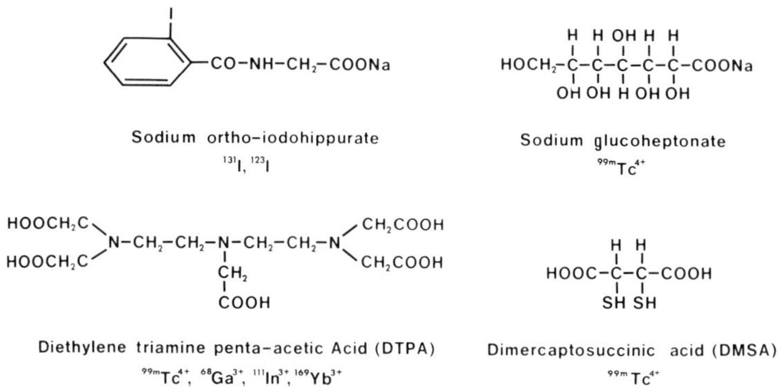

Figure 13–1
Structural formulas for four representative radiopharmaceuticals used in renal studies.

Instead of attempting to discuss all the agents that have ever been used for renal imaging, this chapter will concentrate on four representative agents currently in use. These agents are (1) iodine-131-labeled sodium ortho-iodohippurate ([^{131}I] Hippuran, Hipputope); (2) technetium-99m-labeled diethylenetriamine penta-acetic acid ([^{99m}Tc] DTPA); (3) technetium-99m-labeled dimercaptosuccinic acid ([^{99m}Tc] DMSA); and (4) technetium-99m-labeled glucoheptonate ([^{99m}Tc] GH). The chemical structural formulas for these four compounds are shown in Figure 13–1, and their radiation absorbed doses are listed in Table 13–1. The radiation doses for [^{131}I] Hippuran are from reference 37; the others are from reference 1. Pediatric doses are given in reference 11.

Mercury-197 and mercury-203-labeled chlormerodrin, a diuretic, have been used for renal imaging but have the disadvantage of giving relatively high patient radiation doses. Various labeled forms of gluconate have also been used [7]. However, the use of these and other agents for renal imaging has been superseded to a large extent by the use of one or another of the four representative agents.

In certain renal infections there is an increased concentration of ^{67}Ga in the kidneys [34]. A case of ^{67}Ga localization in renal microabscess has been described [44]; renal localization of ^{67}Ga in renal amyloidosis has also been reported [3].

Another point of interest is that some renal and urological abnormalities may be discovered incidentally in bone scans [36, 58], which adds the bone scan agents to the list of those of use in renal imaging. These agents include ^{99m}Tc-labeled pyrophosphate, diphosphonate, and polyphosphate complexes. Later in this chapter examples will be given of renal abnormalities being discovered through scans performed for other purposes.

Table 13–1. Radiation Absorbed Doses for Agents Used in Renal Imaging (Rads/mCi)

Target Organ	[^{131}I] Hippuran	[^{99m}Tc] DTPA	[^{99m}Tc] Glucoheptonate	[^{99m}Tc] DMSA
Renal cortices	—	—	0.20	0.76
Whole kidneys	0.08	0.042	0.17	0.62
Bladder mucosa	0.29	0.55	0.80	0.28
Ovaries	0.13	0.019	0.020	0.022
Blood	—	—	0.010	0.019
Total body	0.11	0.016	0.007	0.016
Maximum administered dose (mCi)	0.35	5	10	5

Note: The tabulated absorbed radiation doses are calculated for the standard 70-kg man and for an administered dose of 1 mCi. These values are multiplied by the actual administered dose to obtain the absorbed dose in a given individual. A correction for weight may be necessary.

The following sections discuss the four representative renal imaging agents in detail.

SODIUM ORTHO-IODOHIPPURATE. Iodohippurate is a radiopaque substance that has been used as a contrast agent in urology. It is chemically similar to para-aminohippuric acid, an agent traditionally used to evaluate renal function. The use of a labeled form of another contrast agent, [^{131}I] sodium iodopyracet, for the radioisotopic renogram was originally developed by Taplin and colleagues [54]. However, 10 to 15 percent of this agent is collected in the liver, which interferes with studies of the right kidney. Nordyke and co-workers [43] showed the advantage of [^{131}I] sodium ortho-iodohippurate for renograms, and Wenzl and associates [59] began the use of this agent in renal scintigraphy. The kinetics of [^{131}I] sodium ortho-iodohippurate will be discussed subsequently in the section on renograms. The rapid excretion rate of this substance renders it unsuitable for renal imaging by rectilinear scanning. However, good images may be obtained with a gamma scintillation camera. It is now used for the imaging that is incidental to producing renograms, but as a primary renal imaging agent it has largely been replaced by other agents.

DTPA. The use of [^{99m}Tc] DTPA for kidney scanning was initiated by Hauser and co-workers [23]. Their studies indicate that following intravenous injection, [^{99m}Tc] DTPA rapidly becomes uniformly distributed throughout the extracellular space without crossing the normal blood-brain barrier and that it is rapidly and probably almost exclusively eliminated by the kidneys. Other studies show that the mechanism of excretion in the kidney is by glomerular filtration. DTPA has been used to measure the glomerular filtration rate, but because there is some protein binding, the result is lower than that determined by inulin studies [2]. In dynamic flow studies it may be used to demonstrate the quality of renal perfusion.

When [^{99m}Tc] DTPA is used as a kidney scanning agent, the maximum concentration is found in the kidney at 3 to 5 minutes after intravenous injection. The kidneys should be seen in the scan at about the same time as activity appears in the major arteries. There is little or no binding of the chelate to the renal parenchyma, and it is not normally retained in the kidney.

DTPA may also be labeled with other agents such as ^{51}Cr, ^{68}Ga, ^{111}In, ^{113m}In, or ^{169}Yb. In certain applications it may be advantageous to use one of these agents rather than [^{99m}Tc] DTPA.

DMSA. DMSA is a chelate that has organomercurial-like kinetics in that it is selectively extracted from the blood by the kidney, and it is not excreted into the urine in appreciable quantities. When labeled with ^{99m}Tc, DMSA becomes an agent for imaging the renal parenchyma without activity in the urinary collection system [22, 35]. It is commercially available in kit form as an aqueous solution of 2,3-dimercaptosuccinic acid and stannous chloride; the user labels this agent by adding ^{99m}Tc pertechnetate solution and mixing.

GLUCOHEPTONATE. [^{99m}Tc] glucoheptonate has been developed relatively recently as an agent for renal imaging [30, 39]. It is also of use in brain imaging, and it has been proposed that the two procedures be combined in a single study [30]. The renal concentration of [^{99m}Tc] glucoheptonate is not as great as that for [^{99m}Tc] DMSA, but its blood and urinary clearance are much faster, resulting in lower radiation doses to most organs [1]. Glucoheptonate also has a longer shelf life than DMSA. Between the first and fourth hour after injection, about 22 percent of the injected dose is found in the kidneys. Early camera images with [^{99m}Tc] glucoheptonate show both the renal parenchyma and the collecting system, but in later images the parenchyma alone is seen [1]. Glucoheptonate is commercially available in kit form for labeling with ^{99m}Tc by the user.

Applications

The renal scan (Fig. 13–2) shows the size, shape, and location of the kidneys and gives some indication of the relative quality of their blood perfusion and their ability to secrete urine. Space-occupying lesions, including abscesses, cysts, and neoplasms, appear as cold areas if sufficient renal parenchymal tissue has been displaced or replaced [24, 40] (Fig. 13–3). Congenital abnormalities such as fetal lobulation, a pelvic kidney, or horseshoe kidneys are readily detected on a renal scan [24] (Fig. 13–4). The following list* gives the indications for

* Reprinted, by permission, from J. L. Izenstark, Scintillation Scan Techniques in the Evaluation of Renal Disease. In J. L. Quinn (Ed.), *Scintillation Scanning in Clinical Medicine.* Philadelphia: Saunders, 1964. Pp. 245–257.

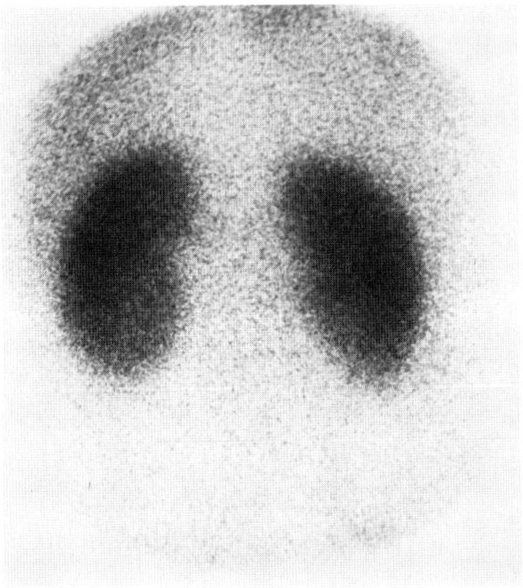

Figure 13–2
Normal kidney images obtained by intravenous administration of 5 mCi of [^{99m}Tc] DMSA in a 36-year-old woman, using a gamma camera.

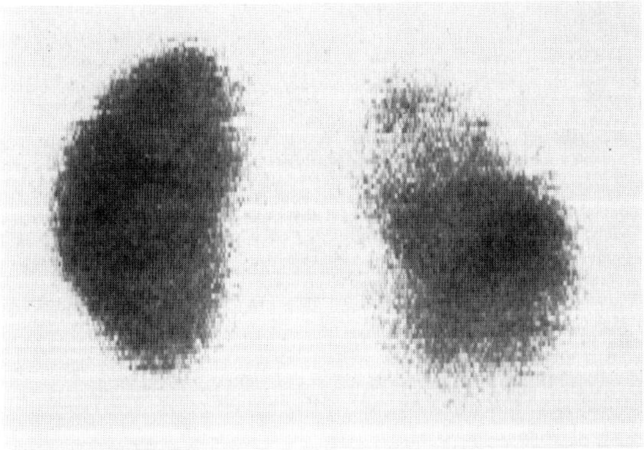

Figure 13–3
Filling defect due to renal abscess in upper pole of right kidney in a 6-year-old boy. Agent: 1.25 mCi of [^{99m}Tc] DMSA. Rectilinear scanner.

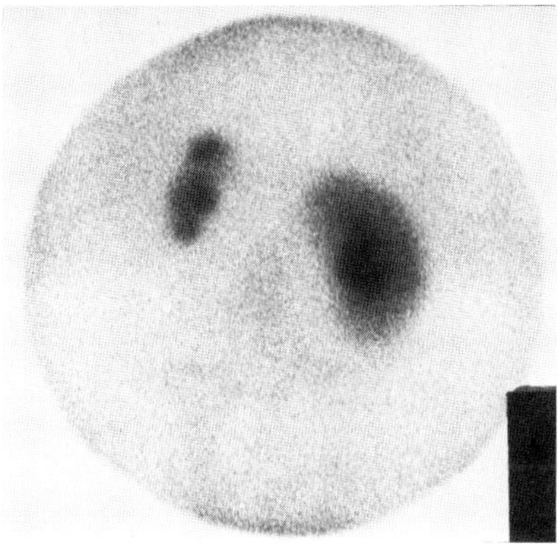

Figure 13–4
Small left kidney with compensatory hypertrophy of the right kidney in a 45-year-old woman. Agent: 22 mCi of [^{99m}Tc] glucoheptonate. With this agent activity is seen in the renal pelvis, in contrast to the case with DMSA.

kidney scanning that were recognized about 15 years ago; to this list may now be added dynamic studies for the evaluation of renal perfusion and the status of renal transplants.

- I. Roentgenographic inadequacy
  - A. Allergy to iodides
  - B. Inadequate roentgenography
    1. Obesity
    2. Repeated failure at adequate bowel cleaning
    3. Inability to visualize renal outlines satisfactorily
- II. Spatial evaluation
  - A. Congenital anomalies
  - B. Tumor
- III. Functional evaluation
  - A. Vascular disorders
  - B. Inflammatory disorders
  - C. Renal insufficiency

The general principles of renal evaluation with radionuclides have recently been reviewed by Blaufox and Bell [5], who discuss some applications in the measurement of glomerular filtration, tubular secretion, renal plasma flow, renal blood flow, and clearance measurements. Bell and Blaufox [4] discuss certain clinical applications including anomalies, urinary tract infection, renal vascular diseases, renal tumors, traumatic lesions, diffuse renal disease, and transplant evaluation. These articles should be consulted for reference to the early literature on renal imaging. Other clinical applications have been reported in urology [29, 50], in renal failure [48], and in trauma [33].

An interesting pitfall to be avoided in the interpretation of renal scans is the appearance of a phantom kidney at the site of a congenitally or surgically absent kidney [25]. Evidently other structures can occupy the renal space and in the perfusion phase can simulate the appearance of the kidney. The distinction is readily made, however, on the basis of the lack of filtration and excretion functions on the affected side.

A rare condition that may be discovered in a renal scan is an ectopic kidney. Strakosch and colleagues [52] report an ectopic kidney that in a ^{99m}Tc macroaggregated ferrous hydroxide liver-lung scan had the appearance of a subphrenic abscess. That this coincided with the location of the kidney was shown in a [^{99m}Tc]-Fe-gluconate renal scan. The kidney had also been seen in a [^{99m}Tc] polyphosphate bone scan.

In another study [19] an upward displacement of the kidney due to the presence of a pheochromocytoma was seen in a myocardial scintigram with ^{99m}Tc stannous pyrophosphate.

Even a normal kidney may produce an abnormality in a liver scan, and it has been suggested that the kidney be considered as a possibility in cases of a "nonspecific periportal defect" [41].

In the diagnosis of angiotensinogenic hypertension, renal imaging with [^{99m}Tc] glucoheptonate and [^{131}I] Hippuran has proved valuable in indicating which patients had a unilateral abnormality [38].

EVALUATION OF RENAL TRANSPLANTS. A major application of renal imaging has developed in the evaluation of renal transplants [16, 26, 60]. Shortly after surgery, a dynamic renal scan is useful in demonstrating the adequacy of the perfusion of the transplant by the blood [16]. In later studies renal imaging is useful in detecting acute tubular necrosis (ATN) and rejection, although the distinction between these two processes is often difficult. Renal imaging also demonstrates the ability of the transplant to excrete urine and is useful in detecting the presence of aberrant urine paths.

The same radiopharmaceuticals that are used in studies of the natural kidneys are useful in renal transplant studies. Our routine for transplant studies is first to obtain a dynamic study with 14 mCi of [^{99m}Tc] DTPA to evaluate the transplant's blood perfusion and the early clearance. For the dynamic study, images are obtained at 2-second intervals for the first minute; second and sixth minute static scans are then obtained. Using computerized data processing, the appearance and disappearance of the [^{99m}Tc] DTPA in the transplant is compared with the simultaneous blood curve produced by flagging an area over one of the iliac arteries, preferably the one supplying the transplant (Fig. 13–5). The DTPA study is followed by a 20-minute study using 0.35 mCi of [^{131}I] Hippuran and producing a camera renogram with static views for the 0 to 3, 10 to 13, and 17 to 20 minute intervals being selected for interpretation. The bladder is usually included in the field of view of the static scans, and the rate

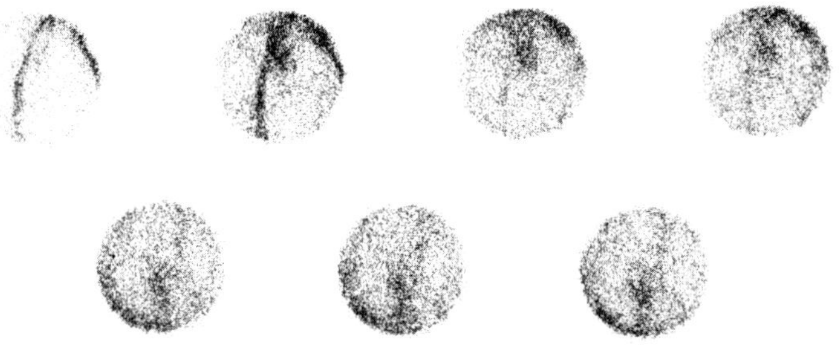

Figure 13–5
Dynamic study with [^{99m}Tc] DTPA in a renal transplant. Activity is seen in the transplant shortly after its appearance in the iliac artery and then rapidly disappears. Frames are at 2-second intervals.

of appearance of activity in the bladder is an aid in evaluating the ability of the transplant to excrete urine.

The normally functioning transplant shows a uniform distribution of [^{99m}Tc] DTPA throughout the renal parenchyma. There is a peak of activity in the transplant at the same time as in the iliac artery, and the [^{99m}Tc] DTPA then washes out to about half of the peak value in a few seconds and certainly within the first minute. In the Hippuran studies the activity goes through a maximum at 3 to 5 minutes, and the distribution is uniform (Fig. 13–6). Next there is a gradual diminution of activity in the parenchyma to about twice the background level at 20 minutes. During the 3- to 20-minute period a relatively increased level of activity may be seen in the collecting system, depending on the rate of urine flow. The Hippuran renogram is very similar to the renograms obtained in normal kidneys in situ, as described in a subsequent section (Fig. 13–7).

As has been mentioned, the distinction between ATN and rejection of a renal transplant may be difficult. However, it is very important to make the distinction, if possible, because the therapy is different for the two conditions.

George and colleagues [17] have studied the problem of distinguishing between ATN and rejection, using [^{99m}Tc] pertechnetate and [^{131}I] Hippuran. In ATN they found the most consistent feature to be a continuous accumulation of Hippuran with no clearance at 20 minutes. Except in delayed studies, there was an absence of bladder activity. The pertechnetate studies showed normal perfusion with poor washout in 83 percent of the patients. In transplants undergoing rejection there was a variable pattern. In 18 percent there was no visualization of the transplant with either Hippuran or pertechnetate; such cases require renal arteriography for differentiation from vascular obstruction. Eighty-two percent of all rejecting transplants showed enlargement on serial examination. Nonhomogeneous uptake was often seen. The renal transit times were normal more often than not, but parenchymal clearance at 20 minutes tended

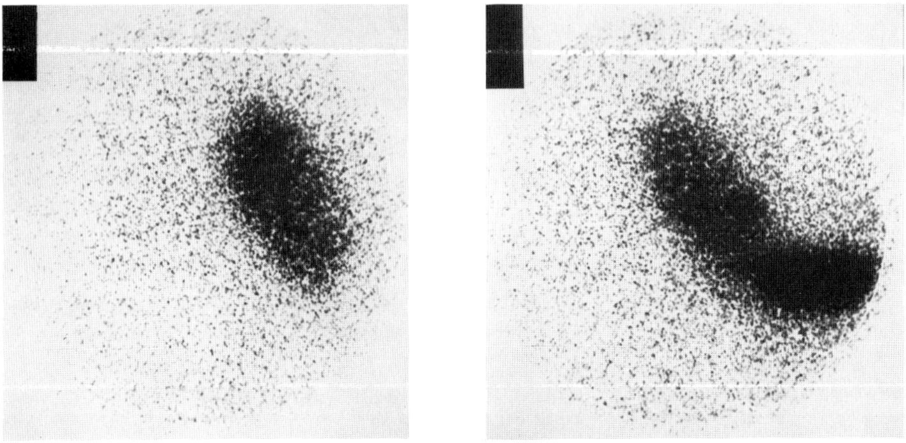

A B

Figure 13–6
Functioning kidney transplant studied with [^{131}I] Hippuran. (A) Scan at 3 to 5 minutes shows uniform distribution in normal size transplant. (B) Scan at 10 to 12 minutes shows excretion from the transplant into the bladder.

to be poor or absent. Twenty-nine percent showed continuous accumulation of activity in the transplant; in these cases it is particularly difficult to exclude ATN.

Of course, the transplant history provides additional information that may be helpful in making the clinical decision. The ischemia associated with the surgical transplant procedure leads to an early ATN. After the first week symptoms of acute rejection may develop, and these symptoms may be superimposed on ATN. Subsequent changes in the perfusion pattern and enlargement of the transplant in a transplant that has been functioning well probably indicate chronic rejection.

Rejection has also been studied with [^{99m}Tc] sulfur colloid ([^{99m}Tc] SC) [18, 32], with mixed results. Kim and associates [32] concluded that [^{99m}Tc] SC accumulation in renal transplants appears to be a useful indicator of rejection in the absence of other causes of renal accumulation, such as sepsis. The

Figure 13–7
Computerized gamma camera studies of a normally functioning renal transplant. (A) [^{99m}Tc] DTPA study showing good perfusion and normal washout. The vertical lines in the graph represent 10-second intervals. At 6 minutes the activity is mostly in the renal pelvis and the bladder. (B) [^{131}I] Hippuran study. There is maximal activity in the transplant at 3 minutes. At 10 and 20 minutes nearly all the activity seen is in the bladder. Normal renogram is obtained by light-penning the transplant area exclusive of the overlying bladder area.

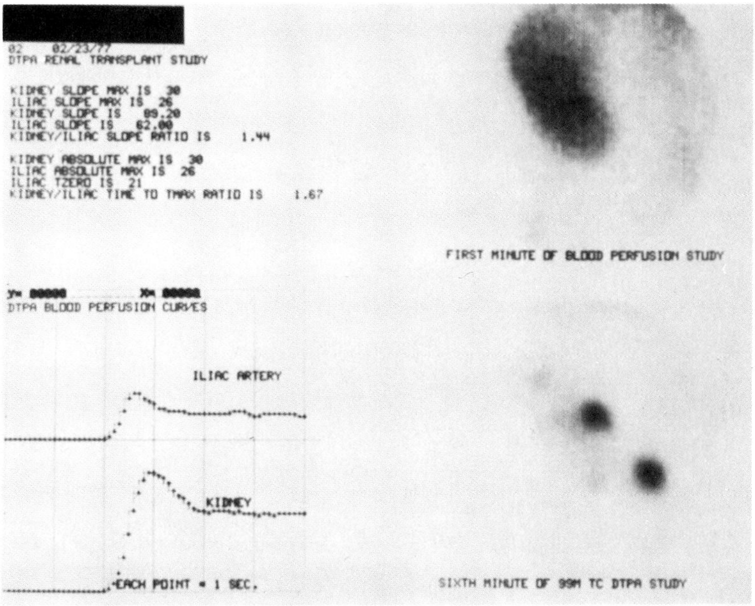
[redacted]
02 02/23/77
DTPA RENAL TRANSPLANT STUDY
KIDNEY SLOPE MAX IS 30
ILIAC SLOPE MAX IS 26
KIDNEY SLOPE IS 89.20
ILIAC SLOPE IS 62.00
KIDNEY/ILIAC SLOPE RATIO IS 1.44
KIDNEY ABSOLUTE MAX IS 30
ILIAC ABSOLUTE MAX IS 26
ILIAC TZERO IS 21
KIDNEY/ILIAC TIME TO TMAX RATIO IS 1.67
FIRST MINUTE OF BLOOD PERFUSION STUDY
DTPA BLOOD PERFUSION CURVES
ILIAC ARTERY
KIDNEY
EACH POINT = 1 SEC.
SIXTH MINUTE OF 99M TC DTPA STUDY

A

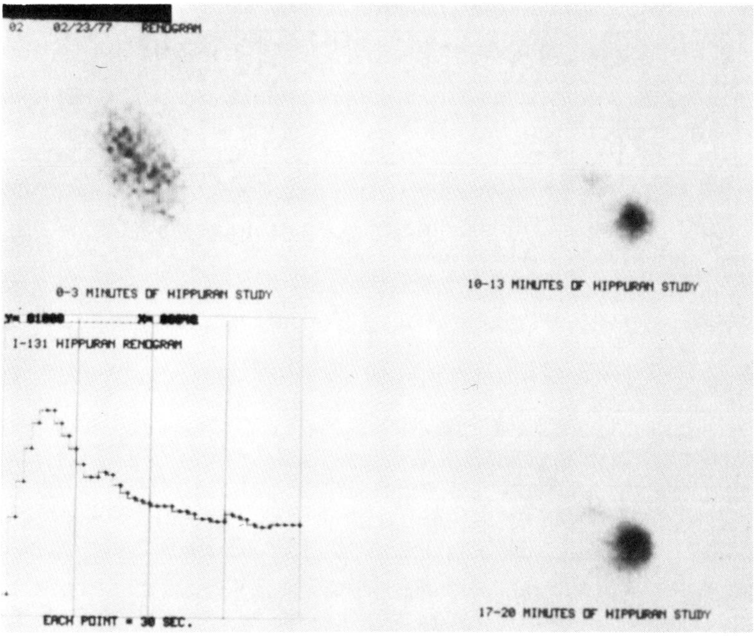
[redacted]
02 02/23/77 RENOGRAM
0-3 MINUTES OF HIPPURAN STUDY
10-13 MINUTES OF HIPPURAN STUDY
I-131 HIPPURAN RENOGRAM
EACH POINT = 30 SEC.
17-20 MINUTES OF HIPPURAN STUDY

B

normal transplant does not accumulate [^{99m}Tc] SC. However, transplants that have recovered from a rejection episode may continue to accumulate [^{99m}Tc] SC.

Renography

Certain radioactive tracers are excreted relatively rapidly from the body into the urine by the kidneys. In this excretion process the amount of radioactivity in each kidney typically rises to a maximum within a few minutes after an intravenous injection of the tracer and then declines as the radioactivity leaves the kidney via the ureter. Through the use of external radiation detectors such as gamma cameras or collimated probes, a serial record of the counting rate over each kidney can be recorded. The curve describing this counting rate as a function of time after intravenous injection of the radioactive agent is referred to as a *renogram*.

In the most simplistic terms, the renogram may be described as the resultant of the interplay between renal uptake and excretory functions. The factors or processes that normally determine renal uptake include the renal blood perfusion rate, glomerular filtration, and tubular secretion. The structure and physiology of the kidney are such that there is necessarily a lag time of a few minutes, the renal transit time, between the entry of a given molecule into the kidney and its appearance in the urine. However, the renal transit time depends in part on the tubular length, which is not uniform from nephron to nephron, so the relationship between uptake and excretion rates is complicated. Pathological processes such as renal infection, urinary tract obstruction, and renal arterial sclerosis may affect one or more of the basic processes and modify the shape of the renogram [49]. In studies of transplanted kidneys, ATN and rejection also affect the shape of the renogram. Largely based on empirical relationships between these and other known diseases and consequent changes in the renogram shape, the renogram has become a widely used renal function test. Clinically, it is more widely used as a diagnostic test based on pattern recognition than for quantitative physiological measurements; however, as will be shown in subsequent sections, a certain amount of quantitative or semiquantitative data can be extracted from the renogram.

Historical Development

In the mid-1950s Taplin had been working with [^{131}I]-labeled rose bengal in studies of liver function. This work suggested similar possibilities for renal studies, and in 1956 Taplin and co-workers [54] described the first "radioisotope renogram" obtained through the use of [^{131}I]-labeled iodopyracet (Diodrast), a radiographic contrast agent excreted by the kidneys and used for intravenous urography. A major difficulty with Diodrast and certain other contrast agents that were tried was that 10 to 15 percent of the injected dose became concentrated in the liver and interfered with the renogram of the right kidney. This obstacle was largely removed in 1960 when Tubis [56] synthesized [^{131}I]o-hippurate (OIH), a substance that is chemically and physiologically quite similar to para-aminohippurate (PAH), a well-established agent for measuring renal tubular function. OIH has remained in use ever since as the principal agent for radioisotope renograms. A very recent development is the use of ^{123}I instead of ^{131}I, with a reduction in the patient's radiation dose.

Concurrent with the development of radiopharmaceuticals suitable for renography was the development of instrumentation. The design features of the collimated probe system described by Nordyke and Tonchen [42] are still applicable. Probe systems have the advantages of simplicity and sensitivity. However, there is often uncertainty in regard to the kidney location. With a gamma camera the kidneys can be positively located, and renograms of selected portions of the kidney are readily obtained.

Tauxe and associates [55] have emphasized the importance of standardization of the renographic procedure. In particular, the renogram is affected by the state of hydration and the position of the patient. The sitting position offers the advantage of having the urine flow assisted by gravity, but the kidney location is more variable. The supine position appears to give the best reproducibility, at least in well-hydrated patients. A wide variety of techniques remain in use, but within a given institution the procedure should be standardized.

Brucer [9] describes picturesquely the evolution of the acceptance of the renogram as a diagnostic aid. The early attempts to relate the renogram to certain diseases were disappointing. Later, recognition of its ability to measure functional changes resulted in a second wave of empirical interpretations.

Many methods of mathematical (or semimathematical) quantifications of the shape of the renogram curve have been suggested [9, 45, 46]. The peak amplitude, the time of maximum amplitude, the time of one-half of maximum amplitude, the slopes at various times, and the 15-minute level of activity are among the more popular parameters that have been invoked [9]. Pircher and colleagues [45] used 28 parameters to describe the renogram, 14 of which were the differences between the first 14 in the left and right kidney.

A more sophisticated mathematical analysis of the renogram has been expounded by Britton and Brown [8]. In this analysis, computerized data-processing methods are used to subtract the blood background from the original renogram and to analyze the resultant curve by a deconvolution program. This procedure yields a spectrum of the renal transit times and gives a more precise relationship between the renogram and the fundamental physiological processes involved in excretion of the tracer.

Interpretation by Pattern Recognition

The normal OIH renogram (Fig. 13–8) has been described many times [5, 9, 14, 57]. In the earlier descriptions the segments of the curve labeled phases I to IV in Figure 13–8 were named by the following descriptive terms: I, vascular; II, secretory; and III and IV, excretory phases [9]. Other terms that have been

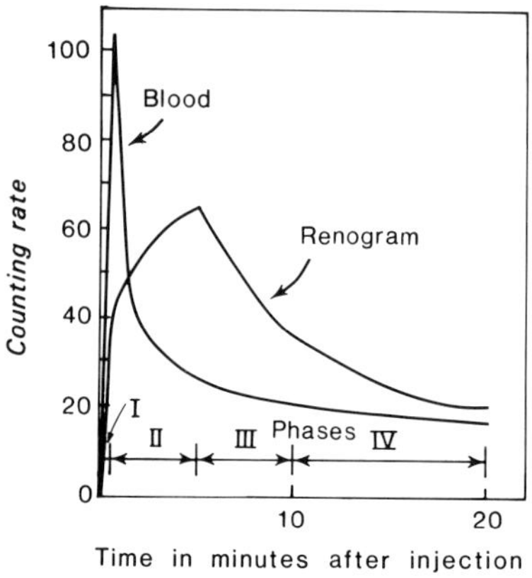

Figure 13–8
Normal renogram. The counting rate is in arbitrary units. (See text for details.)

used [9] are I, initial appearance; II, renal transit time; III, initial drainage; and IV, secondary drainage. Though not entirely inaccurate, the descriptive terms do not adequately reflect the complex interplay of dynamic processes that shape the second and third phases and may be misleading.

Also shown in Figure 13–8 is the blood curve, which serves several useful purposes. In our probe renogram method, the blood curve is obtained through the use of a collimated NaI(Tl) crystal detector placed over the left subclavian artery. The peak amplitude of this curve provides a scale of reference for the renogram. The initial rise should be very rapid, indicating a bolus injection, whereas a less rapid rise may indicate a vascular problem or a defective injection. The shape of the down slope of the blood curve is determined largely by the renal excretory function and should be approximately exponential, leveling off at 20 percent or less of the peak counting rate by 20 minutes. Higher asymptotic values are a sign of renal inadequacy. Use of the blood curve in analysis of the renogram will be discussed subsequently.

Like the blood curve, the phase I portion of the renogram normally is very steep. If the blood curve is steep and the phase I slope is not, this may indicate a renal vascular problem. The height of this portion of the curve is dependent on so many factors, such as the administered dose, the patient's body size, and the counting geometry, as well as the renal blood flow rate, that it does not have absolute significance except that to be normal it should probably fall within the range of 30 to 70 percent of the blood curve peak amplitude. With the blood curve, the phase I height provides a relative scaling factor for comparing the left and right renograms. Although a difference between the heights of phase I in the two renograms may be due to a difference in kidney size, probe position and other extrarenal factors are more likely considerations. If there is a question about the kidney size, it is most easily answered by a camera view of the kidneys.

During the second phase the activity in the kidney continues to rise, but at a decreasing rate. It ends at 3 to 5 minutes, when there is normally a sharp break indicating the beginning of phase III. The peak amplitude is normally about half again the height of the end of phase I. Flattening or complete loss of the second phase suggests severe tubular disease. However, certain other procedures, such as a previous PAH clearance study, may produce a similar result.

The beginning of the third phase coincides with the appearance of activity in the bladder and indicates that activity is leaving the field of view of the renal probe. This portion of the curve is normally concave upward. It appears approximately as the inverse of phase II and should fall to the level of the end of phase I in about the same length of time as that of phase II.

The fourth phase is usually a smooth continuation of the third, and by 20 minutes the counting rate should drop to a level less than twice that of the blood.

Deviations from the normal renogram pattern will be produced by disturbances of any of the processes involved in urinary secretion. Brucer [9] fits these changes into five more or less distinctive patterns:

1. The renal hypertension renogram (or renal arterial stenosis, chronic nephritis, nephrosclerosis).
2. The tubular disease renogram (or depressed renal blood flow, glomerulonephritis, essential hypertension).
3. The pyelonephritis renogram.
4. The urinary obstruction renogram.
5. The nonfunctioning renogram.

In the fifth pattern the renogram rises to meet the blood curve, then falls along a curve with about the same shape as the blood curve. This pattern is also seen after a nephrectomy and represents simply the blood pool in the kidney area. Some of the more striking characteristics of the other four patterns are listed in Table 13–2.

Analysis

As mentioned previously, the renogram represents a complex interplay of dynamic processes in the kidney. The instantaneous counting rate, as usually recorded, also includes activity from other tissues falling in the field of view. Several approaches have been devised for separating the components of the renogram.

Hall and Monks [21] compared the curves obtained with [^{131}I] human serum albumin ([^{131}I] HSA) and [^{131}I] Hippuran by counting over the kidneys. Since [^{131}I] HSA remains in the vascular system, or at least is removed very slowly

Table 13–2. Renogram Patterns

Phase	Renal Hypertension	Tubular Disease	Pyelonephritis	Obstruction
I	Depressed	Depressed	Slightly depressed	Depressed
II	Symmetrically prolonged	Flattened	Slightly prolonged	Markedly prolonged
III	Symmetrically prolonged	Normal time to peak	Erratic	Concave downward
IV	Prolonged	Smooth continuation of phase III	Erratic and prolonged	Continues phase III curve
Comments	May be unilateral	Typically bilateral	Typically unilateral	Typically unilateral

Source: Reprinted, by permission, from M. Brucer, *The Renogram,* Vignettes in Nuclear Medicine, Nos. 35–37. St. Louis: Mallinckrodt Chemical Works, 1968, 1969.

and not primarily by the kidneys, the difference between the two curves is largely attributable to the removal of the Hippuran from the blood by the kidneys. Britton and Brown [8] adopted this concept in a computerized method referred to as CABBS (computer assisted blood background subtraction renography). In this method, the blood curve that is to be subtracted from the conventional renogram is obtained through the use of a third detector placed over the subclavian area. The required correction factors for converting the subclavian area counting rates to the renal area counting are obtained by injecting [^{131}I] HSA and comparing the counting rates from the areas of interest. With camera renograms it may not be feasible to obtain a subclavian area recording, and some other area in the camera field must be used. In any event, the resultant of CABBS or other methods for subtracting the blood component is a curve that more accurately represents the events in the kidney. Secker-Walker and co-workers [51] discuss applications of this method in more than 100 patients.

The corrected renogram may be analyzed further to obtain a spectrum of renal transit times. Before there is any removal of activity from the kidney in the urine, the uptake in the corrected renogram is an integral of the blood curve. The uptake would presumably be linear if the concentration of activity in the blood were maintained at a constant level. However, since the concentration in the blood does in fact fall, the uptake rate falls proportionally and the slope of the uptake curve tends to decrease. A curve proportional to the integral of the blood curve may thus be fitted to the uptake portion of the corrected renogram. When activity starts to leave the field of view via the urine, the fitted blood curve integral diverges from the observed corrected renogram. Extrapolation of this curve beyond the renogram peak may be regarded as representing what the uptake would be if there were no drainage. Subtraction of the observed corrected renogram from the extrapolated uptake curve then yields a derived drainage curve. If the renal transit time (RTT), defined as the time required for a given infinitesimal increment of activity to leave the field of view after being removed from the blood by the kidney, were the same for every nephron, the drainage curve obtained by the above procedure would be like the uptake curve, but displaced in time by the RTT. However, since all nephrons are not alike, the RTT has a spectrum of values instead of a single value.

In principle the spectrum of RTTs could be obtained by presenting a very sharp bolus of activity (ideally a "spike" function) to the kidney by renal arterial injection instead of by the usual blood curve. The resulting spectrum is also referred to as the *impulse response function*, $H(t)$. However, it is not practicable to do this experiment. Instead, we may assume that $H(t)$ exists and may consider the observed corrected renogram $R(t)$ to be the convolution integral of the blood curve, or input function, $I(t)$, by $H(t)$.

Mathematically expressed,

$$R(t) = \int_0^t H(t - \tau)\ I(\tau) d\tau \tag{1}$$

or

$$R = H * I \tag{2}$$

where the * indicates the convolution integration operation as defined by Equation 1.

In the practical situation, $R(t)$ and $I(t)$ are known, by measurement, and the problem is to solve for $H(t)$. This requires a deconvolution procedure, represented as $\overline{*}$. Then

$$H = R \mathbin{\overline{*}} I \tag{3}$$

Britton and Brown [8] developed a computer program to achieve this by an iterative method; Figure 13–9 shows an example of a set of renograms analyzed by this method. The normal renogram curve shows an $H(t)$ spectrum that appears approximately gaussian. The abnormal one shows other components in the spectrum. Such an analysis can enhance the pattern recognition approach, but at present the correlation between the RTT spectrum and clinical conditions remains on more of an empirical than a theoretical basis.

Fleming and Goddard [15] and later Kenny and associates [31] showed that the required deconvolution can be achieved analytically using the Laplace transform, and if the blood curve can be described by a biexponential function, $H(t)$ can be derived without the use of a large computer.

Diffey and colleagues [13] have applied the method of deconvolution analysis to the [^{99m}Tc] DTPA renogram and give an example of how this may be used to distinguish postrenal obstruction from intrarenal disease.

Other methods of analyzing the renogram have been used to obtain values for various physiological parameters, including renal blood flow [47], renal plasma

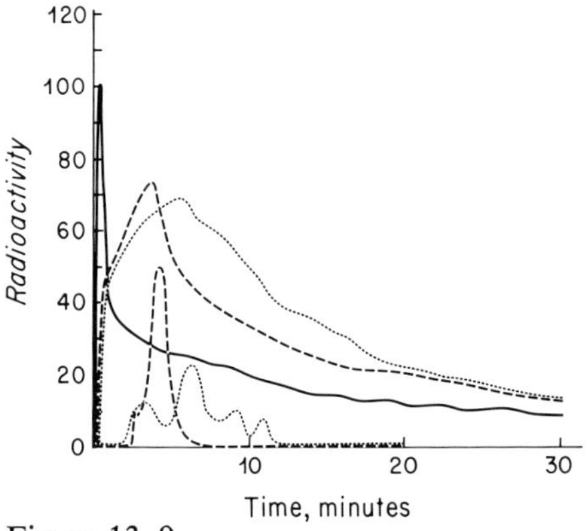

Figure 13–9
Renograms in a 58-year-old woman with mild hypertension analyzed by blood background subtraction and deconvolution. The upper dashed curve is a normal left renogram. The lower dashed curve (approximately gaussian in shape) is the renal transit time spectrum or impulse response function derived from the left renogram. The upper dotted curve is an abnormal right renogram showing marked early outflow delay. The lower dotted curve is derived from the right renogram and shows several peaks, suggesting that the nephron population has several subgroups with different renal transit times. (2–949–665.)

flow [10], and Hippuran clearance [20]. These values are based on estimations of the slope of the phase II portion of the renogram.

References

1. Arnold, R. W., Subramanian, G., McAfee, J. G., et al. Comparison of ^{99m}Tc complexes for renal imaging. *J. Nucl. Med.* 16:357, 1975.
2. Atkins, H. L., Eckelman, W. C., Hauser, W., et al. Evaluation of glomerular filtration rate with ^{99m}Tc-DTPA (abstract). *J. Nucl. Med.* 12:338, 1971.
3. Beckerman, C., and Vyas, M. I. Renal localization of ^{67}Ga-citrate in renal amyloidosis (case report). *J. Nucl. Med.* 17:899, 1976.
4. Bell, E. G., and Blaufox, M. D. Clinical Application of Renal Imaging. In A. Gottschalk and E. J. Potchen (Eds.), *Diagnostic Nuclear Medicine.* Baltimore: Williams & Wilkins, 1976. Chap. 36.
5. Blaufox, M. D., and Bell, E. G. General Principles of Renal Evaluation with Radionuclides. In A. Gottschalk and E. J. Potchen (Eds.), *Diagnostic Nuclear Medicine.* Baltimore: Williams & Wilkins, 1976. Chap. 35.
6. Blaufox, M. D., and Funck-Brentano, J.-L. *Radionuclides in Nephrology.* New York: Grune & Stratton, 1972.
7. Boyd, R. E., Robson, J., Hunt, F. C., et al. ^{99m}Tc-gluconate complexes for renal scintigraphy. *Br. Radiol.* 46:604, 1973.
8. Britton, K. E., and Brown, N. J. G. *Clinical Renography.* Chicago: Year Book, 1972.
9. Brucer, M. *The Renogram.* Vignettes in Nuclear Medicine, Nos. 35, 36, 37. St. Louis: Mallinckrodt Chemical Works, 1968, 1969.

10. Burbank, M. D., Tauxe, W. N., Maher, F. T., et al. Evaluation of radioiodonated Hippuran for estimation of renal plasma flow. *Proc. Staff Meet. Mayo Clin.* 36:372, 1961.
11. Chervu, L. R., Freeman, L. M., and Blaufox, M. D. Radiopharmaceuticals for renal studies. *Sem. Nucl. Med.* 4:3, 1974.
12. Cohen, M. L. Radionuclide clearance technique. *Semin. Nucl. Med.* 4:23, 1974.
13. Diffey, B. L., Hall, F. M., and Corfield, J. R. The ^{99m}technetium dynamic renal scan with deconvolution analysis. *J. Nucl. Med.* 17:352, 1976.
14. Farmelant, M. H., and Burrows, B. A. The renogram: Physiologic basis and current use. *Semin. Nucl.* Med. 4:61, 1974.
15. Fleming, J. S., and Goddard, B. A. A technique for the deconvolution of the renogram. *Phys. Med. Biol.* 19:546, 1974.
16. Freedman, G. S., Schiff, M., Zager, P., et al. The temporal and pathological significance of perfusion failure following renal transplantation. *Radiology* 114:649, 1975.
17. George, E. A., Anderson, C. B., Codd, J. E., et al. Differentiation of acute tubular necrosis and rejection by dual radionuclide transplant renography. *Proc. Clin. Dial. Transplant Forum* 3:77, 1974.
18. George, E. A., Fletcher, J. W., Newton, W. T., et al. Renal accumulation of ^{99m}Tc-sulfur colloid in transplant rejection. *Radiology* 111:465, 1974.
19. Gray, W. R., Oakes, P. L., Lewis, S. E., et al. Renal displacement visualized on myocardial scintigram (case report). *J. Nucl. Med.* 18:350, 1977.
20. Grünfeld, J.-P., Sabto, J., Bankir, L., et al. Methods of measurement of renal blood flow in man. *Semin. Nucl. Med.* 4:39, 1974.
21. Hall, F. M., and Monks, G. T. The renogram: A method of separating vascular and renal components. *Invest. Radiol.* 1:220, 1966.
22. Handmaker, H., Young, B. W., and Lowenstein, J. M. Clinical experience with ^{99m}Tc-DMSA (dimercaptosuccinic acid), a new renal-imaging agent. *J. Nucl. Med.* 16:28, 1975.
23. Hauser, W., Atkins, H. L., Nelson, V. S., et al. Technetium 99m DTPA: A new radiopharmaceutical for brain and kidney scanning. *Radiology* 94:679, 1970.
24. Haynie, T. P., Stewart, B. H., and Kurtz, D. M. Clinical Application of Renal Scanning. In J. L. Quinn (Ed.), *Scintillation Scanning in Clinical Medicine.* Philadelphia: Saunders, 1964. Pp. 231–244.
25. Holmes, E. R., III, Klingensmith, W. C., III, Kirchner, P. T., et al. Phantom kidney in technetium-99m DTPA studies of renal blood flow (case report). *J. Nucl. Med.* 18:702, 1977.
26. Hör, G., Pabst, H. W., Pfeifer, K. J., et al. Radionuclides in renal transplantation. *J. Nucl. Med.* 13:795, 1972.
27. Hosain, F. Quality control of ^{99m}Tc-DTPA by double-tracer clearance technique. *J. Nucl. Med.* 15:442, 1974.
28. Izenstark, J. L. Scintillation Scan Techniques in the Evaluation of Renal Disease. In J. L. Quinn (Ed.), *Scintillation Scanning in Clinical Medicine.* Philadelphia: Saunders, 1964. Pp. 245–257.
29. Joekes, A. M. Obstructive uropathy. *Semin. Nucl. Med.* 4:187, 1974.
30. Kahn, P. C., Dewanjee, M. K., and Brown, S. S. Routine renal imaging after ^{99m}Tc-glucoheptonate brain scans. *J. Nucl. Med.* 17:786, 1976.
31. Kenny, R. W., Ackery, D. M., Fleming, J. S., et al. Deconvolution analysis of the scintillation camera renogram. *Br. J. Radiol.* 48:481, 1975.
32. Kim, Y. C., Massari, P. U., Brown, M. L., et al. Clinical significance of ^{99m}technetium sulfur colloid accumulation in renal transplant patients. *Radiology* 124:745, 1977.

33. Koenigsberg, M., Blaufox, M. D., and Freeman, L. M. Traumatic injuries of the renal vasculature and parenchyma. *Semin. Nucl. Med.* 4:117, 1974.
34. Kumar, B., and Coleman, R. E. Significance of delayed ^{67}Ga localization in the kidneys. *J. Nucl. Med.* 17:872, 1976.
35. Lin, T. H., Khentigan, A., and Winchell, H. S. A ^{99m}Tc-chelate substitute for organomercurial renal agents. *J. Nucl. Med.* 15:34, 1974.
36. Maher, F. T. Evaluation of renal and urinary tract abnormalities noted on scintiscans: A retrospective study of 1,711 radioisotope skeletal surveys performed in an 18-month period. *Mayo Clin. Proc.* 50:370, 1975.
37. Mallinckrodt Nuclear, Inc. Hippuran^{R} I-131 UC I injection package insert, St. Louis, Mo., 1976.
38. McAfee, J. G., Thomas, F. D., Grossman, Z., et al. Diagnosis of angiotensinogenic hypertension: The complementary roles of renal scintigraphy and the saralasin infusion test. *J. Nucl. Med.* 18:669, 1977.
39. McRae, J., Barry, A. C., and Valk, P. E. Renal scintigraphy using technetium-stannous chloride gluconate. *Aust. N.Z. J. Med.* 1:291, 1961.
40. Morales, J. O. Space-occupying lesions of the kidney. *Semin. Nucl. Med.* 4:113, 1974.
41. Myerson, P. J. Focal porta-hepatis defect on nuclide imaging (letter). *J. Nucl. Med.* 18:944, 1977.
42. Nordyke, R. A., and Tonchen, A. The radiohippuran renogram: Enhanced reproducibility by changes in instrumentation and patient position. *J. A. M. A.* 183:440, 1963.
43. Nordyke, R. A., Tubis, M., and Blahd, W. H. Use of radioiodinated Hippuran for individual kidney function tests. *J. Lab. Clin. Med.* 56:438, 1960.
44. Park, H.-M., Forry, A. E., and Sagalowski, R. L. Localization of ^{67}Ga in renal microabscesses. *J. Nucl. Med.* 18:313, 1977.
45. Pircher, F. J., Carr, E. A., and Patno, M. D. Evaluation of quantitative aspects of the radioisotope renogram. *J. Nucl. Med.* 4:117, 1963.
46. Pircher, F. J., Wegst, A. V., and Dodson, V. N. In vitro analysis of the radioisotope renogram test. *J. Nucl. Med.* 4:45, 1963.
47. Raynaud, C. A technique for the quantitative measurement of the function of each kidney. *Semin. Nucl. Med.* 4:51, 1974.
48. Reba, R. C., Poulose, K. P., and Kirchner, P. T. Radiolabeled chelates for visualization of kidney function and structure with emphasis on their use in renal insufficiency. *Semin. Nucl. Med.* 4:151, 1974.
49. Rosenthal, L. Radiotechnetium renography and serial radiohippurate imaging for screening renovascular hypertension. *Semin. Nucl. Med.* 4:97, 1974.
50. Schlegel, J. U. The value of radionuclide studies to the practicing urologist and nephrologist. *Semin. Nucl. Med.* 4:213, 1974.
51. Secker-Walker, R. H., Shepherd, E. P., and Cassell, K. G. Clinical application of computer-assisted renography. *J. Nucl. Med.* 13:235, 1972.
52. Strakosch, C. R., Cooper, R. A., Wiseman, J. C., et al. High ectopic kidney presenting as an abnormal liver-lung scan (case report). *J. Nucl. Med.* 18:274, 1977.
53. Sziklas, J. J., Hoszin, F., Reba, R. C., et al. Comparison of ^{169}Yb-DTPA, ^{113}In-DTPA, ^{14}C-inulin and endogenous creatinine to estimate glomerular filtration. *J. Nucl. Biol. Med.* 15:122, 1971.
54. Taplin, G. V., Meredith, O. M., Jr., Kade, H., et al. The radioisotope renogram: An external test for individual kidney function and upper urinary tract patency. *J. Lab. Clin. Med.* 48:886, 1956.
55. Tauxe, W. N., Hunt, J. C., and Burbank, M. K. The radioisotope renogram

(ortho-iodohipppute ^{131}I): Standardization of technique and expression of data. *Am. J. Clin. Pathol.* 37:567, 1972.
56. Tubis, M., Posnich, E., and Nordyke, R. N. Preparation and use of ^{131}I-labeled sodium iodohippurate in kidney function tests (abstract). *Proc. Soc. Exp. Biol. Med.* 103:497, 1960.
57. Wagner, H. N., Jr., Reba, R. C., and Goodwin, D. A. The Kidney. In H. N. Wagner (Ed.), *Principles of Nuclear Medicine.* Philadelphia: Saunders, 1968. Chap. 13.
58. Wahner, H. W., Maher, F. T., and Hattery, R. R. Prostatakarzinom: Diagnose von Harnabflusstörungen mit Hilfe der Knochenszintigraphie. *Aktuelle Urologie* 8:261, 1977.
59. Wenzl, J. E., Tauxe, W. N., and Hunt, J. C. A single-injection technique for renal photoscanning with ortho-iodohippurate ^{131}I. *Proc. Mayo Clin.* 38:313, 1963.
60. ZumWinkel, K., Harbst, H., Das, K. B., et al. Application of radionuclides in renal transplantation. *Semin. Nucl. Med.* 4:169, 1974.

14. Analysis of Immunoglobulins in Urine

Robert A. Kyle

The study of immunoglobulins in urine requires a description of normal immunoglobulins and their relationship to the overproduction of monoclonal immunoglobulins. This introductory section will be followed by a description of detection of immunoglobulins in urine, including methodology and possibilities of error, and then by a discussion of the clinical significance of immunoglobulins in the urine.

Normal Immunoglobulins

Prior to 1960, the term *gamma globulin* was used to designate those proteins that migrated in the gamma mobility region (toward the cathode) of the electrophoretic pattern. It has long been recognized that these gamma globulins migrate in the beta and alpha-2 mobility regions as well as the gamma, and they are now termed *immunoglobulins*. The five groups presently recognized are designated by capital letters that correspond to the class of their heavy chains, which are designated by Greek letters: gamma (γ) in IgG, alpha (α) in IgA, mu (μ) in IgM, delta (δ) in IgD, and epsilon (ϵ) in IgE (Table 14–1). The properties of the five groups of immunoglobulins are listed in Table 14–2.

IgG

Three-fourths of the immunoglobulin in normal serum is of the IgG type. It has a molecular weight of 150,000 and a sedimentation coefficient of 6.7S. Its electrophoretic mobility ranges from slow gamma (cathodal area) to alpha-2. Many antibodies to both bacteria and viruses are of the IgG class. Reducing agents such as mercaptoethanol disrupt the disulfide bonds linking the polypeptide chains of the IgG molecule. If the reduced protein is alkylated with iodoacetamide and fractionated in the presence of a solvent (such as guanidine or urea) that is capable of dissociating noncovalent bonds, two kinds of polypeptide chains can be recovered: heavy (H) and light (L) (Fig. 14–1).

HEAVY CHAINS. In each immunoglobulin molecule, both heavy chains are of the same class [in IgG, both gamma (γ)] and the two light chains are alike—both kappa (κ) or both lambda (λ). Each gamma heavy chain has a molecular weight of approximately 55,000 and consists of 440 to 450 amino acids. Each has a variable (V_H) region, in which many amino acid substitutes make each chain different from the next, and a constant (C_H) region, in which there are very few amino acid differences from the constant region of any other gamma

This investigation was supported in part by Research Grants CA–4646, CA–16835 and NS–14304K from the National Institutes of Health, U.S. Public Health Service.

Table 14–1. Classification of Immunoglobulins of Normal Human Serum

Immunoglobulin	IgG	IgA	IgM	IgD	IgE
Synonyms	γ, 7Sγ, γ_2, γG	β_x, β_2A, γ_1A, γA	γ_1, 19Sγ, β_2M, γ_1M, γM	γD	γE
Heavy-chain					
Classes	Gamma (γ)	Alpha (α)	Mu (μ)	Delta (δ)	Epsilon (ϵ)
Subclasses	IgG1, IgG2, IgG3, IgG4	IgA1, IgA2	—	? Ja, La	—
Light-chain types	Kappa (κ)	κ	κ	κ	κ
	Lambda (λ)	λ	λ	λ	λ
Molecular formula	$\gamma_2\kappa_2$	$\alpha_2\kappa_2$ *	$(\mu_2\kappa_2)5$	$\delta_2\kappa_2$	$\epsilon_2\kappa_2$
	$\gamma_2\lambda_2$	$\alpha_2\lambda_2$ *	$(\mu_2\lambda_2)5$	$\delta_2\lambda_2$	$\epsilon_2\lambda_2$
Designation	IgGκ	IgAκ	IgMκ	IgDκ	IgEκ
	IgGλ	IgAλ	IgMλ	IgDλ	IgEλ

* May form polymers.

Source: Reprinted, by permission, from R. A. Kyle, Immunoglobulins and syndromes associated with monoclonal gammopathies. In *Tice's Practice of Medicine,* Vol. 1. Hagerstown, Md.: Harper & Row, 1977, p. 2.

Table 14–2. Properties of Immunoglobulins of Normal Human Serum

Property	IgG	IgA	IgM	IgD	IgE
Electrophoretic mobility	γ to α_2	γ to β	γ to γ_2	γ to β	γ to β
Sedimentation coefficient	6.7S	7–15S *	19S	7S	8S
Molecular weight	150,000	170,000–500,000 *	900,000	180,000	200,000
Carbohydrate (%)	2.6	5–10	9.8	10–12	11
T½, days	23	5.8	5.1	2.8	2.3
Serum concentration (mean mg/ml)	11.4	1.8	1.0	0.03	0.0003
Total serum immunoglobulin (%)	74	21	5	0.2	0.002
Total body pool in intravascular space (%)	45	42	76	75	51
Intravascular pool catabolized per day (%) (normal)	6.7	25	18	37	89
Normal synthetic rate (mg/kg/day)	33	24	6.7	0.4	0.02
Fixes complement	Yes (IgG4 via alternate pathway)	Alternate pathway	Yes	No	Alternate pathway
Crosses placenta	Yes	No	No	No	No

* Tends to form polymers of the monomer form.

Source: Modified from R. A. Kyle, R. C. Bieger, and G. J. Gleich. Diagnosis of syndromes associated with hyperglobulinemia. *Med. Clin. North Am.* 54:918, 1970. By permission of the W. B. Saunders Company.

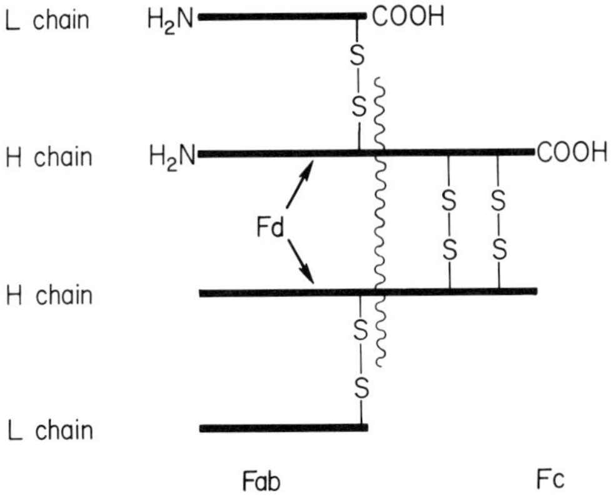

Figure 14–1
IgG molecule, with cleavage of papain into Fab and Fc fragments. Note Fd piece. L = light; H = heavy. (Reprinted, by permission, from R. A. Kyle. Immunoglobulins and Syndromes Associated With Monoclonal Gammopathies. In *Tice's Practice of Medicine*. Hagerstown, Md.: Harper & Row, 1977. Vol. 1, Chap. 48, p. 3.)

chain. The variable region of the gamma chain consists of approximately 110 amino acid residues, beginning at the amino terminal of the chain. The constant region of the gamma chain consists of 310 to 330 amino acids and contains three homology regions or domains, designated $C\gamma_1$, $C\gamma_2$, and $C\gamma_3$. The homology region $C\gamma_1$ is in the Fd fragment and runs from amino acid 110 to 220; $C\gamma_2$ is in the Fc fragment and extends from 220 up to 330; and $C\gamma_3$ extends to the carboxy terminus.

LIGHT CHAINS. Historically, the light chains were encountered first, but their mystery has yielded slowly indeed.

Saturday, Nov. 1st, 1845

Dear Doctor Jones,—The tube contains urine of very high specific gravity. When boiled it becomes slightly opaque. On the addition of nitric acid, it effervesces, assumes a reddish hue, and becomes quite clear; but as it cools, assumes the consistence and appearance which you see. Heat reliquifies it. What is it? [4]

This cryptic message and a urine sample were sent by a leading physician of London, Dr. Thomas Watson, to Henry Bence Jones, a 31-year-old physician at St. George's Hospital who had already established a reputation as a chemical pathologist. A graduate of Cambridge, Jones had studied medicine at St. George's Hospital and chemistry at Giessen under Liebig. Although Henry Bence Jones gained the fame and the eponym for his description of the unusual properties of the urine in the medical journals of the day [3, 5], the credit actually belongs to Dr. William Macintyre. A well-known Harley Street consultant, Dr. Macintyre had been called by Dr. Watson on October 30, 1845 to examine a patient, Thomas Alexander McBean, "a highly respectable tradesman," who complained of excruciating bone pain [42].

Because edema had been observed during the patient's illness, the astute Macintyre personally examined the urine, but he found no evidence of sugar. When heated, the urine was seen to ". . . abound in animal matter. . . ." The urine became clear with the addition of nitric acid but developed a precipitate after an hour. This precipitate ". . . underwent complete solution on the application of heat, but again consolidated on cooling" [42]. After Macintyre's visit, Watson sent the foregoing note and a sample of the urine to Jones.

Having received specimens of the patient's urine from both Watson and Macintyre on November 1, Dr. Jones corroborated the finding of a protein that was precipitated by heating, dissolved by boiling, and reprecipitated by cooling. He concluded that the protein was an oxide of albumin, specifically "hydrated deutoxide of albumen" [5]. Although the heat properties of the urinary protein he described were not his own discovery, Jones certainly deserves credit for emphasizing its place in the diagnosis of myeloma, for he said, "I need hardly remark on the importance of seeking for this oxide of albumen in other cases of mollities ossium" [4].

More than a century later, it was found that the urinary proteins that evoked such interest from Macintyre and Jones were the light-chain components of the immunoglobulin molecule. In 1962, Edelman and Gally [18] demonstrated that the light chains prepared from a serum IgG myeloma protein and the Bence Jones protein from the same patient's urine had the same amino acid sequence, similar spectrofluorometric behavior, the same molecular weight, identical appearance on chromatography with carboxymethylcellulose and on starch gel electrophoresis after reduction and alkylation, and the same ultracentrifugal pattern—as well as the same thermal solubility. They precipitated when heated to between 40 and 60° C, dissolved on boiling, and reprecipitated when cooled to between 40 and 60° C.

The light chains have a molecular weight of 22,500 and contain 210 to 220 amino acids. Two distinct groups of Bence Jones proteins (group I and group II) were recognized by Bayne-Jones and Wilson in 1922 [2a]. Their two major classes are kappa and lambda. Approximately 70 percent of serum IgG monoclonal proteins are of the kappa type, and approximately 30 percent are lambda. In patients with Waldenström's macroglobulinemia, 80 percent are kappa; the opposite occurs in IgD myeloma, where 90 percent are lambda.

Analyses of amino acid sequence in individual light chains have disclosed that the region of the chain from amino acid 107 to the carboxy terminus at position 210 to 220 is very similar in chains of the same type (kappa or lambda), although amino acid substitutions have been found at a dozen different positions in the constant region of human lambda chains [37]. The region from the amino (NH_2) terminus (position 1) to approximately position 110 has been different in every light chain thus far analyzed. Consequently, these two regions are termed the *constant* (C_L) and *variable* (V_L) portions of the light (L) chains. It is the variable half of the light chain that contains the unique thermal solubility characteristics of Bence Jones proteins [67].

The amino acid differences in the constant portions of the light chains can be related to certain markers. In the kappa chains, if the amino acid leucine is at position 191, the protein is Inv(1) or Inv(2), whereas if valine is at this position, it is Inv(3). Inv(1) has valine at position 153; the others have alanine. Of Caucasians who have the Inv(1) antigen, 98 percent also have the Inv(2) antigen. In contrast, no genetic factors have been identified for human lambda chains. These isotypic markers include Oz(+) if lysine is at position 193, whereas if arginine is present, it is Oz(−). Another marker in lambda chains has been designated Kern(+) when glycine is present at position 156 and Kern(−) when serine is there, and another variant, Mcg, has been reported which has threonine at position 103 instead of glycine [21, 65].

Amino acid sequence studies have revealed four basic groups of kappa light chains, designated κI, κII, κIII, and κIV [74]. The frequency of occurrence of κI, κII, κIII, and κIV monoclonal kappa light chains is approximately 60, 10, 28, and 2 percent, respectively, and as one would expect, this reflects the proportion of κI, κII, κIII, and κIV light chains in immunoglobulins of normal serum [66]. The lambda light chains have not been as well delineated, but five subclasses of lambda chains have been reported [19].

Bence Jones proteins are synthesized de novo and are not degradation products of the complete immunoglobulin in the serum. Putnam and Hardy [58] showed that ^{13}C-labeled glycine was incorporated promptly into Bence Jones protein and could not be a breakdown of serum or other tissue protein.

Light chains clearly are metabolized by the kidney. After injection into mice, Bence Jones proteins of humans, labeled with ^{131}I, were cleared rapidly from the circulation. Ligating and severing the ureters lengthened the disappearance time only slightly, but removal of the kidneys greatly prolonged the survival of light chains. Human IgG was not cleared by the kidney in the same experiments [76].

Mogielnicki and colleagues [48] produced tubular proteinuria with the use of sodium maleate, a potent tubular toxin. The urinary proteins had a molecular weight of less than 50,000 but were heterogeneous, comprising serum enzymes, immunoglobulin light chains, and perhaps small protein hormones. The induced damage to the tubules did not alter the rate of disappearance of light chain from the circulation while the glomerular filtration remained normal; however, after a larger dose of maleate had produced both tubular and glomerular damage, the fractional metabolic rate was markedly reduced. In glomerular proteinuria most of the urinary proteins were of large molecular weight, such as albumin and transferrin. It was demonstrated that mice treated with sodium maleate excreted twice as much light chain in the urine as control mice. Turnover of light chain in maleate-treated, ureter-severed animals was considerably slower than in untreated ureter-severed controls. This experiment demonstrated that sodium maleate decreases the fractional metabolic rate of light chains when the effect on endogenous catabolism is not counterbalanced by the effect on proteinuria. Therefore, the renal tubules are the mechanisms for uptake and catabolism of light chains.

Primarily, kappa chains are in the monomeric form (molecular weight 22,500); however, they may exist as noncovalently linked dimers or as a mixture of monomers and dimers, whereas lambda proteins occur as covalently linked dimers (molecular weight 45,000) via their penultimate cysteinyl residues [65]. In addition, kappa light chains precipitate maximally over a narrower range of pH than lambda light chains [56]. Recognition of light chains as kappa or lambda by monospecific antisera depends on the variable and constant domains as well as on the interdomain "switch" region between the variable and constant portions [66].

FAB AND FC FRAGMENTS. Treatment of IgG with the proteolytic enzyme papain cleaves it into three pieces: two Fab fragments, so named because they possess antigen-combining activity, and an Fc fragment, so named because in certain species it can be crystallized (see Fig. 14–1). Each Fab fragment (molecular weight 52,000) consists of the amino terminal portion of a heavy chain and a complete light chain. Three regions of "hypervariability" have been identified in V_L: positions 24 to 34, 50 to 56, and 89 to 97 [77]. This hypervariability and the existence of similar hypervariable regions in the variable portion of the heavy chain (V_H) in positions 30 to 37, 51 to 68, 84 to 91, and 101 to 110 [12] permit the formation of many different antigen-combining sites.

The Fc fragment consists of the C-terminal portion of both heavy chains, which are linked to each other by disulfide bonds. Its molecular weight is 48,000. Biological activities of the Fc fragment include fixation of complement, passive cutaneous anaphylaxis (PCA), binding with rheumatoid factors, binding with receptors on macrophages and lymphocytes, reaction with staphylococcal A protein, and transfer across the placenta. Isotypic specificity (for gamma, alpha, mu, delta, or epsilon) resides in the Fc fragment. The Fc piece is devoid of antibody activity.

IgA

Two heavy alpha chains and two light chains (both kappa or both lambda) form IgA [70]. IgA has a molecular weight of 170,000 and a sedimentation coefficient of 7S, but it also has a propensity to form polymers with sedimentation coefficients of 9 to 15S. Its catabolic rate of 5.8 days (T½) is greater than that of IgG. About 70 percent of serum monoclonal IgA proteins are of the kappa type. Aggregated IgA can fix the late components of complement, beginning with C3 (alternate pathway). There are two subgroups of the alpha chain, α_1 and α_2, resulting in IgA1 and IgA2 immunoglobulins. Almost 95 percent of monoclonal IgA proteins are of the IgA1 class. IgA2 molecules are unique among the immunoglobulins in that their light chains are bound to the α_2 chains by noncovalent forces rather than by disulfide bonds.

SECRETORY IGA. Secretory IgA, or SIgA, is found in high concentration in the secretions of many glands lining the respiratory and gastrointestinal tracts and in tears, colostrum, and urine. SIgA, which has a sedimentation coefficient of 11S and a molecular weight of 390,000, is composed of two IgA molecules attached by disulfide bonds to a glycoprotein (molecular weight 60,000) termed the *secretory component*. The secretory component is synthesized in mucosal epithelial cells; it increases the resistance of the molecules against digestion by trypsin and pepsin. SIgA exhibits antibacterial activity and has a neutralizing effect on viral replication [17]. Production of IgA begins 4 weeks after birth and approaches the adult level at 1 year. No significant changes of concentration occur during childhood.

IgM

A third immunoglobulin, IgM, is composed of subunits linked by disulfide bonds [46]. The heavy chain (mu) of IgM has a molecular weight of approximately 70,000; the subunits, composed of two heavy chains and two light chains, each have a molecular weight of 180,000 to 190,000. Since the molecular weight of IgM is approximately 900,000, it evidently comprises five subunits. The mu chain, recently sequenced, consists of one variable (V_H) and four constant ($C\mu_1$, $C\mu_2$, $C\mu_3$, $C\mu_4$) domains [57]. Low-molecular-weight IgM (sedimentation coefficient 7S) has been found in patients with various pathological conditions, including lupus erythematosus, macroglobulinemia, other lymphoproliferative processes, and cirrhosis [10]. IgM antibodies are the first to be produced in a primary immune response. Cold agglutinins, isoagglutinins, rheumatoid factor, and heterophile and Wasserman antibodies, as well as antibodies to various bacteria, are of the IgM class. Rapid IgM synthesis begins in the first few days of neonatal life, and adult serum levels are attained at 1 year. IgM concentrations have been reported to decrease by the sixth decade. Approximately 80 percent of IgM monoclonal proteins are of the kappa type, as opposed to two-thirds of IgG and IgA monoclonal proteins.

IgD

In 1965, Rowe and Fahey [60] found a myeloma protein containing a heavy chain unlike those of the other immunoglobulins. This class, named IgD, is present in low concentrations in normal serum, is rapidly catabolized, and has a serum half-life of 2.8 days. Approximately 75 percent of IgD is intravascular, a distribution that may be due to irregularities in the shape of the molecule. Although antigen-combining activity associated with IgD has been reported, the functions of the molecule that are attributable to the heavy chain have remained obscure. IgD is frequently found on the surface of lymphocytes [71]. Because 90 percent of the IgD myeloma proteins are lambda, in contrast to the predominance of kappa in IgD found on the surface of lymphocytes, it has been suggested that serum and cell-bound IgD may represent two IgD subclasses [67a]. Others have noted antigenic heterogeneity in IgD heavy chains, and this may be indicative of subclasses (Ja and La). Of patients with IgD myeloma, 90 percent have lambda light chains, in contrast to 30 percent of patients with IgG myeloma.

IgE

The fifth class of immunoglobulins, IgE, has been purified from the serum of allergic patients [25]; approximately a dozen cases of IgE myeloma have been reported. IgE has a molecular weight of 200,000 and a sedimentation coefficient of 8S. The combination of a short biological half-life (2.3 days) and a very low rate of synthesis results in an extremely low serum concentration in normal persons.

IgE mediates the wheal-and-flare reaction associated with reaginic allergies and binds to basophils. IgE is fixed on normal human target cells, and histamine is released when the cell-fixed IgE reacts with the allergen. Many patients with extrinsic asthma and hay fever have elevated concentrations of IgE [78].

Monoclonal Proteins

Relationship to Normal Immunoglobulins

Although monoclonal proteins have long been thought of as abnormal, studies conducted over the past several years have disclosed strong indications that they are only excessive quantities of immunoglobulins that occur normally. The striking feature of monoclonal proteins that led investigators to consider them as abnormal is their homogeneity. Whereas normal IgG in human serum is electrophoretically heterogeneous and is distributed from the α_2 to the slow γ regions, IgG monoclonal proteins are localized sharply in their electrophoretic migration.

Monoclonal antibody activity in humans has been associated with cold agglutinin disease as well as with a wide variety of bacterial antigens [62]. It is almost certain that more monoclonal human proteins will be found to have antibody activity. Indeed, it has been postulated that all myeloma proteins may have antibody activity [51].

As illustrated in Figure 14–2, the normal collection of immunoglobulin molecules comprises minute amounts of highly homogeneous proteins from many diverse single clones of plasma cells and thus is polyclonal. If a single clone escapes the normal control over its multiplication, it reproduces excessively and synthesizes an excess of protein with a single heavy-chain class and subclass and a single light-chain type. Sometimes only light chains are synthesized, with resultant Bence Jones proteinemia and proteinuria. This monoclonal protein is often associated with a neoplastic or potentially neoplastic process.

Patterns of Overproduction

Normally, plasma cells produce heavy chains and a slight excess of light chains that spill over into the urine. In IgG myeloma about three-fourths of patients

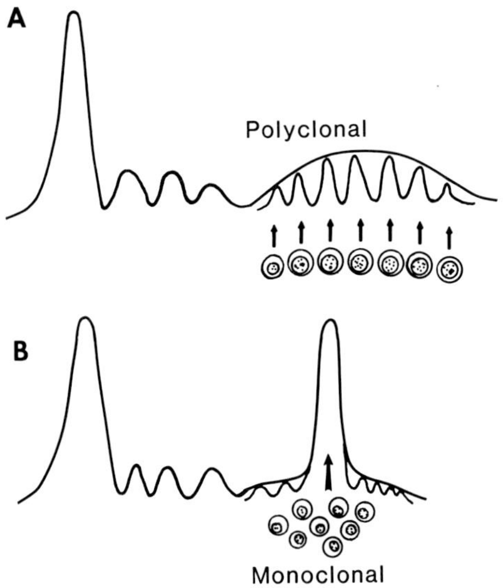

Figure 14–2
Polyclonal and monoclonal electrophoretic patterns. (A) Broad outline comprising small peaks of many different homogeneous proteins (each represented here in normal amount, related by an arrow to its peak) that have been produced by many different plasma cell clones (polyclonal). (B) Tall, narrow peak of homogeneous protein (single heavy-chain and single light-chain type), which represents excessive output of a single clone (monoclonal). (Reprinted, by permission, from R. A. Kyle and P. R. Greipp. The laboratory investigation of monoclonal gammopathies. *Mayo Clin. Proc.* 53:719–739, 1978.)

have an excess of light chains, which may be excreted into the urine (Bence Jones proteinuria) or catabolized [11]. In some instances of myeloma, no heavy chain is produced by the plasma cell and only excessive quantities of light chains are detected ("light-chain disease") [68]. Finally, the plasma cells in a small proportion of myeloma patients do not secrete either heavy or light chains to excess, as a result of either a simple failure of production or blocking of secretion; this type of myeloma is called "nonsecretory" [55].

Laboratory Methods for Study of Immunoglobulins in Urine

The analysis of immunoglobulins in urine requires sensitive, rapid, dependable screening to detect the presence of protein and a specific assay to identify the type of light chain and to determine whether it is polyclonal or monoclonal [32a]. Although there are many qualitative tests—the use of heat with acetic acid, nitric acid (Heller's test), potassium ferrocyanide, sulfosalicylic acid, magnesium sulfate (Roberts' test), and the biuret reaction—we prefer Exton's test (sulfosalicylic acid and sodium sulfate) [20].

Exton's Test for Protein

A fresh morning urine specimen should be collected without a preservative.

REAGENT. Dissolve 200 gm of sodium sulfate in 750 ml of deionized water in a volumetric flask with heating. Cool the solution and add 50 gm of sulfosalicylic acid and dilute to 1 liter with deionized water. This 5% sulfosalicylic acid solution is stable indefinitely and can be stored at room temperature.

PROCEDURE

1. Centrifuge 15 ml of urine for 5 minutes at 2000 rpm.
2. Put 1.5 ml of 5% sulfosalicylic acid in a 15 × 150 mm Pyrex tube.
3. Add 1.5 ml of supernatant fluid from a centrifuged urine specimen to the 1.5 ml of sulfosalicylic acid and mix well.
4. Warm to about 70° C.

INTERPRETATION

Grade	Description	Amount of Protein (est. mg/dl)
1	Faint trace	5–20
2	Definite precipitate (finger is visible behind tube)	30–50
3	"Cannot see finger behind tube"	60–90
4	"Thick with curdle"	>100

If the urine specimen is turbid after centrifugation, this may be due to the presence of phosphates or urates. If the urine is alkaline, phosphates will disappear when it is acidified with 10% acetic acid. Urates will disappear when the specimen is heated to 41° C. Turbidity from chyluria will not clear, and the degree of turbidity should be subtracted from that obtained with the addition of Exton's reagent.

Sulfosalicylic acid precipitates protein in urine and produces turbidity that is approximately proportional to the concentration of protein in the solution. Sulfosalicylic acid detects albumin and globulin as well as Bence Jones protein, polypeptides, and proteases. Penicillin (and its derivatives, nafcillin or oxacillin), tolbutamide metabolites, sulfisoxazole metabolites, and certain organic roentgenological contrast media may produce a false-positive reaction [40]. This reaction usually disappears with subsequent boiling.

Albustix (Ames Company, Miles Laboratory, Elkhart, Ind.) is used in many laboratories as a screening test for protein. The strip contains bromphenol blue indicator and turns yellow-green to blue, depending on the amount of protein. It can detect 20 to 30 mg of protein per deciliter of urine; thus it is less sensitive than sulfosalicylic acid, which detects 5 to 10 mg/dl. However, Albustix does not detect Bence Jones protein and should not be used when a possibility of Bence Jones proteinuria exists.

Normal persons excrete less than 150 mg of protein per day in the urine, the mean value being 40 to 80 mg daily. The protein content of normal urine is 2 to 8 mg/dl [59].

Heat Test for Bence Jones Protein

Almost from the time of the discovery of the unique thermal properties of urinary light chains by Macintyre and Jones, screening tests for their detection have been in use. Although all of these tests have had shortcomings, the heat test of Putnam and colleagues [56] has been the most satisfactory. The sulfosalicylic acid test (Exton's) [20] should be performed first; if it is negative, no detectable Bence Jones protein is present.

REAGENT. The reagent used for the heat test is an acetate buffer consisting of 17.5 gm of sodium acetate trihydrate and 4.1 ml of glacial acetic acid. First, put the sodium acetate trihydrate in a 100-ml volumetric flask and add the glacial acetic acid; then add water to 100 ml (pH 4.9, 2 M).

PROCEDURE

1. Add 1.0 ml of 2 M acetate buffer of pH 4.9 to 4.0 ml of filtered urine and mix. The pH should be 4.9 ± 0.1.
2. Heat the mixture at 56° C in an incubation bath for 15 minutes. Precipitation suggests Bence Jones protein.
3. Heat the same tube for 3 minutes at 100° C and observe while the tube is in the boiling bath. Any decrease in the amount of precipitate or clearing of the opacity is considered confirmatory.
4. Filter the contents of the tube taken directly from the boiling water. If the filtrate is clear and then becomes cloudy as it cools, Bence Jones protein is present.

INTERPRETATION. Turbidity of urine or large amounts of albumin will obscure the dissolution of any Bence Jones protein with heating. The urine specimen should be fresh or refrigerated, because Bence Jones protein may denature if the urine is left at room temperature. A large amount of Bence Jones protein precipitating at 56°C may not redissolve upon boiling, so the test should be repeated with diluted urine. With the Putnam heat test, a protein concentration of 145 mg/dl is required for a positive result [38].

False-positive results with the heat test (no globulin band on electrophoresis of concentrated urine and no monoclonal light chain on immunoelectrophoresis) have been encountered in our experience. Connective tissue diseases were the most frequent cause of this false-positive reaction, followed by chronic renal insufficiency, nonmyelomatous malignancies, and fever of undetermined origin [54]. The results of urine and serum electrophoreses performed in the cases with false-positive results were nearly evenly divided between normal and polyclonal patterns. It appears that the heat test detected an increased quantity of kappa and lambda chains, which is a polyclonal response often seen in connective tissue diseases and neoplasia. Chronic renal insufficiency may cause lessening of the catabolism of light chains by the renal tubules and thus lead to increase of the amounts of kappa and lambda polyclonal chains in the urine. Therefore, the lack of a dense band on electrophoresis of adequately concentrated urine and a reaction to both kappa and lambda antisera on immunoelectrophoresis indicates that the positive result of the Bence Jones heat test is false.

On the other hand, Bence Jones heat test results have been negative in some cases where urinary electrophoresis has shown a dense globulin band or spike and where immunoelectrophoresis has demonstrated a monoclonal light chain. In a study of urines with a monoclonal protein and either positive or negative response to the Bence Jones heat test, we were unable to demonstrate the presence of a substance inhibiting the formation of dimer light chains from monomers. Both positive and negative groups had gel electrophoretic patterns with bands corresponding to the molecular weights of dimer and monomer species. Neither free sulfhydryl groups nor carbohydrates were demonstrable. Isoelectric focusing revealed similar values for both positive and false-negative Bence Jones proteins. Other studies disclosed similar amino acid compositions. There was no correlation between the light chain type or subtype and the thermal properties. The most likely explanation for the false-positive heat test results is an atypical Bence Jones protein with differences in amino acid sequence that produce conformational changes in the variable portion of the light chain [53].

Not all precipitates that form with heating of urine are Bence Jones protein. In one instance when a precipitate formed after heating of the urine and the possibility of Bence Jones proteinuria was suggested, electrophoresis showed a sharp band of α_2 mobility. This band was red-brown when stained with toluidine and subsequently was identified as hemoglobin, which is insoluble at 57°C at a pH of 5.2. Therefore, one must remember that hemoglobinuria can form a dense band on electrophoresis and can appear as a positive response to the heat test [52].

Electrophoresis and Immunoelectrophoresis of Urine

Electrophoresis and immunoelectrophoresis of urine should be performed in all cases with a monoclonal protein in the serum. In addition, both tests should be applied to urine in all instances of multiple myeloma, Waldenström's macroglobulinemia, amyloidosis, monoclonal gammopathy of undetermined significance, heavy-chain diseases, or suspicion of these entities. In addition, immunoelectrophoresis should be performed on a concentrated urine specimen from all adults older than 40 years of age with an apparently idiopathic nephrotic syndrome because the detection of a monoclonal light chain strongly suggests the diagnosis of primary systemic amyloidosis.

First, a 24-hour collection of the urine must be made for determination of the total amount of protein excreted per day. This is a most important factor when one is following the course of a patient being treated for disease.

DETERMINATION OF TOTAL PROTEIN. The biuret solution is prepared by adding 900 ml of 23% NaOH to 300 ml of $CuSO_4 \cdot 5\ H_2O$. Add 100 ml of tungstic acid (10% $Na_2WO_4 \cdot 2\ H_2O$) to 800 ml of 0.083 N H_2SO_4. Then add 0.1 ml of H_3PO_4.

Add 1 ml of filtered and centrifuged urine to 5 ml of tungstic acid and allow to sit for 5 minutes; then centrifuge. Dissolve the precipitate in 5 ml of saline and 5 ml of biuret solution. After 10 minutes, read at 545 nm in a Coleman Junior spectrophotometer. Optical density $\times$ 2.35 = gm/dl. One must run standard curves on known protein concentration to determine the factor.

ELECTROPHORESIS. In 1937, Tiselius [69] used electrophoretic techniques to separate serum globulins into three components that he designated alpha, beta, and gamma. Electrophoretic techniques were applied in the study of multiple myeloma protein by Longsworth and colleagues [41], who demonstrated the tall, narrow-based "church-spire" peak. The method was cumbersome and difficult, so electrophoresis was not readily available until the early 1950s, when filter paper was introduced as a supporting medium (zone electrophoresis). Cellulose acetate now has largely supplanted filter paper in this use [28]. The advantages of cellulose acetate membrane over filter paper for electrophoresis include decreased absorption of urine on the supporting medium, less tailing, and a sharper separation of protein bands. This technique also allows for a smaller amount of urine to be applied and is much faster.

The basic principle of electrophoresis is that charged particles in solution migrate according to their charge—for example, albumin toward the anode (positive pole). Since electrophoresis is performed at pH 8.8, where proteins have a negative charge, all immunoglobulins migrate toward the anode. The size of the molecule and the viscosity of the electrophoresis medium have no influence when the supporting medium is a cellulose acetate membrane.

Many instruments are available for electrophoresis of urinary protein (Beckman Instruments, Fullerton, Calif.; Gelman Instrument Company, Ann Arbor, Mich.). We use a Zip Zone (Helena) electrophoresis chamber, Super Z applicator, Drummond microdispenser, Titan III cellulose polyacetate electrophoresis strips, Ponceau S protein stain, tris (hydroxymethyl) aminomethane-barbital-sodium-barbital buffer (pH 8.8), and a Cliniscan densitometer (Helena Laboratories, Beaumont, Tex.) with a Centronics printer (Hudson, N.H.).

For electrophoresis of urine, it is usually necessary first to concentrate a sample of the 24-hour urine specimen. The ideal concentration of protein for electrophoresis is 3 gm/dl. Urine may be concentrated by dialysis against polyvinylpyrrolidine or dextran or by vacuum. We prefer ultrafiltration with a Minicon-B15 concentrator (Amicon Corp., Lexington, Mass.). First, 5 ml of urine is added to the concentrator; when the volume has decreased, 3 ml more of urine is added. The volume of urine is reduced to 0.1 ml ($\times$ 80) or to 0.04 ml ($\times$ 200). All substances with a molecular weight greater than 15,000 are retained.

The rest of the procedure is as follows.

1. Wet the cellulose acetate strips in the buffer for 20 minutes to 2 hours prior to use.
2. Pour 55 ml of tris-barbital buffer in each of the compartments of the Zip Zone electrophoresis chamber. Wet two disposable paper wicks in the buffer and then drape one over each support bridge, making sure it has buffer contact.
3. Use a Drummond microdispenser; fill each well in the sample well plate with 3 μl of sample.
4. Load the Super Z applicator from the sample well plate.
5. Remove the wetted cellulose acetate plate from the buffer and blot once. Transfer the applicator to the aligning base and apply the specimen to the cellulose polyacetate membrane. The number of applications depends on the protein concentration of the urine: one application if the concentration is $\geq$ 6.5 gm/dl; two if it is 4.0 to 6.5 gm/dl; three if it is 2.0 to 4.0 gm/dl; four if it is 1.0 to 2.0 gm/dl; and five applications if the concentration is $<$ 1 gm/dl. Place the cellulose acetate strip in the electrophoresis chamber, and then set the power supply at 200 volts and run for 11 minutes.
6. Place the cellulose polyacetate membrane in Ponceau S stain for 5 minutes. Destain in four successive washes of aqueous 5% acetic acid for 2 minutes each or until the background is white. Place the strip in dehydrating solution (100% methanol) three times for 1 minute each, and then in the clearing solution (71.5% methanol, 26% acetic acid, 2.5% Clear Aid [polyethylene glycol] 70 ml, acetic acid 650 ml, methanol 1720 ml) for 6 minutes. Air dry for 2 minutes and then place in a 92° to 95°C oven for 3 to 4 minutes.
7. Place the cellulose polyacetate membrane in the Cliniscan for densitometric quantitation.

Ordinarily, controls are not needed for the performance of electrophoresis; if the laboratory does need them, it is advisable to run a specimen known to contain a large amount of monoclonal protein and one known to have a normal pattern. Quality control should be maintained by utilizing sera or urine in

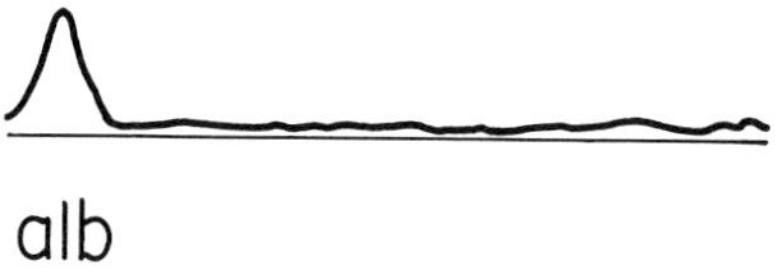

A

B

Figure 14–3
Normal urine. (A) Densitometer tracing. (B) Cellulose acetate electrophoretic pattern. Anode is on the left. Only a small amount of albumin is seen.

which the amounts of component proteins are agreed upon by several laboratories. Instrument standardization is also important, and linearity of response may be checked by use of densitometric standards, such as a step wedge.

In normal persons albumin constitutes about a third of urinary protein, and α_1- and α_2-globulins constitute almost half. The remainder are beta and gamma components [9]. These proteins consist of α_2- and β_2-microglobulins as well as both kappa and lambda light chains [35]. In a study of normal individuals, 15 percent of the gamma globulins had the characteristics of an Fc fragment. More than half of the gamma globulins were kappa and lambda light chains [72]. The mean normal urinary excretion of IgG is 2.9 mg and for IgA is 2.0 mg per 24 hours [23]. In most normal individuals the cellulose acetate tracing shows no bands or only a small albumin band.

Urinary monoclonal protein appears as a dense, localized band on the cellulose acetate strip or a tall, narrow, homogeneous peak on the densitometer tracing (Figs. 14–3 and 14–4). In general, a monoclonal protein in urine makes a wider band than a monoclonal protein in serum. Occasionally two discrete bands may be seen in the cellulose acetate tracing of the urine. These bands may be a monoclonal light chain plus a monoclonal immunoglobulin (from the serum), or the two bands may be monomers and dimers of the monoclonal light chain (Fig. 14–5). A polyclonal increase of light chains is seen as a very broad band extending through most of the gamma area; it has fuzzy, indistinct advancing and trailing edges. The densitometer tracing is broad-based (Fig. 14–6). In the nephrotic syndrome, one sees a large albumin band and prominent α_2 or β bands but minimal amounts of α_1 and γ globulins in the serum electrophoretic pattern and mainly albumin in the urine (Figs. 14–7 and 14–8).

The electrophoretic pattern signifying tubular abnormality is characterized

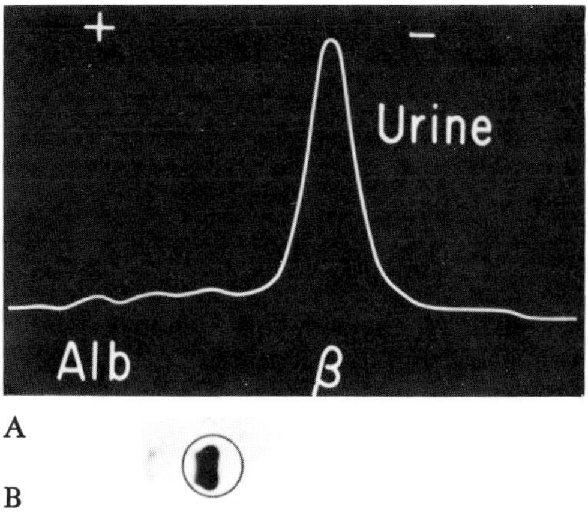

A

B

Figure 14–4
(A) Densitometer tracing. Tall, narrow-based monoclonal peak of beta mobility in patient with monoclonal protein. (B) Cellulose acetate electrophoretic pattern. Dense band of beta mobility represents a monoclonal light chain. (Reprinted, by permission, from R. A. Kyle and P. R. Greipp. The laboratory investigation of monoclonal gammopathies. *Mayo Clin. Proc.* 53:719–739, 1978.)

by a small amount of albumin (10 to 20 percent of total protein, the remainder being globulin fractions), and significant amounts of light chains are always present. The pattern representing glomerular abnormality is characterized by a large amount of albumin (more than 50 percent of the total) and modest amounts of globulin [44].

IMMUNOELECTROPHORESIS OF URINE. Immunoelectrophoresis should be performed on the concentrated urine of all patients who have a monoclonal protein in the serum or a sharp peak or band on the cellulose acetate tracing of the urine, and in all cases where myeloma, macroglobulinemia, amyloidosis, or a related disorder is suspected.

Immunoelectrophoresis is necessary to establish the presence or absence of light chains and to determine whether they are monoclonal or polyclonal. The concentrated urine specimen is placed in a well on a microscope slide covered with 1% agar or agarose and subjected to electrophoresis to separate the various components. A trough is cut into the agar, parallel to the line of migration of the components, and the trough is filled with a specific antiserum. Proteins from the sample that has undergone electrophoresis (antigen) and from the antiserum (antibody) are then allowed to diffuse toward each other and to form precipitin lines or arcs along the line of contact between antigen and antibody.

It is essential to use monospecific antisera to determine whether the light chains consist of either kappa or lambda or both (polyclonal). Polyclonal in-

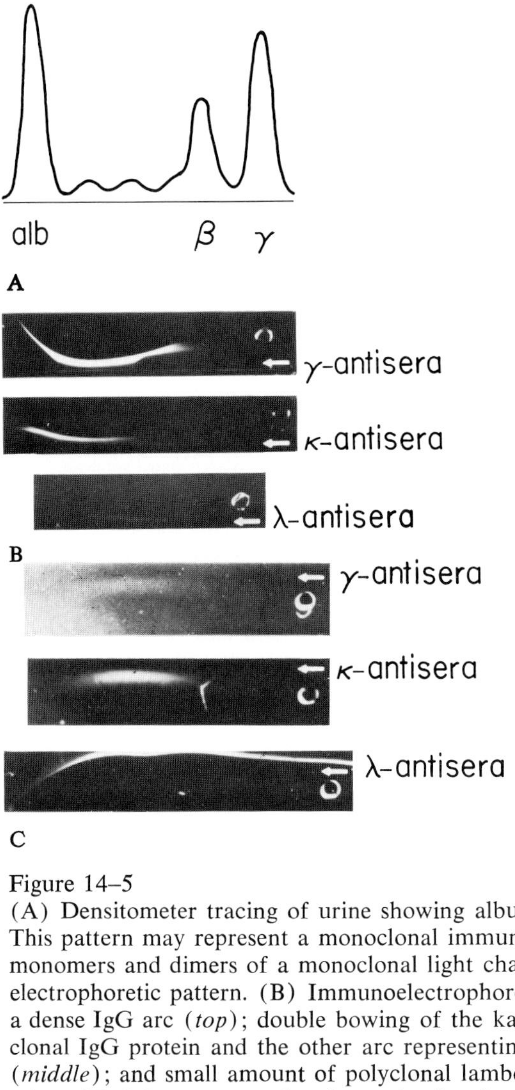

Figure 14–5
(A) Densitometer tracing of urine showing albumin, beta peak, and gamma peak. This pattern may represent a monoclonal immunoglobulin plus free light chain or monomers and dimers of a monoclonal light chain, causing the two peaks in the electrophoretic pattern. (B) Immunoelectrophoresis of concentrated urine showing a dense IgG arc (*top*); double bowing of the kappa arc corresponding to a monoclonal IgG protein and the other arc representing free monoclonal kappa chains (*middle*); and small amount of polyclonal lambda (*bottom*). This pattern is indicative of IgG kappa monoclonal protein plus free monoclonal kappa in the urine. (C) Immunoelectrophoresis of urine, with IgG (*top*) showing no localized arc; antisera to kappa (*middle*) showing a normal-appearing kappa arc; and antisera to lambda (*bottom*) showing a dense, doubly bowed lambda arc overwhelming the antisera. This pattern is consistent with monomers and dimers of a monoclonal lambda light chain. (Reprinted, by permission, from R. A. Kyle and P. R. Greipp. The laboratory investigation of monoclonal gammopathies. *Mayo Clin. Proc.* 53:719–739, 1978.)

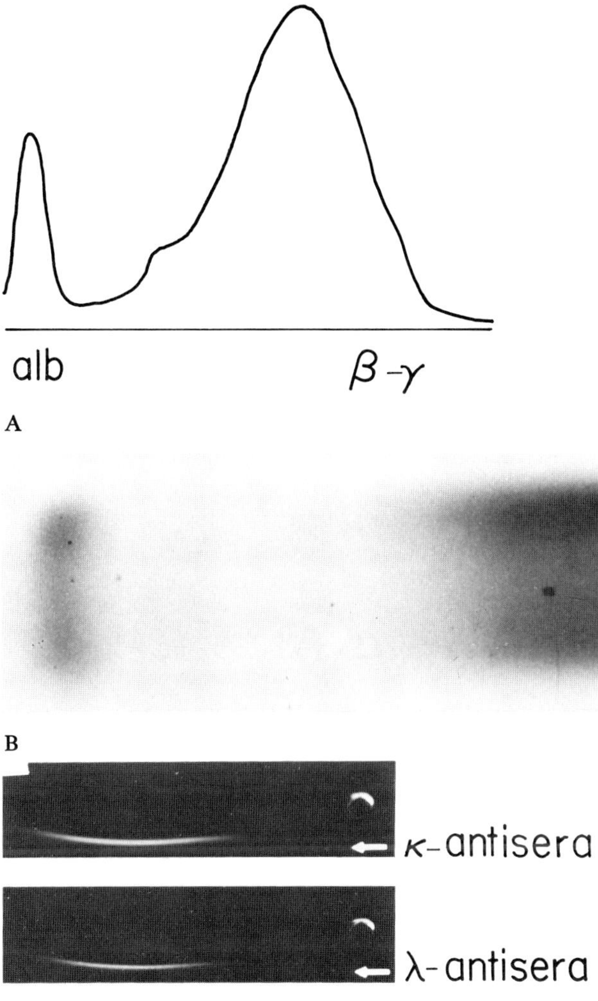

Figure 14–6
Urine with polyclonal increase in light chains. (A) Densitometer tracing. Note broad-based β-γ peak. (B) Electrophoretic pattern on cellulose acetate. Note the small albumin band and broad β-γ band, with advancing and trailing edges diffuse and fading into the background. (C) Immunoelectrophoresis with kappa- and lambda-antisera showing both kappa and lambda arcs, which appear to be normal and represent a polyclonal increase in light chains. (Reprinted, by permission, from R. A. Kyle and P. R. Greipp. The laboratory investigation of monoclonal gammopathies. *Mayo Clin. Proc.* 53:719–739, 1978.)

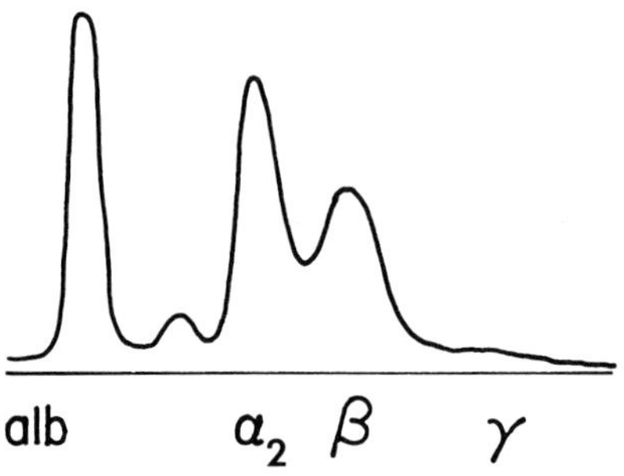

Figure 14–7
Nephrotic syndrome. Serum electrophoretic pattern showing decreased albumin (0.95 gm/dl) and γ-globulin with increased α_2- and β-globulin components. (Reprinted, by permission, from R. A. Kyle and P. R. Greipp. The laboratory investigation of monoclonal gammopathies. *Mayo Clin. Proc.* 53:719–739, 1978.)

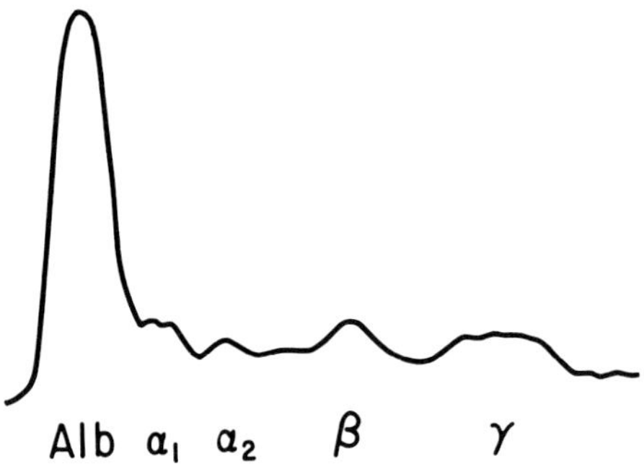

Figure 14–8
Nephrotic syndrome. Urine electrophoretic pattern; most of the protein is albumin. (Reprinted, by permission, from R. A. Kyle, R. C. Bieger, and G. J. Gleich. Diagnosis of syndromes associated with hyperglobulinemia. *Med. Clin. North Am.* 54:917, 1970.)

creases of immunoglobulins are usually associated with an inflammatory process, whereas a monoclonal protein is usually associated with a neoplastic or potentially neoplastic proliferation. Theoretically, it would be best to use antisera that would recognize only free kappa or lambda immunoglobulins rather than light chain antisera that recognize light chains in an intact immunoglobulin. However, such antisera are not readily available. We recently evaluated a kappa antiserum that was considered to be specific for free kappa chains. It recognized 9 of 10 urines with free kappa chains but also gave a positive reaction to 5 of 17 urines containing only lambda chains; in addition, it reacted with 5 sera containing an intact monoclonal globulin. Thus the kappa antisera recognized almost all free monoclonal kappa chains but also reacted to several serum and urine specimens without monoclonal free kappa proteins, so it was not as specific as one would wish. A lambda antiserum from the same source gave no reaction to any of the 9 kappa urines but recognized only 5 of 15 urines containing free lambda chains. None of the sera containing complete immunoglobulins reacted with the lambda antiserum. Thus the lambda antiserum exhibited excellent specificity but was not potent enough for general use. Consequently, we use kappa and lambda antisera that recognize both free and combined light chains but are monospecific and potent.

A monoclonal protein forms an arc that is bowed locally or restricted, whereas a polyclonal increase of light chain causes elongation and fuzziness of the arc. Most important, a monoclonal light chain in the urine produces a characteristic heavy, bowed or restricted arc of a monoclonal protein, whereas the other light-chain class produces a faint, fuzzy, elongated arc. Because of their arc configurations, therefore, we have had little difficulty in distinguishing monoclonal from polyclonal light chains in the urine.

Practical Difficulties. Various difficulties exist in the application of this method. The agar must be free from bubbles and impurities, because they produce distortions in the precipitin arcs. Since unequal depth of agar can cause aberrations of the arcs, the agar must be of uniform depth throughout the plate. Drying or freezing of the agar plates will prevent satisfactory electrophoresis and diffusion of the samples in the agar. In removing the agar from the wells and cutting the troughs, great care must be taken to avoid any irregularity or splitting of the agar because this may allow artifactual bowing or asymmetry of the arcs, suggesting a monoclonal protein. One must avoid pulling the agar away from the microscope slide, since this would allow antiserum to run under the agar. During electrophoresis, the wicks must maintain a good contact between the slide holder and the microscope slides and the buffer, or electrophoresis of the protein will be irregular. Inadvertent dropping of antiserum on the agar slide will produce artifactual distortion of the arcs and make interpretation very difficult.

Reagent. This determination utilizes a reagent prepared in two steps. First, 205.3 gm of barbital sodium and 36.8 gm of barbital (which must be dissolved in hot distilled water) are placed in a 5-liter volumetric container and diluted to 20 liters with distilled water. The barbital buffer (pH 8.2, 0.03 M) is stored at 4° C until use. Next, 4 gm of 1% noble agar is mixed with 400 ml of barbital buffer and heated to dissolve. Nine drops of 1% thimerosal (Merthiolate) are then added.

Procedure. Immunoelectrophoresis involves a more extensive procedure than does electrophoresis. A plastic holder accommodates six glass microscope slides, and the electrophoresis chamber will accept three slide holders; therefore, four sera and six urines can be run at one time. The steps to be followed are given below.

1. Place six new clean microscope slides in a slide holder and put the slide holder on a table that has been previously leveled.
2. Apply several drops of warm agar (1% noble agar in barbital buffer) to the microscope slides to make a seal between the slides, and at both ends of the row of slides to prevent excess loss of agar.
3. After allowing the agar seal to cool, apply a total of 10 ml of warm agar to one row of three slides.
4. Add 10 ml of warm agar to the second row of three slides.
5. Allow the slides to cool at 4° C in a humidity chamber until needed. The agar should be poured at least half an hour before use.
6. Record the name and number of the patient whose urine will be placed in the wells. This is best done on a 21.5 × 28 cm sheet marked with an outline of the six troughs, where the arcs can be drawn and results of interpretation can be recorded.
7. Punch the well-trough pattern, using an LKB die with a 1-mm trough and a diffusion distance of 5.1 mm from the trough.
8. Remove the agar from the wells with only gentle suction.
9. Using Fisher capillary tubes, fill the wells with urine concentrated 80- to 200-fold. Urine from the same patient is put in the top wells of the first two slides in the holder, and urine from a different patient is put in each bottom well.
10. Fill the wells of two more slide holders with the serum or urine specimens of additional patients, and place the three slide holders in the electrophoresis chamber. Be certain that the wicks are in good contact with the agar on all three slide holders. Set the voltage at 150, which produces approximately 30 mA.
11. Apply the current continuously for approximately 1½ hours.
12. Shut the current off and take the slide holders from the electrophoresis chamber.
13. Remove the agar gently from the troughs with suction.
14. Fill the troughs with monospecific antisera to kappa and lambda.
15. Store the slide holders in a humidity chamber at room temperature for 24 hours.

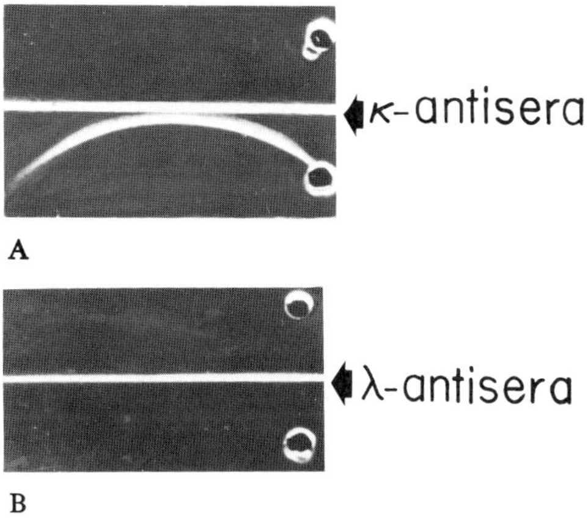

Figure 14–9
Immunoelectrophoresis of urine. (A) Antisera to kappa showing no arcs with normal urine (*top*); for comparison, note monoclonal kappa arc (*bottom*). (B) With antisera to lambda, no arcs are seen in normal urine (*top*), and there is no arc in the urine of a patient with a monoclonal kappa protein (*bottom*). The top portions of (A) and (B) represent normal urine; the bottom portions of (A) and (B) represent urine with a monoclonal kappa protein.

16. Read the immunoelectrophoretic patterns in a view box, and photograph the abnormal patterns. We use a Nikon F-2 camera with a Micro-Nikkor 105-mm f/4 lens, and Kodak high-contrast copy film, black and white, HC 135–36. The negatives are stored in plastic folders.

Interpretation. Potent monospecific antisera to kappa and lambda chains are essential. It is most important for each laboratory to test its antisera. For example, to ascertain the specificity and strength of kappa antiserum, it should be run against known IgA kappa, IgA lambda, IgM kappa, IgM lambda, IgG kappa, and IgG lambda sera as well as several urines containing only kappa or lambda monoclonal light chains. It is always useful to have antisera of various sources available when typing monoclonal proteins because the antigenic determinants of some monoclonal proteins are so restricted that they will not be recognized by all antisera.

Monoclonal protein produces localized thickening or bowing of the arc (Fig. 14–9). Occasionally, a thickened arc appears as if cut off abruptly near the trough. This phenomenon may be caused by overwhelming of the antiserum by the antigen or by formation of a soluble antigen-antibody complex (antigen excess). Consequently, immunoelectrophoresis should then be repeated with unconcentrated urine. Sometimes the monoclonal light chain content of the urine is so high that the unconcentrated urine must be diluted to make an arc visible. Occasionally, the concentrated urine will need to be diluted in order to detect a localized arc. Lesser concentrations of antigen will produce an arc near the well. Most precipitin arcs form within 24 hours. If the diffusion is allowed to continue more than 24 hours, the arcs become diffuse and exaggerated, making interpretation very difficult.

If electrophoresis of the urine reveals a globulin spike but immunoelectrophoresis does not demonstrate a monoclonal light chain, one must suspect the presence of gamma heavy-chain disease. Immunoelectrophoresis of concentrated urine should then be performed with antisera to IgG (gamma heavy chains) (Fig. 14–10).

Immunoelectrophoresis should be performed on the urine of a patient with suspected monoclonal gammopathy, even if Exton's sulfosalicylic acid test [20] is negative for protein. We have seen a number of cases in which urine osmolality was normal or elevated and reaction for protein negative but in which electrophoresis of concentrated urine revealed a small, localized band of protein and immunoelectrophoresis demonstrated a monoclonal light chain. As stated previously, these findings may be the first clue to amyloidosis.

Immunoelectrophoresis with monospecific light-chain antisera should be performed on the urine of all adults who develop the nephrotic syndrome. We have seen a number of patients in whom electrophoresis of urine showed a large amount of albumin and insignificant amounts of globulin, but who actually had a monoclonal light chain in the urine. Many of these patients had primary amyloidosis, although a few had multiple myeloma. A monoclonal light chain in the urine is sometimes the first clue that a patient has amyloidosis with a nephrotic syndrome rather than idiopathic nephrotic syndrome (Figs. 14–7 and 14–8).

The need for collection of a 24-hour urine specimen cannot be overemphasized. First, it allows one to measure the amount of the monoclonal protein excreted in the urine, which is an excellent indication of the effect of chemotherapy or evidence of progession of the disease; it is also very useful in following the course of a patient with amyloidosis and the nephrotic syndrome.

Immunodiffusion

All urines studied by immunoelectrophoresis should also be examined by immunodiffusion, applied to a neat (unconcentrated) specimen as well as to specimens concentrated 80- or 200-fold.

PROCEDURE (OUCHTERLONY)

1. Microscope slides are coated with 1% agar as described for immunoelectrophoresis, except that the agar is dissolved in 0.01 M potassium phosphate-0.15 M sodium chloride.
2. Wells are punched as shown in Figure 14–11. A die that makes six or eight wells around the central well rather than four may be used.
3. The center well is filled with kappa or lambda monospecific antiserum. For

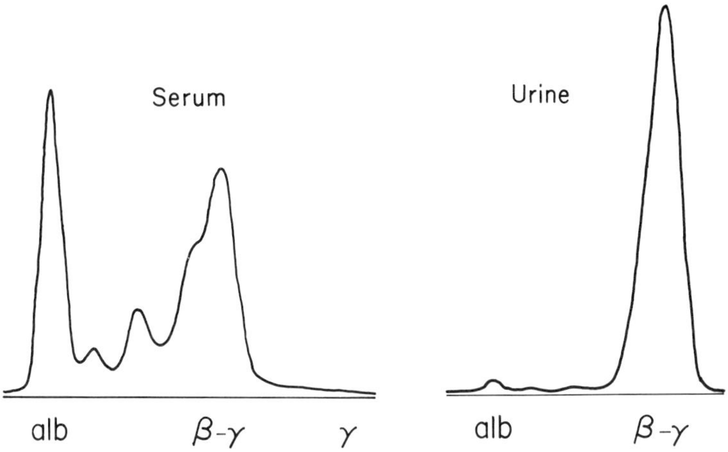

A

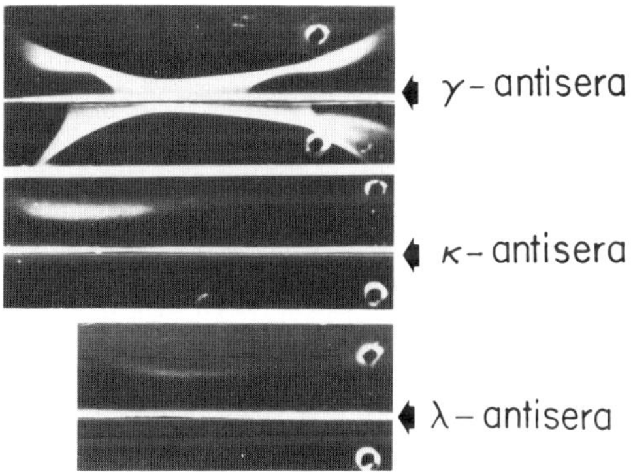

B

Figure 14–10
Gamma heavy-chain disease. (A) Densitometer tracings. Serum: Note the tall peak of β-γ mobility. Urine: Note the dense β-γ band. (B) Immunoelectrophoresis. The top well in each immunoelectrophoretic pattern represents serum, while the bottom well represents concentrated urine. With γ-antisera, a dense, thickened, asymmetrical arc is seen in both serum and urine; with κ-antisera, a faint, fuzzy arc is seen in the serum and no arc is seen in the urine; with λ-antisera, there is a faint, fuzzy lambda arc in the serum and none in the urine. This pattern represents a monoclonal gamma chain in the serum and urine (gamma heavy-chain disease). (Reprinted, by permission, from R. A. Kyle and P. R. Greipp. The laboratory investigation of monoclonal gammopathies. *Mayo Clin. Proc.* 53:719–739, 1978.)

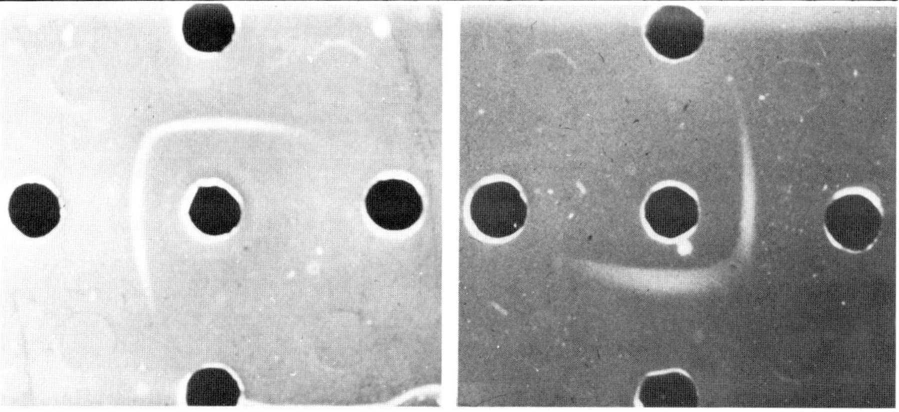

A B

Figure 14–11
Immunodiffusion (Ouchterlony) with antisera to kappa (A) and lambda (B) in center of each slide. The top well and left well show a kappa band and no lambda band in urine; the bottom and right wells show a dense lambda band and no kappa band in urine. (Reprinted, by permission, from R. A. Kyle and P. R. Greipp. The laboratory investigation of monoclonal gammopathies. *Mayo Clin. Proc.* 53:719–739, 1978.)

a control, one of the peripheral wells is filled with the urine of a patient with a known kappa or lambda protein. The urines to be tested are placed in the other wells. We place both undiluted and concentrated urine of each patient in the wells.

4. The slides are read at 24 hours, and photographs may be taken.

INTERPRETATION. The presence of a dense precipitin band confirms the presence of protein of that class. Again, the concentrated urine may overwhelm the antisera without forming a band. Conversely, a very faint band suggests the possibility of a monoclonal protein, and immunoelectrophoresis should be performed with a more concentrated urine specimen to determine whether the band on immunodiffusion represents a monoclonal increase of light chain or merely a polyclonal light chain.

Immunodiffusion is more sensitive than immunoelectrophoresis and is a useful screening test, but it reacts to both monoclonal and polyclonal light chains; therefore, immunoelectrophoresis must always be performed to prove that the protein detected is monoclonal.

Although the heat test for Bence Jones protein is useful as a clinical screening test, one must remember the shortcomings of this test mentioned earlier. For demonstrating a monoclonal protein in the urine, electrophoresis and immunoelectrophoresis of an adequately concentrated specimen are the methods of choice.

Differential Diagnosis of Monoclonal Proteins in Urine

The presence of a monoclonal light chain in the urine suggests the following possibilities:

1. Multiple myeloma (IgG, IgA, IgD, IgE, and free light chains)
   a. Solitary plasmacytoma of bone
   b. Extramedullary plasmacytoma, solitary or multiple
   c. Plasma cell leukemia
   d. Acquired Fanconi's syndrome in adults
2. Waldenström's macroglobulinemia (primary macroglobulinemia; IgM)
3. Amyloidosis
   a. Primary
   b. With myeloma
4. Mu heavy-chain disease (μ HCD)
5. Monoclonal gammopathy of undetermined significance
6. Lymphoma
7. Idiopathic Bence Jones proteinuria

Multiple Myeloma

Multiple myeloma is the most common cause of a monoclonal light chain in the urine (Bence Jones proteinuria). At the Mayo Clinic, 658 of 869 myeloma patients seen between 1960 and 1971 were tested for the presence of Bence Jones proteinuria utilizing the heat test. Of the 658 tested, 47 percent were positive, 48 percent negative, and 5 percent equivocal [29]. Electrophoresis of the urine in 551 myeloma cases at the Mayo Clinic revealed a globulin peak in 75 percent and an albumin peak in 10 percent. No albumin or globulin peak was seen in 15 percent of the cases. The incidence of globulin peaks in the urine is higher than expected in this series; it would be lower if urine electrophoresis had been performed in all 869 cases (since in those with no proteinuria on routine analysis, performance of electrophoresis would have been less likely). Of the 551 patients, 9 percent excreted more than 10 gm of globulin daily. Immunoelectrophoresis of concentrated urine and immunodiffusion of neat urine showed a monoclonal light chain in 80 percent of 198 cases. Of those patients with a monoclonal protein in the urine, 58 percent had kappa light chains.

The finding of Bence Jones protein in the urine of patients with multiple myeloma and renal insufficiency is of interest. All of our patients with multiple myeloma whose creatinine or urea was measured initially were divided into two groups on the basis of normality or insufficiency of renal function (creatinine more than 1.2 mg/dl in males and more than 0.9 mg/dl in females, or blood urea more than 50 mg/dl in either males or females). Bence Jones proteinuria was present (ascertained by heat test) in 58 percent of the 299 patients with renal insufficiency and in 43 percent of the 317 patients with normal renal function; this difference is of borderline statistical significance. Of the patients with

Table 14–3. Multiple Myeloma: Serum Creatinine and Urinary Globulin (Within One Month of Diagnosis) in Patients With Monoclonal Light Chains in Urine

Parameters	Urinary protein	
	Kappa	Lambda
Serum creatinine, mg/dl	(N = 64)	(N = 55)
Mean	1.9	2.3
$\geq$ 2.0	20%	29%
Urinary globulin, gm/24 hr	(N = 60)	(N = 53)
Mean	3.8	4.2
$\geq$ 2.0	45%	55%
$\geq$ 4	32%	32%
$\geq$ 6	20%	25%
$\geq$ 10	10%	11%

Source: From R. A. Kyle and E. D. Bayrd. *The Monoclonal Gammopathies: Multiple Myeloma and Related Plasma-Cell Disorders,* 1976. Courtesy of Charles C Thomas, Publisher, Springfield, Illinois.

renal insufficiency (elevated creatinine or urea), 80 had a monoclonal light chain in the urine—kappa in 54 percent and lambda in 46 percent. Of the patients with normal renal function, 79 had a monoclonal light chain in the urine, which was kappa in 63 percent and lambda in the remainder [32]. The presence of a single light-chain class was not associated with an excessive incidence of renal insufficiency.

In a group of 64 patients with kappa monoclonal protein in the urine, the mean serum creatinine concentration was lower than in 55 patients with lambda, but the difference was not significant [32]. The same is true of the amount of urinary globulin excretion (Table 14–3). The serum creatinine was 2 mg/dl or more in 20 percent of the patients with kappa monoclonal protein in the urine and in 29 percent of those with lambda. We found no convincing evidence that a monoclonal lambda protein was significantly more nephrotoxic than kappa.

Whether or not the prognosis is related to the type of immunoglobulin abnormality is not clear. A report stating that patients producing only the lambda type of Bence Jones protein did not respond to melphalan, whereas those producing only kappa Bence Jones protein did respond [7], was later refuted [36, 49]. It has been said that patients with lambda light chains have briefer survival than those with kappa light chains and that those producing only Bence Jones proteins survive for the shortest period [2]; and in a reported study [1], patients with lambda Bence Jones protein did not survive as long as those with kappa. In a recent study the median survival from diagnosis was 30 months for 52 patients with kappa light-chain disease and 10 months for 45 patients with lambda light-chain disease [63].

SOLITARY PLASMACYTOMA OF BONE. The diagnosis of solitary plasmacytoma depends on histological proof that the tumor consists of plasma cells identical to those seen in myeloma and that no other evidence of multiple myeloma exists. Most patients with apparent solitary plasmacytoma of bone eventually develop widespread disease (multiple myeloma) [47]. Electrophoresis and immunoelectrophoresis of an adequately concentrated urine specimen are helpful in recognizing the development of multiple myeloma. Although Bence Jones proteinuria has been reported with solitary plasmacytoma [6], its occurrence strongly suggests multiple myeloma.

EXTRAMEDULLARY PLASMACYTOMA. Plasma cell tumors that arise outside the bone marrow are termed *extramedullary plasmacytomas.* They may be extensions of already existing multiple myeloma, or they may appear to be primary and disseminate later to produce widespread disease. The upper respiratory tract, including the nasal cavity and sinuses, nasopharynx, and larynx, is the most frequent location of lesions [75]. Periodic testing of the urine for monoclonal light chains is helpful in following the patient.

PLASMA CELL LEUKEMIA. Increased numbers of plasma cells in the peripheral blood characterize plasma cell leukemia (more than 20 percent plasma cells in the peripheral blood and an absolute plasma cell content of at least $2000/mm^3$). This disease should be considered as a form of multiple myeloma and not as a separate entity [34].

IgD MYELOMA. Since the discovery of IgD immunoglobulin in 1965, more than 130 cases of IgD myeloma have been reported [27]. Bence Jones proteinuria is present in more than 90 percent of cases. Monoclonal lambda light chains are found in 90 percent, whereas only 30 percent of IgA and IgG myelomas are of the lambda type.

ACQUIRED FANCONI'S SYNDROME IN ADULTS. Adult patients with acquired Fanconi's syndrome have dysfunction of the proximal renal tubules, which produces glycosuria, aminoaciduria, phosphaturia, and acidosis. Of 17 reported cases, 11 included Bence Jones proteinuria; typing in 7 patients showed that the Bence Jones protein was of the kappa class [43]. The amount of monoclonal light chain in the urine must be checked periodically, because patients with acquired Fanconi's syndrome may develop symptomatic multiple myeloma or amyloidosis. One of our 3 patients with adult Fanconi's syndrome developed multiple myeloma, and amyloidosis was found in another after 17 years.

In one instance, a patient with monoclonal kappa protein in his urine had proximal renal tubular dysfunction (glycosuria, phosphaturia, uricosuria, aminoaciduria, and proximal renal tubular acidosis), which is characteristic of the adult Fanconi's syndrome, but this patient also had distal tubular dysfunction manifested by distal renal tubular acidosis and nephrogenic diabetes insipidus [64].

Waldenström's Macroglobulinemia

Waldenström's macroglobulinemia is a malignant lymphoplasmoproliferative disorder characterized by a large amount of monoclonal IgM protein in the serum. Renal failure occurs ultimately in one-third of the patients. Approximately one-fourth of patients have Bence Jones proteinuria [14, 45].

Primary Amyloidosis

The diagnosis of primary amyloidosis is given in patients with histological proof of amyloidosis but no preceding or coexisting disease. The recognition of amyloidosis is facilitated by the presence of a monoclonal protein in the serum or urine. In fact, the presence of a monoclonal protein with the nephrotic syndrome, congestive heart failure, carpal tunnel syndrome, peripheral neuropathy, or orthostatic hypotension requires the exclusion of amyloidosis. Since adopting this policy, we have doubled the annual number of new diagnoses of amyloidosis at our institution. Almost half of patients with primary amyloidosis have renal insufficiency when the diagnosis is made, and proteinuria is present in 90 percent. Electrophoresis of the urine frequently shows a large albumin peak, since almost a third of these patients have a nephrotic syndrome. Not infrequently, a small monoclonal light chain is found in the patients with a nephrotic syndrome. The globulin spike in these instances is usually very small and easily overlooked. Among cases in which immunoelectrophoresis of the serum and urine was performed, 88 percent had a monoclonal protein [31]. Other investigators have also noted a high incidence of monoclonal proteins in patients with amyloidosis [26, 50]. Amyloidosis may be associated with multiple myeloma.

Heavy-Chain Diseases

Heavy-chain diseases (HCD) are characterized by the presence of a portion of a monoclonal immunoglobulin heavy chain in the serum or urine or both.

GAMMA HEAVY-CHAIN DISEASE. The abnormal protein in gamma HCD is the heavy chain of IgG (gamma)—mainly the Fc fragment of this chain, since the monoclonal protein usually includes a deletion of the variable portion of the heavy chain. This abnormal protein produces a lymphoma-like illness that usually progresses. The most significant laboratory features are a dense globulin band or spike on electrophoresis of the urine, a negative response to the Bence Jones heat test, and lack of light-chain identification on immunoelectrophoresis. In such cases, immunoelectrophoresis of the concentrated urine discloses a monoclonal gamma heavy chain. Serum electrophoresis usually reveals a band in the beta or gamma region, but often the band is broad and appears heterogeneous and more suggestive of a polyclonal than a monoclonal protein. Bence Jones proteinuria is not a feature of the disease [8].

ALPHA HEAVY-CHAIN DISEASE. Alpha HCD has become the most frequently reported type of HCD, with more than 80 cases in the literature [58a]. It is characterized by severe malabsorption with weight loss, diarrhea, and steatorrhea. There is diffuse and extensive infiltration of the gastrointestinal tract with lymphocytes and plasma cells. The amount of alpha chain in the urine is small, and the urine must be concentrated before it can be detected. Bence Jones proteinuria has never been reported in alpha HCD.

MU HEAVY-CHAIN DISEASE. Most instances of mu HCD have occurred in patients with chronic lymphocytic leukemia [22], but association with typical lymphoma has been reported also. Most patients have large amounts of Bence Jones protein in the urine, but mu chain fragments are rarely seen.

Monoclonal Gammopathy of Undetermined Significance

We have observed 241 patients with a monoclonal protein in the serum who initially had no evidence of multiple myeloma, macroglobulinemia, amyloidosis, or lymphoma [30]. At the conclusion of the study the patients were classified as follows: group 1, without significant increase in monoclonal protein, 57 percent; group 2, with more than 50 percent increase in monoclonal serum protein or development of monoclonal urine protein, 9 percent; group 3, died without five-year serum studies, 23 percent; and group 4, having developed myeloma, macroglobulinemia, or amyloidosis, 11 percent.

Retrospective analysis of age, sex, presence of organomegaly, hemoglobin level, amount and type of serum monoclonal protein, presence of small amounts of monoclonal light chain in the urine, serum albumin level, levels of uninvolved immunoglobulins, IgG subclass, and level of plasma cells in the bone marrow did not show how to distinguish initially between stable benign disease and progressive disease.

Immunoelectrophoresis demonstrated a monoclonal light chain in the urine of 12 patients out of 45 tested in group 1 (no significant increase of serum monoclonal protein). In the 6 patients in whom it was discovered at the time when the serum monoclonal protein was diagnosed, the monoclonal urine protein disappeared from 1 after removal of the parathyroid adenoma and remained stable in the other 5. In the 6 patients in whom the urinary monoclonal protein was discovered during the period of observation, the monoclonal serum protein diminished in 4, increased 0.1 gm/dl in 1, and remained the same in 1. Among all 12 patients, the 24-hour urinary excretion was 0.5 gm or less in 8. In 3 of the remaining 4, the amount of urinary light chain had remained stable for more than 10 years, and in the fourth it disappeared after removal of a parathyroid adenoma.

Of 17 urine studies in group 2 (more than 50 percent increase of monoclonal serum protein from initial value, or appearance of monoclonal urine protein), 8 disclosed a monoclonal light chain, although the amount exceeded 0.5 gm per 24 hours in only 1 patient. The urinary monoclonal protein was discovered at the same time as the serum monoclonal protein in 2 patients. The urine protein increased during the observation period in 1 of these patients, and the serum monoclonal protein increased in the other 7; thus either the urinary protein peak or the serum protein peak increased in all 8.

The association of Bence Jones proteinuria with a monoclonal serum protein usually indicates a neoplastic process. Waldenström [73] stated that excretion of a demonstrable amount of Bence Jones protein in the urine of a patient with a monoclonal serum protein was strong evidence of malignancy. Hobbs [24] said that Bence Jones proteinuria of more than 1.0 mg/dl (10 mg/L) was of "sinister significance" and suggestive of malignant plasmacytic disease. Seligmann and Basch [61] noted that a Bence Jones protein level of 30 mg/dl (300 mg/L) or more in a patient with a pathological serum immunoglobulin and decreased normal immunoglobulins strongly suggested malignant proliferation. Dammacco and Waldenström [16], from a study of 42 patients with benign monoclonal gammopathy, reported weakly positive results of the heat test for Bence Jones protein in 1 patient and small amounts of light chains in 10. None of these patients had more than 60 mg/L of Bence Jones protein. The presence of a monoclonal light chain in the urine is very suggestive of a neoplastic process, and such a patient must be followed closely for the development of multiple myeloma, amyloidosis, or other serious disease.

Idiopathic Bence Jones Proteinuria (Benign Monoclonal Light-Chain Gammopathy)

The possibility of a benign monoclonal gammopathy of the light-chain type must be considered, despite the fact that Bence Jones proteinuria is a recognized feature of multiple myeloma, Waldenström's macroglobulinemia, primary amyloidosis, and occasionally lymphoma. We have followed two patients who have maintained a stable amount of monoclonal serum protein and excreted 0.8 gm or more of Bence Jones protein daily for more than 12 years without evidence of the development of myeloma, amyloidosis, or similar malignant diseases. One of these patients had documented proteinuria 10 years before the recognition of Bence Jones proteinuria, making a total duration of proteinuria of 22 years [33]. Currently we are following two additional patients who have excreted more than 1 gm per 24 hours of a monoclonal light chain for 4 and 7 years and who have no monoclonal protein in the serum, no anemia, no lytic bone lesions, and no evidence of multiple myeloma. Cronstedt and colleagues [15] reported a patient in whom decreased IgG and IgA protein had persisted for 5 years and then Bence Jones proteinuria had appeared (175 mg/L), still without myeloma. Therefore, appreciable Bence Jones proteinuria may be benign or idiopathic and is not always an ominous finding.

Lymphoma

We have seen a rare patient with the histological and clinical features of lymphoma but who had a large monoclonal light chain in the urine.

Although urinary light chain excretion may be increased in lymphoma, it is usually polyclonal [39]. The presence of a monoclonal kappa protein was found in the serum and urine of a patient with an atypical lymphoma [13].

In a study of 30 patients with non-Hodgkin's lymphoma, Lindström and coworkers [39] found that 7 patients excreted more than 100 mg of light chains per 24 hours. None of these were monoclonal.

References

1. A Cooperative Study by Acute Leukemia Group B. Correlation of abnormal immunoglobulin with clinical features of myeloma. *Arch. Intern. Med.* 135:46, 1975.
2. Alexanian, R., Haut, A., Khan, A. U., et al. Treatment for multiple myeloma: Combination chemotherapy with different melphalan dose regimens. *J. A. M. A.* 208:1680, 1969.

2a. Bayne-Jones, S., and Wilson, D. W. Immunological reactions of Bence-Jones proteins. II. Differences between Bence-Jones proteins from various sources. *Bull. Johns Hopkins Hosp.* 33:119, 1922.

3. Bence Jones, H. On a new substance occurring in the urine of a patient with mollities ossium. *Proc. R. Soc. Lond.* 5:673, 1847.
4. Bence Jones, H. Papers on chemical pathology: Lecture III. *Lancet* 2:88, 1847.
5. Bence Jones, H. On a new substance occurring in the urine of a patient with mollities ossium. *Philos. Trans. R. Soc. Lond.*, p. 55, 1848.
6. Benedict, K. T., Jr. Destructive lesion of the proximal radius. *J. A. M. A.* 212:464, 1970.
7. Bergsagel, D. E., Migliore, P. J., and Griffith, K. M. Myeloma proteins and the clinical response to melphalan therapy. *Science* 148:376, 1965.
8. Bloch, K. J., Lee, L., Mills, J. A., et al. Gamma heavy chain disease: An expanding clinical and laboratory spectrum. *Am. J. Med.* 55:61, 1973.
9. Boyce, W. H., Garvey, F. K., and Norfleet, C. M., Jr. Proteins and other biocolloids of urine in health and in calculous disease: I. Electrophoretic studies at pH 4.5 and 8.6 of those components soluble in molar sodium chloride. *J. Clin. Invest.* 33:1287, 1954.
10. Bush, S. T., Swedlund, H. A., and Gleich, G. J. Low molecular weight IgM in human sera. *J. Lab. Clin. Med.* 73:194, 1969.
11. Buxbaum, J. N. The biosynthesis, assembly, and secretion of immunoglobulins. *Semin. Hematol.* 10:33, 1973.
12. Capra, J. D., and Kehoe, J. M. Hypervariable regions, idiotypy, and the antibody-combining site. *Adv. Immunol.* 20:1, 1975.
13. Chenais, F., Virella, G., Young, C. D., et al. Atypical B cell dyscrasia with Bence-Jones proteinuria and intracellular retention of γ-chains. *Acta Haematol. (Basel)* 58:166, 1977.
14. Creyssel, R. Diagnostic Value of Bence-Jones Protein. In Y. Manuel, J. P. Revillard, and H. Betuel (Eds.), *Proteins in Normal and Pathological Urine.* Basel: Karger, 1970. Pp. 100–110.
15. Cronstedt, J., Carling, L., and Östberg, H. Idiopathic light chain dyscrasia—a new distinct entity? Report of a case. *Acta Med. Scand.* 196:445, 1974.
16. Darnmacco, F., and Waldenström, J. Bence Jones proteinuria in benign mono-

clonal gammapathies: Incidence and characteristics. *Acta Med. Scand.* 184:403, 1968.
17. DeCoteau, W. E. The role of secretory IgA in defense of the distal lung. *Ann. N.Y. Acad. Sci.* 221:214, 1974.
18. Edelman, G. M., and Gally, J. A. The nature of Bence-Jones proteins: Chemical similarities to polypeptide chains of myeloma globulins and normal γ-globulins. *J. Exp. Med.* 116:207, 1962.
19. Eulitz, M. A new subgroup of human L-chains of the λ-type: Primary structure of Bence-Jones protein DEL. *Eur. J. Biochem.* 50:49, 1974.
20. Exton, W. G. A simple and rapid test for albumin and other urinary proteins. *J. A. M. A.* 80:529, 1923.
21. Fett, J. W., and Deutsch, H. F. Primary structure of the Mcg λ chain. *Biochemistry* 13:4102, 1974.
22. Franklin, E. C. μ-Chain disease. *Arch. Intern. Med.* 135:71, 1975.
23. Hicks, E. J., Nordschow, C. D., and Griep, J. A. Multiple myeloma and macrogammaglobulinemia: I. Urinary protein excretions and serum interrelationships. *Am. J. Clin. Pathol.* 64:1, 1975.
24. Hobbs, J. R. Paraproteins, benign or malignant? *Br. Med. J.* 3:699, 1967.
25. Ishizaka, K., Ishizaka, T., and Hornbrook, M. M. Physicochemical properties of reaginic antibody: V. Correlation of reaginic activity with γE-globulin antibody. *J. Immunol.* 97:840, 1966.
26. Isobe, T., and Osserman, E. F. Patterns of amyloidosis and their association with plasma-cell dyscrasia, monoclonal immunoglobulins and Bence-Jones proteins. *N. Engl. J. Med.* 290:473, 1974.
27. Jancelewicz, Z., Takatsuki, K., Sugai, S., et al. IgD multiple myeloma: Review of 133 cases. *Arch. Intern. Med.* 135:87, 1975.
28. Kohn, J. A cellulose acetate supporting medium for zone electrophoresis. *Clin. Chim. Acta* 2:297, 1957.
29. Kyle, R. A. Multiple myeloma: Review of 869 cases. *Mayo Clin. Proc.* 50:29, 1975.
30. Kyle, R. A. Monoclonal gammopathy of undetermined significance: Natural history of 241 cases. *Am. J. Med.* 64:814, 1978.
31. Kyle, R. A., and Bayrd, E. D. Amyloidosis: Review of 236 cases. *Medicine (Baltimore)* 54:271, 1975.
32. Kyle, R. A., and Elveback, L. R. Management and prognosis of multiple myeloma. *Mayo Clin. Proc.* 51:751, 1976.
32a. Kyle, R. A., and Greipp, P. R. Laboratory medicine—series on clinical testing. 3. The laboratory investigation of monoclonal gammopathies. *Mayo Clin. Proc.* 53:719–739, 1978.
33. Kyle, R. A., Maldonado, J. E., and Bayrd, E. D. Idiopathic Bence Jones proteinuria—a distinct entity? *Am. J. Med.* 55:222, 1973.
34. Kyle, R. A., Maldonado, J. E., and Bayrd, E. D. Plasma cell leukemia: Report on 17 cases. *Arch. Intern. Med.* 133:813, 1974.
35. Laurell, C.-B. Composition and variation of the gel electrophoretic fractions of plasma, cerebrospinal fluid and urine. *Scand. J. Clin. Lab. Invest.* 29 (Suppl. 124): 71, 1972.
36. Lee, B. J., Korngold, L., and Weiner, M. J. Melphalan and antigenic type of Bence Jones proteins in myeloma. *Science* 149:564, 1965.
37. Lieu, T.-S., Deutsch, H. F., and Tischendorf, F. W. Human λ-chain sequence variations and serologic associations. *Immunochemistry* 14:429, 1977.
38. Lindström, F. D., Williams, R. C., Jr., Swain, W. R., et al. Urinary light-chain excretion in myeloma and other disorders: An evaluation of the Bence-Jones test. *J. Lab. Clin. Med.* 71:812, 1968.

39. Lindström, F. D., Williams, R. C., Jr., and Theologides, A. Urinary light chain excretion in leukemia and lymphoma. *Clin. Exp. Immunol.* 5:83, 1969.
40. Line, D. E., Adler, S., Fraley, D. S., et al. Massive pseudoproteinuria caused by nafcillin. *J.A.M.A.* 235:1259, 1976.
41. Longsworth, L. G., Shedlovsky, T., and MacInnes, D. A. Electrophoretic patterns of normal and pathological human blood serum and plasma. *J. Exp. Med.* 70:399, 1939.
42. Macintyre, W. Case of mollities and fragilitas ossium, accompanied with urine strongly charged with animal matter. *Med. Chir. Trans. Lond.* 33:211, 1850.
43. Maldonado, J. E., Velosa, J. A., Kyle, R. A., et al. Fanconi syndrome in adults: A manifestation of a latent form of myeloma. *Am. J. Med.* 58:354, 1975.
44. Manuel, Y., and Revillard, J. P. Study of Urinary Proteins by Zone Electrophoresis: Methods and Principles of Interpretation. In Y. Manuel, J. P. Revillard, and H. Betuel (Eds.), *Proteins in Normal and Pathological Urine.* Basel: Karger, 1970. Pp. 153–171.
45. McCallister, B. D., Bayrd, E. D., Harrison, E. G., Jr., et al. Primary macroglobulinemia: Review with a report on thirty-one cases and notes on the value of continuous chlorambucil therapy. *Am. J. Med.* 43:394, 1967.
46. Metzger, H. Structure and function of γM macroglobulins. *Adv. Immunol.* 12:57, 1970.
47. Meyer, J. E., and Schulz, M. D. "Solitary" myeloma of bone: A review of 12 cases. *Cancer* 34:438, 1974.
48. Mogielnicki, R. P., Waldmann, T. A., and Strober, W. Renal handling of low molecular weight proteins: I. L-chain metabolism in experimental renal disease. *J. Clin. Invest.* 50:901, 1971.
49. Osserman, E. F. Melphalan and antigenic type of Bence Jones proteins in myeloma. *Science* 149:564, 1965.
50. Osserman, E. F., Takatsuki, K., and Talal, N. The pathogenesis of "amyloidosis": Studies on the role of abnormal gamma globulins and gamma globulin fragments of the Bence Jones (L-polypeptide) type in the pathogenesis of "primary" and "secondary amyloidosis," and the "amyloidosis" associated with plasma cell myeloma. *Semin. Hematol.* 1:3, 1964.
51. Osterland, C. K., and Espinoza, L. R. Biological properties of myeloma proteins. *Arch. Intern. Med.* 135:32, 1975.
52. Payne, R. B. A red herring in the detection of Bence-Jones protein (letter to the editor). *J. Clin. Pathol.* 25:183, 1972.
53. Perry, M. C. Personal communication, 1978.
54. Perry, M. C., and Kyle, R. A. The clinical significance of Bence Jones proteinuria. *Mayo Clin. Proc.* 50:234, 1975.
55. Preud'homme, J. L., Hurez, D., Danon, F., et al. Intracytoplasmic and surface-bound immunoglobulins in "nonsecretory" and Bence-Jones myeloma. *Clin. Exp. Immunol.* 25:428, 1976.
56. Putnam, F. W., Easley, C. W., Lynn, L. T., et al. The heat precipitation of Bence-Jones proteins: I. Optimum conditions. *Arch. Biochem. Biophys.* 83:115, 1959.
57. Putnam, F. W., Florent, G., Paul, C., et al. Complete amino acid sequence of the mu heavy chain of a human IgM immunoglobulin. *Science* 182:287, 1973.
58. Putnam, F. W., and Hardy, S. Proteins in multiple myeloma: III. Origin of Bence-Jones protein. *J. Biol. Chem.* 212:361, 1955.
58a. Rambaud, J. C., and Seligmann, M. Alpha-chain disease. *Clin. Gastroenterol.* 5:341, 1976.
59. Relman, A. S., and Levinsky, N. G. Clinical Examination of Renal Function.

In M. B. Strauss and L. G. Welt (Eds.), *Diseases of the Kidney* (2nd ed.). Boston: Little, Brown, 1971. Vol. 1, pp. 87–138.

60. Rowe, D. S., and Fahey, J. L. A new class of human immunoglobulins: I. A unique myeloma protein. *J. Exp. Med.* 121:171, 1965.
61. Seligmann, M., and Basch, A. The clinical significance of pathological immunoglobulins. In Twelfth Congress of the International Society of Hematology, New York, 1968. Pp. 21–31.
62. Seligmann, M., and Brouet, J. C. Antibody activity of human myeloma globulins. *Semin. Hematol.* 10:163, 1973.
63. Shustik, C., Bergsagel, D. E., and Pruzanski, W. κ and λ light-chain disease: Survival rates and clinical manifestations. *Blood* 48:41, 1976.
64. Smithline, N., Kassirer, J. P., and Cohen, J. J. Light-chain nephropathy: Renal tubular dysfunction associated with light-chain proteinuria. *N. Engl. J. Med.* 294:71, 1976.
65. Solomon, A. Bence-Jones proteins and light chains of immunoglobulins. *N. Engl. J. Med.* 294:17, 91, 1976.
66. Solomon, A. Bence Jones proteins and light chains of immunoglobulins: XIV. Conformational dependency and molecular localization of the kappa (κ) and lambda (λ) antigenic determinants. *Scand. J. Immunol.* 5:685, 1976.
67. Solomon, A., and McLaughlin, C. L. Bence-Jones proteins and light chains of immunoglobulins: I. Formation and characterization of amino-terminal (variant) and carboxyl-terminal (constant) halves. *J. Biol. Chem.* 244:3393, 1969.

67a. Spiegelberg, H. L. The structure and biology of human IgD. *Immunol. Rev.* 37:3, 1977.

68. Stone, M. J., and Frenkel, E. P. The clinical spectrum of light chain myeloma: A study of 35 patients with special reference to the occurrence of amyloidosis. *Am. J. Med.* 58:601, 1975.
69. Tiselius, A. Electrophoresis of serum globulin: II. Electrophoretic analysis of normal and immune sera. *Biochem. J.* 31:1464, 1937.
70. Tomasi, T. B., Jr. Human immunoglobulin A. *N. Engl. J. Med.* 279:1327, 1968.
71. Van Boxel, J. A., Paul, W. E., Terry, W. D., et al. IgD-bearing human lymphocytes. *J. Immunol.* 109:648, 1972.
72. Vaughn, J. H., Jacox, R. F., and Gray, B. A. Light and heavy chain components of gamma globulins in urines of normal persons and patients with agammaglobulinemia. *J. Clin. Invest.* 46:266, 1967.
73. Waldenström, J. G. *Diagnosis and Treatment of Multiple Myeloma.* New York: Grune & Stratton, 1970.
74. Wang, A. C., Fudenberg, H. H., Wells, J. V., et al. A new subgroup of the kappa chain variable region associated with anti-Pr cold agglutinins (letter to the editor). *Nature* [*New Biol.*] 243:126, 1973.
75. Wiltshaw, E. The natural history of extramedullary plasmacytoma and its relation to solitary myeloma of bone and myelomatosis. *Medicine (Baltimore)* 55: 217, 1976.
76. Wochner, R. D., Strober, W., and Waldmann, T. A. The role of the kidney in the catabolism of Bence Jones proteins and immunoglobulin fragments. *J. Exp. Med.* 126:207, 1967.
77. Wu, T. T., and Kabat, E. A. An analysis of the sequences of the variable regions of Bence Jones proteins and myeloma light chains and their implications for antibody complementarity. *J. Exp. Med.* 132:211, 1970.
78. Yunginger, J. W., and Gleich, G. J. The impact of the discovery of IgE on the practice of allergy. *Pediatr. Clin. North Am.* 22:3, 1975.

15. Microbiology in Nephrology

John A. Washington II

The microbiological examination of urine provides a sensitive and specific means of establishing the presence of urinary tract infection, provided certain precautions are taken in the process of collecting the urine and transporting it to the laboratory.

Collection of Urine

Clean-Voided Midstream Collection

The clean-voided midstream collection procedure is the one that is most frequently employed and usually recommended. Unfortunately, it is often performed by poorly trained personnel under suboptimal conditions. The quality and validity of specimens collected by this method can usually be improved by training a special team of technicians with responsibility for catheter care and urine collection. By establishing uniform practices in catheter care and by ensuring the proper collection of urine specimens for culture, such a team not only serves to improve patient care but also proves to be cost-effective. Ambulatory patients are most efficiently handled in a centralized urine collection station; however, a specially equipped cart must be available for the team to use with bedridden patients.

Urine is best collected from adequately hydrated ambulatory female patients by placing them on a modified gynecological examining table with an opening where the patient sits and a sliding tray with a removable pan beneath the opening to collect excess urine (Fig. 15–1). Supplies include a pair of examining gloves, two sterile packets of sponges, a sterile screw-capped specimen container, and a dilute hexachlorophene solution (3 parts of the solution to 1 part water). The labia are separated, and the labia minora and the meatus are cleaned by a single downward stroke with each of five sponges soaked with diluted hexachlorophene solution. The area is then dried by single downward strokes with each of several dry sponges. With the labia still held apart, the patient is instructed to void. The initial stream (approximately 30 ml) is discarded, and a midstream specimen is collected in the sterile container. This procedure is modified for the bedridden female by placing a bedpan under the patient. For males, the glans is washed with diluted hexachlorophene solution and dried with sterile sponges. In uncircumcised males the foreskin is retracted during preparation and voiding.

Urethral Catheterization

Urine should not be collected for culture by urethral catheterization unless there is no other way to collect the specimen or unless the catheter is being inserted as

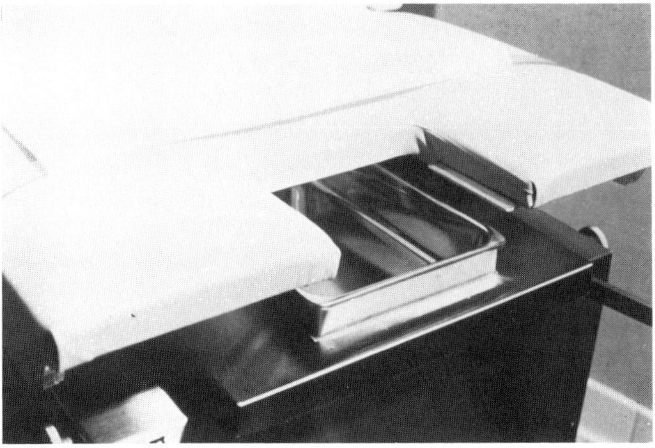

Figure 15–1
Modified gynecological examining table with sliding tray and removable pan for clean-voided midstream urine collection.

part of a urological evaluation or to relieve obstruction. Since catheterization is associated with a small but definite risk of urinary tract infection, measures should be taken to adhere to careful aseptic technique when the catheter is inserted [28].

In patients with chronic indwelling catheters, urine for culture should be collected by needle aspiration through a disinfected portion of the catheter wall itself. Specimens should not be collected by disconnecting the catheter from the drainage tube, nor should they be collected from the drainage bag itself.

Suprapubic Aspiration

The procedure of suprapubic aspiration (Fig. 15–2) is preferred for the collection of urine from infants and small children. It is the only acceptable method for collecting urine from patients with suspected anaerobic bacteriuria, and it is sometimes useful in resolving the question of whether or not significant bacteriuria is present in patients with low or borderline bacterial counts in repeated cultures of midstream specimens. This procedure should be performed only on patients with full bladders. The puncture site in the skin should be prepared with a suitable antiseptic solution and should be locally anesthetized. Once the bladder has been punctured, a volume of urine adequate for urinalysis and culture is aspirated. Suprapubic bladder punctures rarely lead to serious complications.

Localization Studies

Specimen collections may be modified in an attempt to localize the infection to the prostate or to distinguish between upper and lower tract disease. Segmented

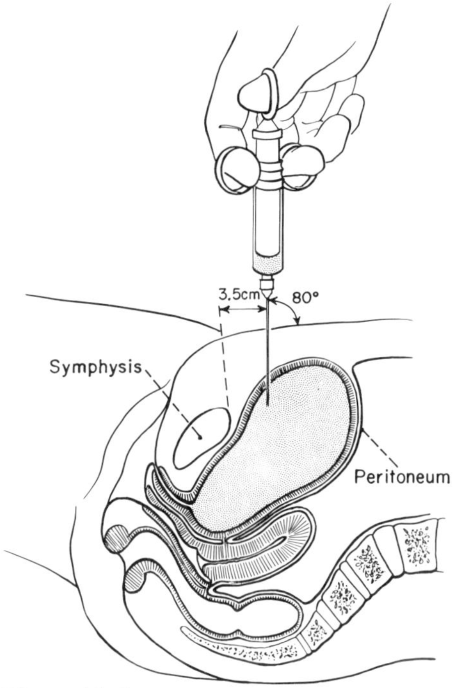

Figure 15–2
Anatomical structures (sagittal view) and technique of suprapubic aspiration in the female. (Courtesy J. W. Segura, M.D., Mayo Clinic.)

urine cultures have been used to diagnose chronic bacterial prostatitis [39]. In this procedure quantitative cultures are made of an initially voided 10 ml of urine, a midstream specimen, secretions following prostatic massage, and a final 10-ml voided specimen following massage. Urethritis results in a higher colony count in the first specimen than in the prostatic secretions or the final voided specimen, and no growth in the midstream specimen. In prostatitis, higher colony counts appear in the prostatic secretions and the final voided specimen.

Bladder washout is used to differentiate lower from upper tract infection [13]. In this procedure a catheter is inserted through the urethra into the bladder and left in place. Residual urine is cultured. Then 50 ml of sterile normal saline solution containing neomycin (40 mg), polymyxin (20 mg), and a mixture of fibrinolysin and deoxyribonuclease (Elase) is instilled into the bladder, and the catheter is clamped for 30 minutes. After bladder washout with 2 liters of sterile water, three urine collections are made at successive 10-minute intervals. Patients with upper tract disease will have persistent or increasing bacteriuria in cultures of the postwashout specimens. In bladder bacteriuria, the prewashout residual urine should contain at least 10^5 colony-forming units (CFU) per milliliter, and the postwashout collections should be negative bacteriologically.

Transport of Urine

Urine is an excellent culture medium when stored at room temperature or above [1, 5]. Therefore, spurious results may occur if its storage at these temperatures exceeds 2 to 4 hours [20, 46]. On the other hand, the numbers of colony-forming units per milliliter will remain constant for at least 6 hours and, in many instances, for at least 5 days [33] in urine that has been refrigerated. Urine should therefore be transported to the laboratory within 2 hours of its collection, or it should be refrigerated following its collection if delays in transport to the laboratory are anticipated. At the Mayo Clinic urine specimens are transported to the laboratory in insulated boxes that have been rendered cold by storage under refrigeration.

As an alternative to these transport requirements, it has been suggested that the specimen be inoculated upon its collection onto bacteriological media [11]. This approach will be discussed in greater detail later in the chapter in the section devoted to microbiological devices or kits for the detection of significant bacteriuria.

Processing the Specimen

Once the urine specimen has arrived in the laboratory, it should be processed promptly or stored under refrigeration until processing. All the elaborate precautions taken to ensure its proper collection and prompt transport to the laboratory will have been in vain if the laboratory is negligent on receipt of the specimen.

Microscopic Examination

The presence of significant bacteriuria ($\geq 7 \times 10^4$ CFU/ml) can be established in at least 90 percent of instances by the finding of at least one organism per oil immersion field (1000×) in a drop of well-mixed urine that has been allowed to dry on a clean glass slide and gram-stained (Fig. 15–3). The procedure for performing a Gram stain is outlined in Table 15–1. A similar degree of correlation between microscopic examination and the presence of significant bacteriuria can be obtained when at least 20 organisms are observed per high-dry field (400×) under reduced light in a wet mount of centrifuged urinary sediment, with or without methylene blue [28].

Urine from patients with suspected renal tuberculosis requires decontamination and concentration [43]. The decontaminated and concentrated sediment is then used for preparing smears that are stained with a carbolfuchsin stain, such as Kinyoun's, or a fluorochrome dye, such as auramine-rhodamine [43].

Phase-contrast microscopy can be helpful in identifying the presence of fungi in urine [35]. A drop of centrifuged sediment is placed on a glass slide, covered with a glass coverslip, and examined with a 40× phase-contrast objective.

Microbiological Procedures

BACTERIOLOGICAL STUDIES. The most essential component of urine bacteriology is quantitation, reflecting the now classic studies performed by Kass [26] of

Table 15–1. Gram Stain Reagents and Procedure

1. Reagents	
a. Stock Crystal Violet	
Crystal violet, 90% dye content	10 g
Methyl alcohol, absolute	500 ml
b. Gram's Iodine Solution	
I_2 crystals	6 g
KI	12 g
Distilled water	1800 ml
c. Decolorizer	
Acetone	400 ml
Ethyl alcohol, 95%	1200 ml
d. Counterstain	
Safranin, 99% dye content	10 g
Distilled water	1000 ml

2. Procedure
   a. Thoroughly flame one side of a clean glass slide to be used for the smear and allow to cool before smearing.
   b. Using fresh tap water to emulsify colonies or portions thereof, prepare a thin smear on the previously flamed side of the slide and allow to air-dry.
   c. Fix the smear by passing the slide through a flame several times.
   d. Flood the slide with crystal violet solution.
   e. After at least 10 seconds, pour off the crystal violet and gently wash the slide in tap water.
   f. Flood the slide with iodine solution.
   g. After at least 10 seconds, rinse off the iodine solution with tap water.
   h. Decolorize with one of the following:
      (1) 95% alcohol—decolorize until no more stain comes off slide, then rinse in tap water.
      (2) acetone-alcohol—wash off immediately with tap water.
   i. Flood with safranin solution for 10 seconds, and rinse off with tap water.
   j. Blot the slide dry with clean, unused filter paper.
   k. Examine the smear under oil immersion.

Source: Reprinted, by permission, from J. A. Washington II (Ed.), *Laboratory Procedures in Clinical Microbiology*. Boston: Little, Brown, 1974.

bacterial counts in urines of various population groups. In these studies it was found that patients with pyelonephritis had urinary bacterial counts of at least 100,000 per milliliter, and that counts between 0 and 10,000 per milliliter represented contamination. Contamination is a result of the bacterial flora indigenous to the urethra [19]. With careful techniques of urine collection and transport, colony counts of at least 10,000 per milliliter are often clinically significant. In fact, the urines of most patients with significant bacteriuria contain at least 1,000,000 CFU/ml. There are, however, circumstances in which the number of colony-forming units per milliliter may be decreased in patients with urinary tract infection [34]: (1) high urinary flow rates; (2) diurnal variation, with low or indeterminate rates in late afternoon or evening specimens; (3) when urine pH and specific gravity are below 5.0 and 1.003, respectively; (4) when

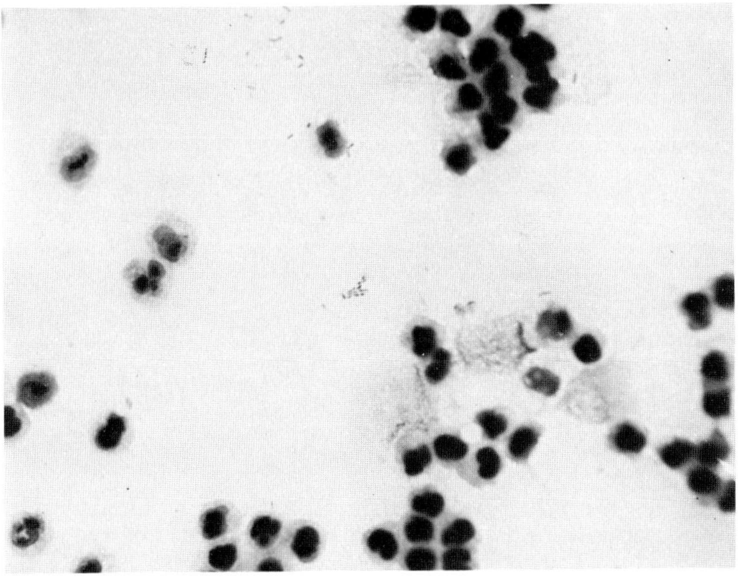

A

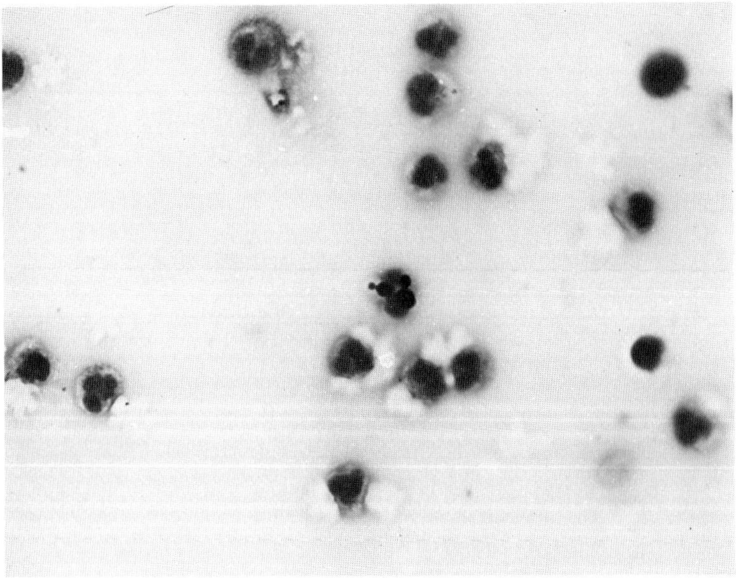

B

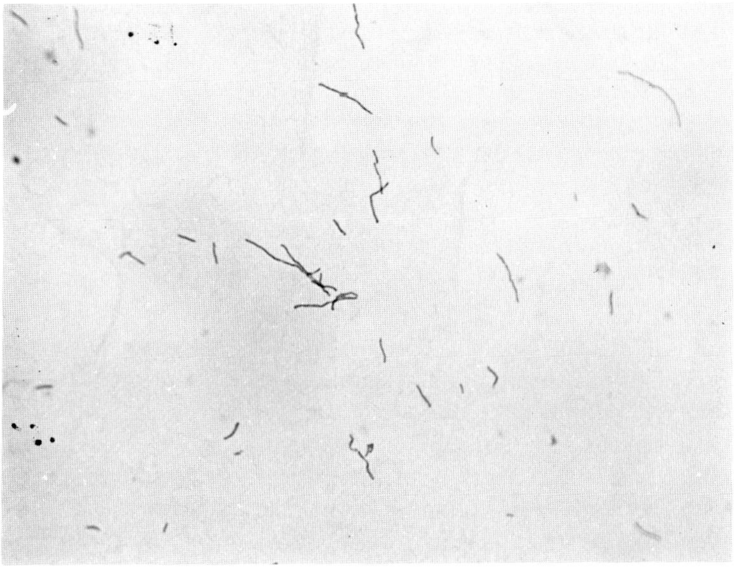

C

Figure 15–3
Gram-stained smears of drops of well-mixed urine specimens: (A) gram-negative bacilli, pus cells; (B) yeasts, pus cells; and (C) gram-negative bacilli, no pus cells ($\times 1000$).

an antimicrobial agent is in the urine; and (5) in patients with chronic, active pyelonephritis. Other examples of infections in which conventional bacterial urine cultures are negative include anaerobic bacteriuria and renal tuberculosis.

Kunin [28] has published minimal diagnostic criteria for bacteriuria in asymptomatic males and females. These criteria are based on the reliability of cultures obtained by the clean-voided specimen. In the male the reliability of a single culture is virtually 100 percent, provided proper care has been taken during preparation for and collection of the specimen. In the female, however, the reliability of a single culture is approximately 80 percent; of two consecutive cultures, approximately 90 percent; and of three consecutive cultures, approximately 100 percent. Based on these figures, Kunin [28, 29] has recommended that the diagnosis of significant bacteriuria in screening programs of high-risk groups be based on finding $\geq 10^5$ CFU/ml in three consecutive cultures. Obviously, in symptomatic females therapy is usually initiated after collection of a single urine specimen.

The diagnosis of anaerobic bacteriuria may be suspected when bacteria are seen microscopically but fail to grow in conventional cultures of voided urine. Because anaerobes are normally present in the urethra [14], clean-voided midstream specimens are not suitable for anaerobic culture, and a suprapubic aspiration must be performed. Anaerobic bacteriuria is very rare [14]. Segura and colleagues [38] examined 5781 midstream urine specimens of which 795 (13.8 percent) contained bacteria microscopically. Of these 795 patients, all but 25 had positive cultures. Seventeen of these 25 patients had suprapubic bladder aspirations, and 10 of the 17 had positive anaerobic cultures. Of the total population studied, the incidence of anaerobic bacteriuria was about 0.2 percent; of those with significant bacteriuria, the incidence of cases with anaerobes was 1.3 percent.

Media. Blood agar and a gram-negative differential medium, such as eosin-methylene blue (EMB) or MacConkey agar, are suitable for conventional bacteriological cultures of urine. These media may be contained separately in Petri dishes or in opposite halves of biplates. Broth cultures should never be inoculated with clean-voided midstream urine specimens, since overgrowth by the normal urethral flora will occur.

Although urine specimens are generally cultured quantitatively on solid media, it is necessary with suprapubic aspirations to ensure the recovery of small numbers of bacteria, as well as of fastidious bacteria such as anaerobes, since urethral contamination is averted and since any bacteria that may be present are likely to be significant. Consequently, in addition to the culture media mentioned above, the following media should be inoculated with urine specimens obtained by suprapubic aspiration: thioglycollate medium supplemented with vitamin K_1 and hemin, blood agar, laked blood agar with vitamin K_1 and hemin, and phenylethyl alcohol blood agar. These media are incubated anaerobically at 35° C; if the cultures are negative after 48 hours, the Petri dishes are discarded, but the thioglycollate medium is reincubated for five days.

Quantitation. Quantitation may be accomplished in two ways: (1) by the pour-plate procedure, in which 0.1 ml of a 1:10 dilution of urine is mixed in 10 to 20 ml of molten (45° C) nutrient agar which is then poured into an empty Petri dish, or (2) by directly inoculating and streaking a measured volume of urine onto the surface of the culture media [21]. The latter approach is preferable for routine purposes because of its simplicity and rapidity of performance. Commercially available 0.001- or 0.01-ml calibrated platinum milk dilution loops are ordinarily used for this purpose. The volume of urine delivered by such loops should be checked at regular intervals [6], since it may change with ordinary wear and tear. Although Hoeprich [21] recommended using both loop sizes for routine cultures, satisfactory results can be obtained by using only one. The 0.01-ml loop is preferred at the Mayo Clinic because it is easier to use and more durable. Regardless of which loop size is used, however, it is important to realize that the volume that the loop is specified to deliver onto the agar surface is accurately delivered only if the loop is dipped into the urine vertically [18] and rapidly [3].

Inoculation of the culture media by the calibrated loop streak-plate technique is performed as shown in Figure 15–4. If the 0.01-ml loop is used, it is recommended that the two previously mentioned media be contained in separate Petri

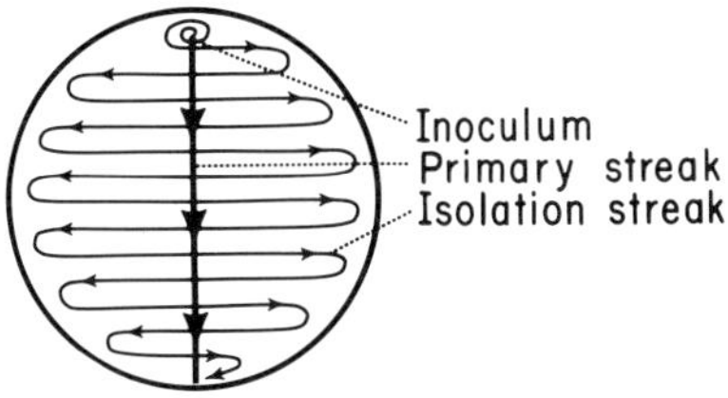

Figure 15–4
Streak plate method using a calibrated (0.01-ml) platinum wire loop. (Reproduced by permission from J. A. Washington, II (Ed.), *Laboratory Procedures in Clinical Microbiology*. Boston: Little, Brown, 1974.)

dishes in order to obtain well-isolated colonies on each. If biplates containing both media are used, it is recommended that the 0.001-ml loop be used. Once inoculated, these media are incubated at 35° C for 16 to 24 hours. Incubation of Petri dishes without growth beyond 24 hours is unnecessary.

The blood agar plate permits an assessment of the total number of organisms present and, more specifically, of the numbers of gram-positive organisms. The differential medium provides for the differentiation and enumeration of different morphological types of gram-negative bacilli. Because such media are inhibitory to certain bacteria and particularly to gram-positive organisms, colony counts of gram-negative bacilli may be slightly lower on these media than they are on a nutrient medium like blood agar. When such discrepancies occur, the higher colony count should be reported. The number of colonies of each kind of organism present on one of the plates should be multiplied by the appropriate dilution factor to obtain the actual colony-forming units per milliliter (e.g., 100 colonies of an organism on EMB equals 10,000 CFU/ml if the 0.01-ml loop was used to inoculate the plate). Because the precise number of colonies per milliliter is clinically unimportant, it is satisfactory to report approximate colony counts (e.g., $< 10^3$, 10^3 to 10^4, 10^4 to 10^5, $\geq 10^5$ CFU/ml).

The question of how to handle cultures of voided urines yielding mixed flora is not readily resolved. In general, mixtures of organisms, each in counts of $< 10^3$ CFU/ml, should be reported as "mixed flora." Any organisms present in counts of at least 10^5 CFU/ml should be reported. Gross and colleagues [16] have reported a series of bacteremias in association with polymicrobial (at least 10^5 CFU/ml of each of two or more species) bacteriuria. The major problem area is with mixtures of organisms in the range of 10^3 to 10^5 CFU/ml. It has been suggested that if there is a mixture of two or more kinds of organisms in this range, they may be reported as mixed flora and a repeat specimen may be requested [6]. Because of the aforementioned precautions taken by the urine collection team at the Mayo Clinic, counts of 10^4 CFU/ml are usually regarded as representing significant bacteriuria; therefore, any organisms in counts exceeding 10^3 CFU/ml are identified. This problem may sometimes be resolved by examining the gram-stained smear of a drop of the urine specimen. The presence of many squamous epithelial cells and the absence of leukocytes strongly suggest improper collection of the specimen. It should be remembered, however, that urine cultures from patients with obstructive uropathies or chronic indwelling urethral catheters frequently do yield more than one kind of organism.

Identification. Identification of significant isolates may be accomplished by a variety of methods. The Enterobacteriaceae, of which *Escherichia coli, Proteus mirabilis,* and *Klebsiella pneumoniae* are the most frequently isolated from urine, can be identified reliably with conventional biochemical tests or with any one of several commercially available kits [44]. Further simplification and speed of identification of *E. coli* and *P. mirabilis* can be achieved with the indole spot test [42]. This test is rapid and generally accurate, provided certain precautions are observed: its use should be limited to swarming strains of *Proteus* (*P. mirabilis* is indole-negative) and to nonmucoid strains of *E. coli* (*E. coli* is indole-positive) producing a metallic sheen on EMB agar; colonies to be tested should be taken from blood agar.

The gram-positive cocci may be differentiated according to procedures outlined elsewhere by Facklam and Smith [12]. The catalase test distinguishes between staphylococci and streptococci, the coagulase test separates *Staphylococcus aureus* from *Staphylococcus epidermidis,* and the bile-esculin test differentiates the group D streptococci from other groups of streptococci.

Pseudomonas aeruginosa can be readily identified by its characteristic odor, colonial morphology, positive oxidase reaction, and pigmentation of various media, including triple sugar iron agar (TSIA). The identification of other nonfermentative gram-negative bacilli is more complex and is described elsewhere [7].

Rapid or Simplified Methods for Detecting Bacteriuria: Chemical and Culture Screening Devices. Chemical Screening Devices. There are a number of chemical methods for detecting bacteriuria. Their principal advantages are economy, speed, and simplicity of performance; their disadvantages are that they often lack sensitivity, they sometimes lack specificity, and they never provide any indication of an organism's identity. Therefore, they are primarily useful as screening procedures.

The nitrate reduction test (Griess test) is based on the principle that most bacteria incubating overnight in the bladder reduce nitrate to nitrite, which can be detected colorimetrically. This test lacks sensitivity when (1) specimens that have been randomly collected during the day are tested, (2) the patient is taking antimicrobial agents, (3) the urine is infected with bacteria lacking or deficient in nitrate reductase, (4) the patient is on a low-nitrate diet, (5) the urine is not heavily infected, (6) the urine is from a patient with a chronic indwelling urethral catheter, or (7) the urine contains a red dye or blood. Recently, this test has become available in a dip-strip combination containing a nitrite reagent pad and two dehydrated media pads (Microstix, Ames Division, Miles Laboratories, Elkhart, Ind.); the test has been found to be fast (30 seconds), convenient, and reliable when used as a screening device with first-voided morning urine specimens. It would, therefore, seem to be useful for screening purposes in the home and in the physician's office.

The glucose oxidase test is based on the principle that small amounts (2 to 20 mg/dl) of glucose found normally in urine are metabolized by the presence of large numbers of bacteria incubating overnight in the bladder. The lack of development of a blue color in the test part of the dip-strip is indicative of a positive test. This test lacks sensitivity if performed on (1) urine specimens randomly collected during the day, (2) urine collected from diabetics, or (3) urine collected from patients receiving antimicrobial agents. Even when these specific qualifications are considered, the glucose oxidase test appears to have a significantly lower level of sensitivity than the Griess test.

Other chemical tests with generally poor levels of sensitivity and specificity for detecting bacteriuria are those based on tetrazolium reduction, catalase production, and the measurement of bacterial adenosine triphosphate (ATP) by the firefly luciferase reaction [9].

Another test that has been evaluated for detecting bacteriuria is based on the principle that small quantities of endotoxin produced by gram-negative bacilli will cause gelation of lysates of amebocytes from the horseshoe crab, *Limulus polyphemus* [24]. Although the *Limulus* assay is highly sensitive and specific in detecting gram-negative bacilluria, it will not detect gram-positive bacteriuria. Another limitation of this test is its requirement for pyrogen-free glassware.

Culture Screening Devices. There are also a number of culture screening devices, which are based on filter paper, dip-slide, and roll tube techniques. With all these devices quantitation is determined by comparing the density of colonies on an agar surface with the manufacturer's graphic representation of colonies in known quantities on the same agar. The advantages of these methods include immediate inoculation of the specimen, simplicity, good correlation of results with standard quantitative techniques, preliminary identification of isolates, and the capacity to proceed with definitive identification and antimicrobial susceptibility testing of isolates. Their disadvantages include a requirement for overnight incubation, difficulties in recognizing mixtures of bacteria when large numbers of organisms are present, and delays imposed by subculture requirements in identification and susceptibility testing.

In the filter paper method a standard volume of urine absorbed into a filter paper strip is delivered onto agar, which is then incubated overnight. All dip-slide methods are based on the procedure described by Cohen and Kass [8] of coating each side of an ordinary glass microscopic slide with bacteriological media. The slide is inoculated by dipping it into urine. After overnight incubation, growth is quantitated by comparison with graphic standards. Several versions of this technique have become available commercially, with the media being contained in paddles or spoons or in dehydrated form on pads. In the roll tube method, the interior of a plastic tube is covered with a thin layer of a transparent agar medium. Urine is poured into the tube and then poured off prior to its incubation. Preliminary identification of isolates in these systems may be obtained because of their growth and morphological characteristics on nutrient and differential agar media.

Most of these culture screening methods are extremely reliable, with falsely positive and negative results falling below the 5 percent level. In the dip-strip nitrite and dehydrated culture media pad combination (Microstix), falsely negative cultures have been observed in patients receiving antibiotics [32].

Although primarily useful for screening purposes, these devices have been successfully used in one major hospital for routine cultures of urine in order to obviate the problems associated with suboptimal practices of urine collection and transport [11]. It has also been suggested that culture screening devices provide accurate results when they are inoculated at home and mailed to the laboratory; however, there are studies showing a significant frequency of unreliable results with devices incubated at room temperature and transported in the mail [2, 4].

Antimicrobial Susceptibility Tests. The indications for performing antimicrobial susceptibility tests are (1) that the organisms have unpredictable susceptibility to the antimicrobial agents of choice and (2) that the organisms are clinically significant. Therefore, susceptibility tests of isolates from the urine should ordinarily be limited to those present in counts of at least 10^4 CFU/ml. Whether or not such isolates require testing routinely is debatable. Uncomplicated first or second episodes of urinary tract infection in females are commonly due to *E. coli,* which is usually susceptible and responds clinically to a variety of antimicrobial agents (e.g., sulfonamides, ampicillin, tetracyclines). Since initial therapy in such cases is often empirical, routine testing of these *E. coli* probably represents an unnecessary expense to the patient. Organisms responsible for persistent or recurrent bacteriuria, those acquired in the hospital, and those involved in complicated infections should be tested. The agents to be tested against urinary tract isolates are listed in Table 15–2. Sulfonamides have not been included on this list because their principal ultilization is in the treatment of uncomplicated first or second episodes of infections which, as has already been stated, are usually due to susceptible strains of *E. coli.*

Essential to the management of urinary tract infection is the determination of the in vivo response by reculturing the urine 2 to 3 days after an antimicrobial agent has been started. If bacteriuria of $\geq 10^4$ CFU/ml with the same organism has persisted, antimicrobial susceptibility testing, if not performed with the original isolate, should certainly be carried out and the therapy altered accordingly.

Susceptibility testing may be carried out by dilution [45] or disc diffusion techniques [31]. In the former procedure, the lowest or minimal concentration (MIC) of antimicrobic required to inhibit the growth of the organism is determined. In the latter method, the diameter of a zone of inhibition about an antimicrobic-impregnated disc is determined. Because this zone relates approxi-

Table 15–2. Selection of Antimicrobial Agents for Susceptibility Testing in Urinary Tract Infection

Agent	Gram-positive Cocci	Gram-negative Bacilli
Amikacin	—	X
Ampicillin	X [b]	X
Carbenicillin	—	X
Cephalothin	X	X
Erythromycin	X	—
Gentamicin	—	X
Kanamycin	—	X
Methicillin [a]	X	—
Nalidixic acid	—	X
Nitrofurantoin	—	X
Penicillin G	X	—
Tetracycline	—	X
Tobramycin	—	X
Trimethoprim-sulfamethoxazole	—	X

[a] Acceptable alternatives are oxacillin and nafcillin.
[b] Tested against group D streptococci only.

mately linearly to the $\log_2$ MIC, it can be translated into susceptible, intermediate, or resistant categories according to published interpretative criteria [31]. Disc diffusion methods are generally more easily performed in most clinical laboratories than are dilution procedures; however, the latter are more efficient and convenient for testing large numbers of isolates [43].

Although these procedures are usually used for testing standardized inocula of colonies of bacteria isolated from cultures, it has been suggested that susceptibility tests be performed directly with urine that is microscopically positive for bacteria on initial examination [29]. This approach is valid provided (1) the urine is microscopically positive and (2) it contains no more than one kind of organism, a determination that is difficult to make reliably by microscopic examination [22]. The principal advantage of direct susceptibility testing is the elimination of the customary 24-hour delay in receiving the results when testing is performed with isolated colonies. Although not yet critically evaluated, the combination of direct testing with a rapid technique [30, 41] may permit reporting of results within several hours after the specimen is received by the laboratory.

Objections have been raised by Stamey [39] concerning the fact that commercially available antimicrobic discs, approved by the Food and Drug Administration (FDA), provide results that are applicable only to antimicrobic levels attainable in serum and do not reflect the much higher levels occurring in urine. He has, therefore, advocated the use of discs with higher antimicrobic content for urinary isolates and has published regression lines relating zone diameters obtained with these discs to MIC. It is without question that urinary tract infections can often be treated successfully with antimicrobics to which isolates appear resistant when tested by the standard disc method [31]; however, there is naturally a considerable degree of reticence on the part of the FDA in approving additional discs because of all the difficulties that were experienced in establishing the standard single disc method. For the time being, therefore, susceptibility testing of urinary isolates at higher concentrations is limited to dilution techniques.

MYCOBACTERIAL STUDIES. It should be emphasized that for the diagnosis of mycobacterial diseases, multiple, fresh, early morning, clean-voided midstream specimens are preferable to 24-hour urine collections. The latter often become overgrown with bacteria other than mycobacteria and with fungi that are difficult to eradicate with the usual decontamination procedures. Specimens are optimally processed on the day of their collection, or after their storage under refrigeration or frozen conditions, since storage at room or higher temperatures will result in higher rates of contamination and in lower rates of recovery of mycobacteria.

These considerations are important to bear in mind because not all the laboratory services that are required for the diagnosis of mycobacterial diseases are performed in all clinical laboratories. Different extents of laboratory service have been suggested by the College of American Pathologists. Briefly, at the first level the laboratory performs no mycobacterial procedures but is responsible for the collection and rapid transport of adequate clinical specimens to specialized laboratories for processing. At the second level of service, the laboratory performs acid-fast stains, inoculates cultures, and transmits these cultures to a reference laboratory. At the third level the laboratory isolates and identifies *Mycobacterium tuberculosis* and makes a preliminary identification of other mycobacterial species. The fourth and most complete level of service involves the definitive identification of mycobacteria; drug susceptibility testing may or may not be performed in such laboratories.

Specimen Processing. The degree of contamination of urine with organisms other than mycobacteria should be established in order to determine the amount of decontamination required. Quantitative inoculation of a blood agar and EMB or MacConkey agar is suitable for this purpose. It may be impossible to decontaminate adequately specimens with greater than 10^3 CFU/ml of gram-negative bacilli, particularly *Pseudomonas aeruginosa.* In such instances, inoculation of the material into guinea pigs may have to be considered.

Assuming the specimen is not heavily contaminated with gram-negative bacilli, it is concentrated by centrifugation and the sediment is then treated with a decontaminant (e.g., NaOH) [43]. Smears are prepared from the sediment to be stained with auramine-rhodamine or with a carbolfuchsin stain, such as Kinyoun's. Screening of smears for acid-fast bacilli is much more rapidly accomplished with the former stain.

Media. It is recommended that tubes or Petri dishes containing egg-based (e.g., Löwenstein-Jensen) and clear agar (e.g., Middlebrook 7H10) be inoculated. The incorporation of antibacterial and antifungal agents into mycobacteriological media, such as Gruft's Löwenstein-Jensen, may be helpful in culturing grossly contaminated specimens.

Inoculated media are incubated at 35° C in an atmosphere containing 10 percent carbon dioxide. They are examined at least once weekly for eight weeks for evidence of growth.

Identification and Drug Susceptibility Tests. The growth after at least 14 days of incubation of slowly growing, nonpigmented, rough colonies is strongly suggestive of *Mycobacterium tuberculosis* and may be confirmed as such by a positive niacin test. The identification of other species of mycobacteria is beyond the scope of this chapter and is described in detail elsewhere along with techniques for drug susceptibility testing [43].

MYCOLOGICAL STUDIES. Fungal infection of the urinary tract usually reflects hematogenous or disseminated spread of the disease. Dissemination with renal involvement has been reported in histoplasmosis, coccidioidomycosis, cryptococcosis, blastomycosis, paracoccidioidomycosis, aspergillosis, and phycomycosis. The isolation of one of these fungi from a urine culture generally poses no great problem in interpretation. A much more difficult problem, however, is the isolation of *Candida* from urine. This occurs frequently and may be indicative of systemic candidiasis, lower urinary tract infection, or simple colonization. Further complicating this picture is the fact that in systemic candidiasis the kidneys are the organs that are most frequently involved.

Candiduria may be secondary to overgrowth of *Candida* in the bowel due to antibiotic therapy; it may occur in immunologically deficient hosts, including poorly controlled diabetics and patients with leukemia and lymphoma; and it may occur in patients with indwelling urethral catheters. According to Schönebeck [37], the finding of *Candida* in cultures of a properly collected urine is always pathological. *Candida albicans* is the species most frequently involved; however, other species of *Candida* rarely cause serious disease, as may *Torulopsis glabrata.* Although it has been suggested that candiduria, like bacteriuria, be quantitated and that levels of 10^3 or 10^5 CFU/ml be considered significant, Schönebeck [37] feels that quantitation is not only unnecessary but is also potentially misleading. On the other hand, Wise and colleagues [47] concluded on the basis of a study of 20 patients with renal pathology due to *Candida* that a count of $\geq$ 15,000 CFU/ml in a clean-voided midstream or single urethral catheterized specimen was significant, but that the colony count of *Candida* in urine from patients with indwelling urethral catheters had no bearing on whether or not upper urinary tract disease was present. As emphasized by Schönebeck [37], neither candiduria nor candidemia should be evaluated as an isolated finding but rather should be evaluated in relation to the total clinical picture. Krick and Remington [27] have defined two reliable criteria for the diagnosis of invasive fungal infection: (1) the demonstration of fungi in tissue, and (2) the isolation of fungi from cerebrospinal fluid, intraocular fluid, or other body fluid—excluding blood and urine—where the fungus is never normally present and when contamination of any sort can be excluded. They also stressed the unreliability of both positive cultures in establishing the diagnosis of opportunistic fungal infection and of negative cultures, antemortem or postmortem, in excluding the diagnosis of certain fungal diseases.

It should be apparent from these comments that the diagnosis of fungal infection by urine culture and the interpretation of cultures yielding *Candida* are fraught with considerable difficulty.

Specimen Processing. Well-mixed urine is inoculated onto media with a 0.01-ml calibrated platinum loop in a manner similar to that described for bacteriological cultures (see Fig. 15–4).

Media. Urine is inoculated onto brain-heart infusion agar containing sheep blood (10%), chloramphenicol (16 μg/ml), and gentamicin (5 μg/ml), with and without cycloheximide (500 μg/ml); inhibitory mold agar (IMA); and Sabouraud's dextrose agar (Emmons' modification).

All cultures are incubated at 30° C for 30 days and examined three times weekly for growth of yeasts and filamentous fungi.

Identification. Yeasts and fungi are identified as described in detail elsewhere [36, 43]. *Candida albicans* is most easily and rapidly identified with the germ-tube test. In our laboratory yeasts are reported quantitatively in ranges similar to those used for bacteria.

OTHER MICROBIOLOGICAL PROCEDURES. *Antibody-Coated Bacteria.* Thomas and colleagues [40] and Jones and co-workers [23] have demonstrated that an immunofluorescence test for the presence or absence of antibody-coated bacteria in the urinary sediments of patients with active infection can be correlated with the site of infection. With the notable exception of urines from males with prostatitis, antibody-coated bacteria are present only when the upper urinary tract is involved. The antibody coating the bacteria is usually IgG.

In this procedure, washed urinary sediment is incubated with fluorescein-conjugated antihuman globulin, smeared, and then examined for fluorescence of bacteria. Careful attention must be paid to the potency of the antiglobulin used in this test, since Forsum and associates [15] have noted a significant frequency of apparently falsely positive tests with one particular Swedish preparation in testing urines from children; these workers felt that staphylococcal protein A was a more satisfactory antiglobulin preparation. This problem has not been commented on by investigators in the United States who, in contrast to the Swedish investigators, compared the results of their tests with those of localization studies.

Harding and Merz [17] investigated the possibility of using antibody coating of yeasts to determine the site of infection. They found, however, that yeasts from all urine specimens and from all specimens examined from other superficially infected or colonized sites were coated with antibodies.

The antibody-coated bacteria (ACB) test, therefore, appears to be a useful investigative tool in differentiating upper from lower urinary tract infection, except in males with prostatitis. Certainly, the ACB test is simpler to perform than localization studies requiring urethral catheterization and bladder washout techniques or those requiring cystoscopy and ureteral catheterization. Further studies of the ACB test in various subpopulations of patients with complicated urinary tract infections are probably indicated in order to define the limitations of the test. The studies by Forsum and colleagues [15] suggest that certain test variables should be investigated more closely.

Critical to the evaluation of this and other localization studies is the reference standard with which they are compared. The most definitive method is probably the cystoscopic one with ureteral catheterization described by Stamey [39]; however, there are obvious limitations to its use in routine clinical evaluations.

Serological classification of Escherichia coli. As has already been discussed, most simple or uncomplicated urinary tract infections are caused by *Escherichia coli,* are susceptible to commonly employed antimicrobics, and are cured with a 10- to 14-day course of these agents. Urine cultures should be sterile within 2 to 3 days after initiating therapy and should remain sterile after the completion of therapy. In some instances, however, bacteriuria will recur due to the presence of either the original organism (relapse) or, more frequently, to the presence of a new serotype of *E. coli* or a new species of bacteria (reinfection). Differentiating between these two types of recurrent infections can be important in the patient's management.

Distinguishing between strains of *E. coli* is most reliably performed by serological means. Biotypes defined by octal codes derived from biochemical reactions of Enterobacteriaceae have been promoted by various kit manufacturers to facilitate identification and for epidemiological purposes. However, it is important to realize that although the reproducibility of reactions and, therefore, of the octal codes in the kits has been satisfactory for species or generic identifications, it has been unsatisfactory for epidemiological purposes.

Complete serological typing of the Enterobacteriaceae requires the determination of somatic (O) antigens, O antigen factors, flagellar (H) antigens, H antigen factors, and capsular or envelope (K) antigens. The complexity of typing clinical isolates of *E. coli* was highlighted in 1972 by Edwards and Ewing, who wrote that 148 O antigen groups had been characterized and that 92 K and 51 H antigens were known [10]. Fortunately, these and other investigators have found that about 70 percent of urinary tract isolates are limited to nine O antigen groups (01, 2, 4, 6, 7, 11, 15, 62, and 75). Typing of urinary isolates is, therefore, usually limited to O antigen testing for these groups, with the recognition that strains of the same O antigen group may not be identical because of potential differences in their H and K antigens.

It is important to recognize that these O antigenic groups possess no properties that render them uniquely pathogenic to the urinary tract and that their prevalence in urinary infections reflects their prevalence in the colon. Attempts have been made to correlate capsular (K) antigens with strains of *E. coli* causing acute pyelonephritis, since the K_1 antigen has been shown to be a virulence factor for strains associated with neonatal meningitis. One recent study did find that five K antigens (1, 2, 3, 12, and 13) accounted for 70 percent of such isolates [25].

Serological grouping of *E. coli* remains an investigative tool. Antisera for all nine O antigen groups most frequently involved in urinary infection are not available commercially and therefore must be obtained from a reference laboratory or prepared in the investigator's laboratory.

References

1. Aascher, A. W., Sussman, M., Waters, W. E., et al. Urine as a medium for bacterial growth. *Lancet* 2:1037, 1966.
2. Alwall, N. Factors affecting the reliability of screening tests for bacteriuria: II. Dip-slide: false positive results following postal transport and false negatives owing to incubation at room temperature. *Acta Med. Scand.* 193:505, 1973.
3. Anhalt, J. P. Personal communication, 1976.
4. Arneil, G. C., McAllister, T. A., and Kay, P. Detection of bacteriuria at room-temperature. *Lancet* 1:119, 1970.
5. Aurelius, G. Bacterial growth in urine. *Acta Pathol. Microbiol. Scand.* 55:201, 1962.
6. Barry, A. L., Smith, P. B., and Turck, M. Laboratory Diagnosis of Urinary Tract Infections. In T. L. Gavan (Ed.), *Cumitech 2.* Washington, D.C.: American Society for Microbiology, 1975.
7. Blazevic, D. J. Current taxonomy and identification of nonfermentative gram-negative bacilli. *Hum. Pathol.* 7:265, 1976.
8. Cohen, S. N., and Kass, E. H. A simple method for quantitative urine culture. *N. Engl. J. Med.* 277:176, 1967.
9. Conn, R. B., Charache, P., and Chappelle, E. W. Limits of applicability of the firefly luminescence ATP assay for the detection of bacteria in clinical specimens. *Am. J. Clin. Pathol.* 63:493, 1975.
10. Edwards, P. R., and Ewing, W. H. *Identification of Enterobacteriaceae* (3rd ed.). Minneapolis: Burgess, 1972.
11. Ellner, P. D., and Papachristos, T. Detection of bacteriuria by dip-slide: Routine use in a large general hospital. *Am. J. Clin. Pathol.* 63:516, 1975.
12. Facklam, R. R., and Smith, P. B. The gram-positive cocci. *Hum. Pathol.* 7:187, 1976.
13. Fairley, F. K., Carson, N. E., Gutch, R. C., et al. Site of infection in acute urinary-tract infection in general practice. *Lancet* 2:615, 1971.
14. Finegold, S. M. *Anaerobic Bacteria in Human Disease.* New York: Academic, 1977. Pp. 314–349.
15. Forsum, U., Hjelm, E., and Jonsell, G. Antibody-coated bacteria in the urine of children with urinary tract infections. *Acta Paediatr. Scand.* 65:639, 1976.
16. Gross, P. A., Flower, M., and Barden, G. Polymicrobic bacteriuria: Significant association with bacteremia. *J. Clin. Microbiol.* 3:246, 1976.
17. Harding, S. A., and Merz, W. G. Evaluation of antibody coating of yeasts in urine as an indicator of the site of urinary tract infection. *J. Clin. Microbiol.* 2:222, 1975.

18. Haugen, J., Strøm, O., and Østervold, B. Bacterial counts in urine: I. The reliability of the loop technique. *Acta Pathol. Microbiol. Scand.* 74:391, 1968.
19. Helmholz, H. F. Determination of the bacterial content of the urethra: A new method, with results of a study of 82 men. *J. Urol.* 64:158, 1950.
20. Hindman, R., Tronic, B., and Bartlett, R. Effect of delay on culture of urine. *J. Clin. Microbiol.* 4:102, 1976.
21. Hoeprich, P. D. Culture of the urine. *J. Lab. Clin. Med.* 56:899, 1960.
22. Hollick, G. E., and Washington, J. A., II. Comparison of direct and standardized disk diffusion susceptibility testing of urine cultures. *Antimicrob. Agents Chemother.* 9:804, 1976.
23. Jones, S. R., Smith, J. W., and Sanford, J. P. Localization of urinary-tract infections by detection of antibody coated bacteria in urine sediment. *N. Engl. J. Med.* 290:591, 1974.
24. Jorgensen, J. H., and Jones, P. M. Comparative evaluation of the limulus assay and the direct Gram stain for detection of significant bacteriuria. *Am. J. Clin. Pathol.* 63:142, 1975.
25. Kaijser, B., Jodal, U., Hanson, L. A., et al. Frequency of *E. coli* K antigens in urinary-tract infections in children. *Lancet* 1:663, 1977.
26. Kass, E. H. Asymptomatic infections of the urinary tract. *Trans. Assoc. Am. Physicians* 69:56, 1956.
27. Krick, J. A., and Remington, J. S. Opportunistic invasive fungal infections in patients with leukemia and lymphoma. *Clin. Haematol.* 5:249, 1976.
28. Kunin, C. M. *Detection, Prevention and Management of Urinary Tract Infections* (2nd ed.). Philadelphia: Lea & Febiger, 1974.
29. Kunin, C. M. Urinary tract infections: Flow charts (algorithms) for detection and treatment. *J.A.M.A.* 233:458, 1975.
30. Lorian, V. A Five Hour Disc Antibiotic Susceptibility Test. In V. Lorian (Ed.), *Significance of Medical Microbiology in the Care of Patients.* Baltimore: Williams & Wilkins, 1977. Pp. 203–212.
31. Matsen, J. M., and Barry, A. L. Susceptibility testing: Diffusion test procedures. In E. H. Lennette, E. H. Spaulding, and J. P. Truant (Eds.), *Manual of Clinical Microbiology* (2nd ed.). Washington, D.C.: American Society for Microbiology, 1974. Pp. 418–427.
32. Moffat, C. M., Britt, M. R., and Burke, J. P. Evaluation of miniature test for bacteriuria using dehydrated media and nitrite pads. *Appl. Microbiol.* 28:95–99, 1974.
33. Mou, T. W., and Feldman, H. A. The enumeration and preservation of bacteria in urine. *Am. J. Clin. Pathol.* 35:572, 1961.
34. Pryles, C. V., and Lustik, B. Laboratory diagnosis of urinary tract infection. *Pediatr. Clin. North Am.* 18:233, 1971.
35. Roberts, G. D. Detection of fungi in clinical specimens by phase-contrast microscopy. *J. Clin. Microbiol.* 2:261, 1975.
36. Roberts, G. D. Laboratory diagnosis of fungal infections. *Hum. Pathol.* 7:161, 1976.
37. Schönebeck, J. Studies on *Candida* infection of the urinary tract and on the antimycotic drug 5-fluorocytosine. *Scand. J. Urol. Nephrol.* [*Suppl.*] 11:1, 1972.
38. Segura, J. W., Kelalis, P. P., Martin, W. J., et al. Anaerobic bacteria in the urinary tract. *Mayo Clin. Proc.* 47:30, 1972.
39. Stamey, T. A. *Urinary Infections.* Baltimore: Williams & Wilkins, 1972. Pp. 31–53.
40. Thomas, V., Shelokov, A., and Forland, M. Antibody-coated bacteria in the urine and the site of urinary-tract infection. *N. Engl. J. Med.* 290:588, 1974.

41. Thornsberry, C., Gavan, T. L., Sherris, J. C., et al. Laboratory evaluation of a rapid, automated susceptibility testing system: Report of a collaborative study. *Antimicrob. Agents Chemother.* 7:466, 1975.
42. Vracko, R., and Sherris, J. C. Indole-spot test in bacteriology. *Am. J. Clin. Pathol.* 39:429, 1963.
43. Washington, J. A., II (Ed.). *Laboratory Procedures in Clinical Microbiology.* Boston: Little, Brown, 1974.
44. Washington, J. A., II. Laboratory approaches to the identification of Enterobacteriaceae. *Hum. Pathol.* 7:151, 1976.
45. Washington, J. A., II, and Barry, A. L. Dilution Test Procedures. In E. H. Lennette, E. H. Spaulding, and J. P. Truant (Eds.), *Manual in Clinical Microbiology* (2nd ed.). Washington, D.C.: American Society for Microbiology, 1974. Pp. 410–417.
46. Wheldon, D. B., and Slack, M. Multiplication of bacteria in urine and interpretation of delayed culture. *J. Clin. Pathol.* 30:615, 1977.
47. Wise, G. J., Goldberg, P., and Kozinn, P. J. Genitourinary candidiasis: Diagnosis and treatment. *J. Urol.* 116:788, 1976.

16. Pathology and Immunopathology of Renal Diseases

Jorge A. Velosa * and Keith E. Holley

Immunological Mechanisms in Renal Diseases

The evidence that immunological mechanisms participate in the pathogenesis of human renal diseases has been derived from serological and immunopathological studies as well as by correlation with certain experimentally induced renal diseases [27, 106, 167, 168]. Two immunological mechanisms have been well established. In one, antibodies react with endogenous antigens present in the glomerular basement membrane (GBM) [88, 112, 166]. In the other mechanism, antibodies react with either exogenous or endogenous antigens and form immune complexes that localize in the glomerulus [27, 31, 78, 118]. When the antibodies react with the GBM or when the immune complexes localize in the glomerulus, tissue injury ensues, which results in physiopathological alterations of the glomerular capillary filter, the mesangium, or both [21, 23, 26, 59]. The antibodies and immune complexes can induce the injury either directly or by recruiting other biological systems that function as mediators for the immune injury, such as the complement system, the kinin-forming system, and the coagulation system [5, 40, 81, 173].

Understanding of the immunological mechanisms that participate in renal disease has been facilitated by studies in animal models. In fact, both antibody-mediated and immune complex–mediated renal diseases were defined initially in experimental animals and subsequently in man. Thus the acute and chronic serum sickness models became the prototype of circulating immune complex glomerulonephritis [27]; the heterologous nephrotoxic serum nephritis [86, 143, 149] as well as the autoimmune [141, 142, 150] form of this disease provided the model for anti-GBM injury.

Immune Complex–Mediated Renal Injury

The mechanism of immune complex–mediated renal injury is probably involved in more than 90 percent of renal diseases that are thought to be of immunological origin. Immune complexes produce renal injury after they localize in the glomerulus. The factors that determine localization are only partially understood [24, 27]; the predominant view is that antigens react with antibodies in the circulation and form soluble immune complexes that deposit in the glomerulus [27, 31]. An alternative proposed mechanism for immune complex localization is initial deposition of the antigen in the capillary wall or the mesangium, followed by in situ reaction with circulating antibodies [63, 103].

* Recipient of Clinical Investigation Award NIAMDD AM 00662–01

Several important factors have been demonstrated to play a role in glomerular deposition of circulating immune complexes, including the size of the immune complex [25, 94, 159, 165]; the antibody avidity [102, 140, 171]; the phagocytic activity of the reticuloendothelial system [165] and the renal mesangium [47, 101, 102]; the variable response of the complement system and other vasoactive mediators that affect the permeability of the capillary walls; and local hemodynamics [12, 43, 46, 72].

Immune complexes that are bound to glomerular structures have been shown to be in dynamic equilibrium with the circulation. Therefore, circulating antigen or antibody can combine with localized immune complexes or can dissociate from them [80, 164].

The hallmark of immune complex renal disease is the demonstration of granular or large lumpy deposits of immunoglobulins and complement in the glomerulus by fluorescence microscopy [75, 105, 108, 118, 127, 157, 167]. The amount of tissue available from human renal biopsy specimens makes this technique the most widely applied in clinical practice. Additional analyses of the glomerular immune deposits have revealed important information; thus elution studies of isolated glomeruli from kidneys obtained at autopsy or after nephrectomy in patients with immune complex renal disease have revealed concentrations of specific antibodies many times higher than those present in serum [74, 113, 167]. Initially, this procedure was used in lupus nephritis and demonstrated high concentrations of antibodies to single-stranded and native DNA in the glomerulus [74, 77–79]. Similar findings have been reported in other glomerulopathies [168].

Known antigens in the glomerular deposits have been demonstrated by the use of fluoresceinated specific antibodies to those antigens. Again, this technique was first applied in kidneys with lupus nephritis for showing the presence of single-stranded and native DNA in the glomerular deposits [78]. Similar methods have demonstrated the presence of other antigens in immune deposits [168]. Antigens responsible for inducing immune complex renal disease may be multiple and of diverse origin. They can be either endogenous or exogenous, and this latter group can originate from living or nonliving products. There are few well-characterized endogenous antigens responsible for immune complex renal disease. Examples of this category include thyroglobulin [77], renal tubular epithelial antigens [124, 145], tumor-associated antigens [29, 92], and systemic lupus erythematosus antigens (perhaps the most common example of this type); however, some investigators believe that the lupus antigens are of viral origin.

There are two renal diseases in which granular immune deposits are characteristically localized in the mesangium or centrilobular regions of the glomerulus: anaphylactoid purpura and recurrent hematuria [156]. The clinical situation in both diseases may represent a different mechanism of immune complex deposition. The mesangial cells of the glomerulus have been shown to be phagocytic in a manner analogous to that of the reticuloendothelial system [39,

101, 116, 156]. Furthermore, an experimental model was developed in which circulating antibodies reacted with a foreign macromolecular antigen that was "planted" in the mesangium [103]. Therefore, this mechanism possibly operates in the localization of immune complexes and other macromolecules within the mesangium, with subsequent production of injury.

The pathogenetic significance of immune complexes in human tubulointerstitial diseases of the kidney is not clear. In lupus nephritis, a considerable number of patients have evidence of tubulointerstitial deposits of immune complexes, as demonstrated by the presence of deposits of IgG and complement [18, 47, 68, 85]; reportedly, the deposits correlate with the histological findings [18, 85]. In other immune complex glomerular diseases, however, tubulointerstitial deposits are seldom found [68].

Anti-GBM Disease

Anti-GBM disease is an important but clinically infrequent immunological mechanism of renal injury that accounts for less than 5 percent of cases of human glomerulonephritis [166]. Antibodies against endogenous GBM antigens develop spontaneously, react with the GBM, and lead to glomerulonephritis. In about half of the patients, the glomerulonephritis is associated with pulmonary hemorrhage (Goodpasture's syndrome) [13, 34, 133, 166]. The typical finding in these patients is the fixation of IgG in a fine, smooth, linear pattern of fluorescence along the glomerular capillary wall of the affected kidney [1, 34, 76, 88, 91, 137, 166, 167]. When the antibody is eluted, it can be shown to fix to normal GBM and to induce severe glomerulonephritis in subhuman primates [88]. The demonstration of anti-GBM antibodies in the circulation of patients with this type of glomerulonephritis is of practical clinical value [112]; these antibodies can be demonstrated by indirect immunofluorescence techniques in 60 to 80 percent of such patients and by radioimmunoassay in most of these patients [166].

The diagnosis of anti-GBM disease is based on the demonstration of both the typical immunofluorescence pattern in renal biopsy tissue and the circulating antibodies to GBM [88, 112, 167]. A more definite method is the elution of the anti-GBM antibodies and demonstration of their activity by indirect immunofluorescence in normal tissue or by radioimmunoassay [98, 100, 167, 169]. The circulating or eluted anti-GBM antibodies frequently react with lung and renal tubular basement membranes [85, 166, 167]. Pulmonary disease, however, does not develop in all cases. Conversely, overt pulmonary disease with circulating anti-GBM antibodies may be associated with only minimal renal disease. Furthermore, the sequence of organ involvement is variable, as is the time interval between the two clinical events; in addition, the disease can be recurrent with self-limited episodes, a concept that is not widely appreciated. It is not known at present what triggers the antibody response or the factors responsible for the variability of the organ involvement. Nevertheless, there are speculations linking this disease to influenza A2 virus [166, 170], exposure to hydrocarbon solvents

[10], potential autoimmunogenicity of urinary basement membrane fragments [87, 107], and other factors responsible for GBM injury that may render it immunogenic [17, 69, 70].

The relevance of antitubular basement membrane antibodies in clinical nephrology is not well established. Evidence is accumulating, however, that suggests the participation of this mechanism in renal injury as a secondary event in anti-GBM glomerulonephritis [4] and in association with immune complex glomerulonephritis [119, 148], methicillin toxicity [7, 17], and renal transplantation [4, 70, 106]. Within the past few years, several experimental models of antitubular basement membrane antibody disease have been demonstrated in guinea pigs [83, 144] and rats [84, 146] by the use of heterologous tubular basement membrane preparations.

Mediators of Immune Renal Injury

The complement system is an important mediator of immune injury in human renal disease [16, 40, 81, 82, 127]. It provides a primary link between the initial immune process and the events leading to tissue damage. A critical function of the complement system in this regard is the attraction of polymorphonuclear leukocytes to the site of tissue injury [23, 57]. These leukocytes in turn release hydrolytic enzymes from their lysosomes, which provides the final step of structural injury [26, 59].

Two pathways of complement activation and the sequential steps have been defined [52, 122, 123, 136]. The classic pathway involves three functional units: the recognition unit (C1), the activation unit (C2, C3, and C4), and the membrane-attack unit (C5, C6, C7, C8, and C9). The alternative pathway of complement is initiated by activation of properdin, which, by utilizing cofactors (factor B, factor D, and Mg^{++}), interacts with the C3 component of the classic pathway [53]. One important aspect of the alternative pathway is that it may not require antibodies for its activation. Substances such as polysaccharides, lipopolysaccharides, and aggregated IgA are known to activate this pathway [50, 130]. Nephritic factors (C3 NeF) also interact with and cleave C3 by utilizing the same cofactors as properdin [138]. C3 NeF is formed in the sera of some patients with hypocomplementemic membranoproliferative glomerulonephritis [152, 162], but the pathogenetic significance of this phenomenon has not been established.

Effective mechanisms of injury other than the complement system participate in renal immune damage [58, 71, 166]. For instance, in anti-GBM nephritis in man, many patients do not show changes of complement component in the serum or deposition on the GBM [166]. The kinin-forming, coagulation, and fibrinolytic systems may participate in renal tissue injury, but their importance has yet to be determined. Hageman factor of the coagulation cascade system plays a central role in linking the coagulation with the kinin-forming and complement systems [5, 67, 99, 158, 173].

Immunological Approach to Human Parenchymal Renal Disease

The patient with parenchymal renal disease can now be studied from the standpoint of the immune mechanism involved, in addition to the more traditional evaluation of the histological tissue response by light and electron microscopy [105, 117, 157, 161, 167]. Thus the presence, distribution, and pattern of renal immune deposits can easily be determined and the results can be interpreted in terms of the nature, prognosis, and treatment of the pathological process. Determination of the presence or absence of anti-GBM antibodies in the renal biopsy tissue or serum (or both) is critical in the patient with the pulmonary renal syndrome or the rapidly progressive form of glomerulonephritis. Participation of the complement system is usually assessed by tissue immunofluorescence and serum level determinations [105, 110, 167]. Currently, efforts are under way to determine the relevance of circulating immune complexes to renal disease [9, 89].

Tissue Immunofluorescence

Tissue immunofluorescence remains the mainstay of immunopathological diagnosis, in terms of both the information derived and the practicality. The fact that the reaction takes place in situ allows detection of not only the presence of immune reactants but also the distribution patterns. Thus the type of immunoglobulin and complement component, their topographical localization, and the pattern that emerges constitute a clinically valuable immunofluorescence profile [105, 108, 117, 161, 167]. Recent application of dual-label antibody immunofluorescence to renal tissue has improved better resolution of topographical localization of immune reactants [155].

Caution should be exercised when human renal tissue is examined. Many renal diseases are focal, both histologically and in regard to immune deposits. Advanced renal damage from various causes, including congenital diseases, shows an immunofluorescence pattern similar to that in glomeruli undergoing sclerosis, which makes etiological interpretations very difficult [153]. Granular deposition of immunoglobulins and complement is difficult to interpret when present in the same topographical location as fibrin-reacting antigens [167]. The linear fluorescence pattern of anti-GBM staining is common in situations other than anti-GBM disease; it is consistently present in diabetic renal disease with IgG and albumin stainings [160]. Many kidneys obtained after autopsy in patients without renal disease, as well as kidneys perfused in preparation for transplantation, show linear fluorescence of capillary walls [35]. Less frequently, this finding has been reported in systemic lupus erythematosus [73]. Normal renal biopsy specimens may occasionally show "accentuation" of GBM staining with IgG.

Complement Studies

The complement system may be activated by immune complexes starting at C1 [122] and by certain immunological and nonimmunological stimuli starting at C3 [52]. There is evidence that both mechanisms operate to various degrees in human glomerulonephritis [27, 117, 167]. Deposition of early complement components and immunoglobulins in the glomeruli is indicative of the classic pathway of complement activation [157], whereas deposition of properdin probably reflects activation of the alternative pathway [161]. Thus classic pathway activation with recruitment of the alternative pathway is thought to operate in systemic lupus erythematosus, acute poststreptococcal glomerulonephritis, and other instances of postinfectious glomerulonephritis such as shunt nephritis and subacute bacterial endocarditis. Predominant involvement of the alternative pathway may occur in membranoproliferative glomerulonephritis, focal glomerulonephritis with cold activation of C3, and some cases of glomerulonephritis in patients with deficiency of complement components such as C1r and C2 [30, 117, 129]. The participation of the complement system in human glomerulonephritis is assessed by measurement of serum complement components and immunofluorescence of renal tissue [49, 105, 117, 167].

Complement profiles of several important clinical entities are given in the following sections.

LUPUS GLOMERULONEPHRITIS. In most cases of lupus glomerulonephritis, there are decreased serum levels of both early and late complement components (C1, C4, C2, and C3) [49, 110]. Immunofluorescence studies of the kidney show glomerular deposition of C3 and C4 in 100 percent of the patients, C1q in about 75 percent, and properdin in about 40 percent [110].

ACUTE POSTSTREPTOCOCCAL GLOMERULONEPHRITIS. In the early phase, acute poststreptococcal glomerulonephritis shows a considerable decrease in all complement components except C1. Later, there is a persistent decrease in C3 [49, 110]. Immunofluorescence demonstrates C3 deposition in all patients, properdin in 80 percent, and C4 in 33 percent [109]. It has been suggested that the alternative pathway plays a role in this disease because C3 and properdin are consistently shown in renal tissue by immunofluorescence and frequently are decreased in the serum. Limited information is available in other types of postinfectious glomerulonephritis, but decreased levels of complement components and deposition of C3 by immunofluorescence seem to be consistent.

MEMBRANOPROLIFERATIVE GLOMERULONEPHRITIS. In membranoproliferative glomerulonephritis (MPGN) (mesangiocapillary glomerulonephritis), hypocomplementemia is frequently but not always present. Two histological types are well recognized; type I MPGN is characterized by subendothelial deposits and type II MPGN by intramembranous deposits [15, 55]. The predominant concept is that the alternative pathway of the complement system is activated in this condition [49, 109, 110, 117, 128]; thus early serum complement components (C1, C4, and C2) are usually normal, but late components (C3 and C5) are decreased. Recently, moderate reductions of serum levels of early complement components C1q and C4 have been reported in type II MPGN [126, 162]. By immunofluorescence study, consistent peripheral lobular deposition of C3 and properdin and, less frequently, of C1q and C4 has been seen in type I MPGN [161, 162]. In type II MPGN, C3 is found in the mesangium and along the basement membrane [44].

ADVANCED RENAL DISEASE. In advanced renal disease, there is evidence suggestive of simultaneous activation of classic and alternative complement pathways [153, 157]. Some cases of chronic glomerulonephritis [157], as well as other end-stage renal diseases of multiple causes, show deposition of C3 and properdin, which suggests alternative pathway activation only [153].

OTHER CONDITIONS. There are several clinical conditions that consistently show complement deposition by immunofluorescence study, but only scattered cases have been reported with decreased serum complement components. These conditions include glomerulonephritis associated with idiopathic mixed cryoglobulinemia; glomerulonephritis associated with hapten-complex (D-penicillamine); membranous glomerulonephropathy; some cases of rapidly progressive glomerulonephritis and most cases of vasculitis; and glomerulonephritis associated with neoplasia [110].

There are two conditions characterized by mesangial proliferation that show C3 and properdin in the mesangium—IgA nephropathy and anaphylactoid purpura. In addition, they show striking deposition of IgA in the same loci [56, 62, 151]. In anti-GBM glomerulonephritis, complement deposition is shown by immunofluorescence in 75 percent of the patients [167].

Circulating Anti-GBM Antibodies

Detection of circulating anti-GBM antibodies is an important step in the confirmation of the presence of anti-GBM glomerulonephritis with or without pulmonary involvement (Goodpasture's syndrome) [112, 167]. Most commonly, this is done by indirect immunofluorescence because this technique is readily available in many immunopathology laboratories. The technique involves detection of IgG in the serum, which reacts with the GBM of normal human kidneys. The major problem with this technique is finding adequate normal renal tissue without any IgG "accentuation" of the capillary wall. Probably the best way to obtain the controlled normal tissue is from in situ biopsy of nonnephritic nephrectomy specimens. The frequency of positive circulating anti-GBM antibodies by indirect immunofluorescence is about 80 percent in patients with Goodpasture's syndrome and 60 percent in patients with other anti-GBM glomerulonephritis [167]. A radioimmunoassay has been developed and applied to detect and quantify circulating anti-GBM antibodies and eluted antibodies to

GBM [98, 169]. It has been reported to be more sensitive than indirect immunofluorescence, yielding positive results in almost all patients with Goodpasture's syndrome and in 80 percent of patients with other anti-GBM glomerulonephritis [167].

Tissue Elution Studies

Elution studies of specific antibodies have been of clinical value in anti-GBM glomerulonephritis [113, 114, 167] and of importance in pathogenic studies of immune complex renal disease, discussed above. The limiting factor in these studies is the quantity of tissue, but techniques have been developed for small renal biopsy specimens, which may be applied in some situations at least [41, 45]. The details of this procedure are beyond the scope of this chapter and can be found elsewhere [74, 78, 88, 113].

Circulating Immune Complexes

Recently, methods have been developed for the detection and measurement of circulating immune complexes in blood and other body fluids. Three different categories of tests are available, based on the interaction of immune complexes with C1q [125], rheumatoid factor [97], and cell surface receptors [139, 147]. The clinical relevance of measuring circulating immune complexes in patients with glomerulonephritis is under active investigation, but little published information is available. Some correlation has been shown between lupus nephritis and circulating immune complexes [9, 89], but more information is necessary. Thus determination of the presence of serum immune complexes in parenchymal renal disease remains experimental, and its clinical relevance in the management of patients has not been proved.

Procedures for Immunofluorescence Studies and Light and Electron Microscopy

Processing of Renal Biopsy Tissues

Ideally, renal tissues obtained from open or closed biopsy should be placed in appropriate fixatives or solutions immediately upon removal. This necessitates sectioning of the renal tissues and selection of appropriate blocks to be used for light microscopy, immunohistology, and electron microscopy. The goal is to have glomeruli in each tissue block. To prevent confusion in the use of the fixatives and solutions, color coding of the bottles is of assistance.

Selection of tissue from open renal biopsy does not present much of a problem in regard to providing glomeruli in each tissue block. In comparison, needle biopsy specimens often prove to be more difficult. Occasionally it is necessary to place tissue in only two containers because of limitation of the tissue sample. It is our practice always to provide a specimen for immunohistology. If the amount of tissue is sufficient for only one additional examination, we fix the tissue in glutaraldehyde. After fixation, a portion is processed for light microscopy by the paraffin technique. If the sample size precludes this,

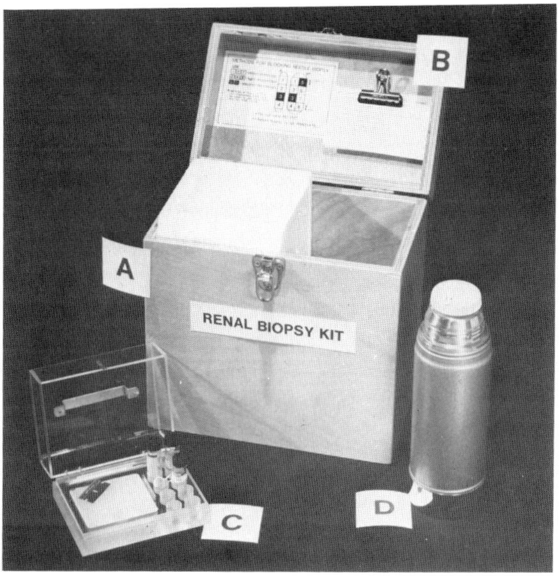

Figure 16–1
Renal biopsy kit. (A) Transportation box. (B) Instructions and clinical data card. (C) Appropriate solutions and fixatives with paraffin cutting surface. (D) Container of liquid nitrogen.

use of light microscopy would be dependent on a review of survey sections of the epon blocks. Similarly, if a specimen is received only in buffered formalin, we cut a portion of this tissue block and process it for electron microscopy. For each biopsy specimen, it is important to use a new razor blade that has been cleaned with alcohol and to cut the tissue rather than crush it. Thickness should be no more than 3 to 4 mm for blocks used for light microscopy and immunohistology; blocks used for electron microscopy should be 1 mm^3. Cutting is facilitated by using a dental wax surface or a paraffin block. Care should always be taken to prevent crushing when these tissue blocks are handled; the use of atraumatic forceps or a saline-moistened wooden applicator stick has proved to be satisfactory.

A biopsy kit (Fig. 16–1) may be prepared; it should include all appropriate fixatives and solutions, a container of liquid nitrogen, applicator sticks, razor blades, and an appropriate surface on which to cut the tissue blocks. Written and diagrammed instructions for tissue handling (Fig. 16–2) should also be included.

Immunofluorescence Microscopy

The quality of tissue immunofluorescence and the reliability of information obtained from it depend primarily on the quality of the reagents and the tissue. In

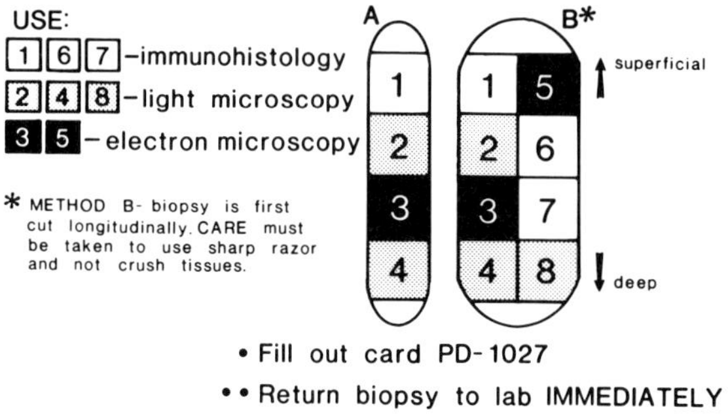

Figure 16–2
Methods for blocking renal biopsy tissue.

addition, the appropriate equipment is important, as is the expertise for interpretation. Fluorochromes containing chemically active groups such as isothiocyanate can be conjugated to antibodies. The conjugate retains the antibody specificity, and the attached fluorochrome acts as a tracer, which allows in situ identification of the corresponding antigen. The fluorochrome most widely used is fluorescein, but rhodamine is coming into more general use.

The objectives in tissue immunofluorescence, such as for renal tissue, are to maximize the fluorescence produced by specific binding of the fluorochrome present in the tissue and to minimize the nonspecific background. Two factors are important in regard to the equipment used: the combination of filters chosen for each fluorochrome and the type of illumination [65, 167]. Recently, epi-illumination obtained by the vertical illuminator system has improved the more traditional transmitted illumination; this new technique provides a better fluorescence at high magnifications and avoids the use of oil-immersion objectives. Epi-illumination is clearly the method of choice for surface membrane immunofluorescence, such as for lymphocyte studies.

Interference filters transmit wavelengths in the range of 490 to 500 nm, which is optimal for fluorescein, or 546 nm, which is optimal for rhodamine. These filters increase the intensity of fluorescence and are superior to older filter systems. Because different filter combinations have different sensitivities, notation of the filters used in immunofluorescence studies is necessary.

REAGENTS. The quality of the reagent used is an important factor, particularly for the detection of less conspicuous immune reactants. Labeled antisera should have potent antibody activity, specificity, and minimal background fluorescence [65]. For routine immunofluorescence, satisfactory commercial reagents are available [167]. In general, those fluoresceinated reagents having an optimal fluorescein-to-protein ratio are obtained by selecting the appropriate antibody fraction by means of ion-exchange chromatography or, less frequently, by elution from immunoabsorbents. Compared with other reagents, these reagents produce greater intensity of fluorescence with less background staining [172].

Specificity of the commercial reagents should be demonstrated [167]. The best method is by absorption with the specific antigen, which shows that the immunofluorescence reaction is abolished. Absorption of antiserum with specific antigen usually is performed by adding small amounts (100 to 200 mg) of antigen to 0.5 to 1.0 ml of antiserum, followed by incubation at 56°C for 1 hour and then centrifugation, preferably at about 30,000 rpm, for 30 minutes. The supernate is tested on tissue under study (the procedure may be repeated), and absence of specific staining should be demonstrated. Testing by immunodiffusion is useful but not sufficient; absorption should demonstrate absence of the precipitating reaction by this technique. Another way to show specificity is by blocking with unlabeled antibody of identical reactivity. The tissue to be examined is incubated first with the unlabeled antibody, which will saturate the available binding sites. When the labeled antibody is added, no specific binding sites are available and the specific tissue fluorescence is abolished.

When antiserum for immunofluorescence is prepared, many problems of background fluorescence can be avoided if the antiserum is very potent. This allows the use of preparations of low-protein (immunoglobulin) concentration [65]. If the antiserum is contaminated with unwanted antibodies, the absorption method of choice to purify the antiserum is the use of insolubilized antigens, preferably immunoabsorbent columns [167].

PREPARATION OF TISSUE. Renal biopsy material should be snap-frozen without delay. A common problem is letting the tissue air-dry. A commonly used snap-frozen method makes use of liquid nitrogen; better results are obtained when isopentane is used as a quenching agent. The following steps have been helpful in securing good quality of tissue. Once the tissue is removed from the biopsy needle, a segment of cortex is cut, mounted in a small piece of wet paper sponge, and usually held by a pin for convenience. The sponge with the tissue adhered to it is then dropped into the bottle of isopentane that has been previously cooled by immersion in liquid nitrogen (−196°C). If liquid nitrogen is not available, snap-freezing may be accomplished by immersion of the tissue in acetone-dry ice slush (≅−70°C). However, some disruption of tissue and formation of ice crystals may be experienced with this method. Tissue may be transported to the laboratory in appropriate containers. If tissue is to be transported some distance, it should be kept frozen in dry ice; convenient shipping containers are available that can hold sufficient dry ice to keep a specimen frozen for 48 to 72 hours.

SECTIONING AND STAINING. Before frozen sections are cut, the tissue should be placed in a cryostat to allow temperature equilibration. Multiple sections should be cut at 4 to 5 μm and placed on acetone-cleaned slides of good quality with a frosted end; appropriate identification should be included on each slide. Appropriate controls include known positive-staining and negative-staining tissue.

The following instructions are currently used in our laboratory.

1. Cut frozen tissue sections on a cryostat at 4 to 5 μm and place them on appropriately labeled high-quality glass slides.
2. After air-drying for 10 minutes, wash the tissue three times in phosphate-buffered saline (PBS; pH 7.2) to remove unbound proteins.
3. Fix the tissue in ether–95% ethyl alcohol (50 : 50) for 10 minutes and 95% ethyl alcohol for 20 minutes.
4. Wash the tissue in PBS three times. Blot excess fluid, but keep the tissue damp.
5. Place several drops of appropriate monospecific fluorescein-conjugated antiserum on the tissue (be sure tissue is covered). Place the slide upright in a moist chamber and incubate for 30 minutes to 1 hour at room temperature.
6. Wash slides in PBS three times (10 to 15 minutes each), with continuous agitation to remove nonbound antiserum.
7. After the final wash, remove excess buffer but prevent tissue from drying before coverslipping. For mounting media, use a glycerol-buffer (PBS) mixture (9 : 1) or, as Wilson [163] recommends, a 0.01 M tris-buffered glycerol (1 : 9). The high pH of 9.6 is said to stabilize the luminescence of fluorescein.
8. Seal the coverslips with clear nail polish.
9. The slides are now ready for examination by fluorescence microscopy.

Light Microscopy

FIXATION. Many fixatives are available for light microscopy; the most common fixative used is 10% buffered formalin. The availability of this fixative and the experience of most laboratories with it make it a good choice. It is particularly useful when transportation necessitates fixation periods exceeding 24 hours. Other fixatives commonly used for renal biopsy specimens include Bouin's, Helly's (Zenker's-formalin), paraformaldehyde, and glutaraldehyde. These last two fixatives allow use of one solution for tissue blocks for examination by both light and electron microscopy. Standard staining procedures for light microscopy may need alteration when glutaraldehyde is used; an additional step in the standard staining process is required with the periodic acid–Schiff stain in order to prevent the entire tissue from staining strongly positive.

PROCESSING. After adequate fixation, which may range from 3 to 7 hours for Bouin's or glutaraldehyde or from 12 to 24 hours for 10% buffered formalin, the tissue is dehydrated and embedded in paraffin. General principles for tissue processing apply [96]. The time periods required for dehydration and infiltration with paraffin for needle biopsy specimens are shorter than for larger blocks of tissue; longer processing times may result in a tissue block that is overly hard

Table 16–1. Procedures for Processing Renal Biopsy Specimens *

Fixative or Solution	Time (min) Technicon-Ultra	Manual
70% alcohol	6	20
80% alcohol	5	20
95% alcohol	5	20
95% alcohol	5	20
Absolute alcohol	5	20
Absolute alcohol	5	20
Absolute alcohol	5	20
Absolute alcohol	5	20
Xylene	5	20
Xylene	5	20
Paraffin (62°C melting point)	5	30
Paraffin (62°C melting point)	12	20 (under vacuum)

* The times listed are for needle biopsy tissues.

and dry. This lack of pliability makes it difficult to obtain serial 2-μm sections that are free of tissue tears and folds.

The use of the Technicon-Ultra processor, which utilizes temperature (37° C) and vacuum, yields satisfactory results. A processing time of 100 minutes for needle biopsy specimens and 3 hours for open biopsy specimens of 2- to 3-mm thickness has proved to be satisfactory in our laboratory. In addition, the use of paraffin waxes of different melting temperatures provides optimal tissue support of thin-section preparations. We have found that a paraffin with a melting point of 62° C has been satisfactory.

Biopsy specimens may be processed satisfactorily by hand, and indeed this may prove to be the best method when the number of biopsies precludes the use of an automatic processor. Small vacuum paraffin units are available that greatly enhance tissue-block preparation. Table 16–1 outlines methods that have proved to be satisfactory for processing renal biopsy specimens. Individual laboratories may vary the times in several steps and still achieve satisfactory results.

SECTIONING. A stable microtome and a sharp microtome knife are essential in the preparation of serial 2- to 3-μm sections. It is generally advisable to have one technician cut and stain these sections, since the art of thin-tissue sectioning and staining is developed by experience. General techniques for paraffin sectioning are applicable. The addition of a few drops of a 30% alcohol solution to the warm glass slide or to the water bath assists in removing wrinkles from the tissue sections.

STAINING. General staining techniques are applicable to renal biopsy specimens, with the exception that thin sections require longer periods of staining with most dyes. Thicker sections (4 to 6 μm) prove useful in demonstrating the presence of certain substances such as amyloid. Most current textbooks on staining list appropriate procedures for use in routine evaluation of renal biopsy specimens. These routine stains include hematoxylin and eosin, periodic acid–Schiff, periodic acid–methenamine silver, and Masson's trichrome. Other special stains may be useful (e.g., cresyl violet, Congo red, and Verhoeff's elastic tissue stain for evaluation of blood vessels).

Electron Microscopy

FIXATION. Prompt fixation of renal biopsy tissue is necessary for ideal cytological and membrane preservation. This is not always possible, but fortunately, in many renal diseases the membranous changes and immune deposits are preserved for some time as long as the tissues are not allowed to dry. The most widely used primary fixative for electron microscopy is buffered glutaraldehyde. This solution is usually used in 3 to 4% concentration, with fixation at 4° C for 3 to 7 hours. Some buffered glutaraldehyde solutions will allow fixation at room temperature and have a reported shelf life of up to one month. Glucose is sometimes added to some solutions to increase the osmolality of the fixative. After primary fixation, the tissue is rinsed in buffer and may be stored in buffer for several days at 4° C before further processing. Buffered osmium tetroxide in 1 to 2% concentration may also serve as a primary fixative; penetration of tissue is less than with use of glutaraldehyde. Care must be taken to have tissue blocks no larger than 1 mm^3.

PROCESSING. Most tissues are postfixed in 1% buffered osmium tetroxide for 1 hour, rinsed, and dehydrated through graded alcohols. En bloc staining with 2% aqueous uranyl acetate may be accomplished at this point. After infiltration with propylene oxide, propylene oxide–epon mixture, and epon, the tissue is embedded in a capsule with epon. Final polymerization takes 24 to 48 hours at 60° C.

SECTIONING AND STAINING. The tissue blocks are shaped by using razor blades, and survey sections (0.5 to 1.0 μm) are cut on an ultramicrotome with a glass or diamond knife. These sections may be stained with 0.5% toluidine blue or 1% azure II and viewed by light microscopy. Grids are then prepared, with sections 500 to 600 Å thick. Staining of grids with 3% uranyl acetate (if not done en bloc) and 3% lead citrate enhances the contrast of tissue structures. Appropriately prepared grids may be viewed by using a variety of electron microscopes.

In some cases, glutaraldehyde or paraformaldehyde fixatives may not be available. Renal tissue fixed in buffered 10% formalin has proved to be satisfactory in many instances; fixatives containing mercury salts are less satisfactory. Similarly, if no tissue has been saved for possible examination by electron microscopy, a portion of paraffin block can be used for ultrastructural examination. The paraffin is removed from the tissue block, and the tissue is rehydrated. After postfixation in 1% osmium tetroxide, the tissue is processed in the usual fashion. We have satisfactorily demonstrated subepithelial deposits in postinfectious glomerulonephritis from paraffin tissue blocks prepared 30 years previously.

Immunopathological Patterns and Morphological Correlations of Parenchymal Renal Disease

The following classification is a modification of the one presented elsewhere by Germuth and Rodriguez [47].

Anti-GBM Glomerulonephritis

The light microscopic findings in anti-GBM glomerulonephritis range from a focal and segmental proliferative lesion to the more devastating picture of extracapillary proliferation (Fig. 16–3A) [60, 63]. There are documented cases of anti-GBM glomerulonephritis with few abnormal manifestations. Electron microscopy shows only gaps and discontinuities of the basement membrane [21].

The typical immunofluorescence picture is a smooth, often delicate, linear staining of the GBM with IgG, less frequently with C3, and occasionally with IgM (Fig. 16–3B, C) [77, 88, 166, 168]. Fibrin is frequently present in the glomerular crescents [166]. Pulmonary tissue shows similar linear deposits of IgG along the alveolar capillary membranes [11, 124].

Immune Complex Deposit Glomerular Disease

SUBEPITHELIAL DEPOSITS. The characteristic feature is the presence of deposits along the capillary walls, involving all glomeruli. Morphologically, there is diffuse and generalized glomerular disease.

In diffuse proliferative glomerulonephritis, there is usually diffuse, scattered glomerular IgG along with C3 and the variable presence of IgM, IgA, C1, C4, and properdin [32, 42, 93]. This pattern is seen in poststreptococcal glomerulonephritis (Fig. 16–4) and in other types of postinfectious glomerulonephritis. Morphologically, the acute stage is characterized by endothelial and mesangial proliferation, with polymorphonuclear infiltration. Both the immunofluorescence and morphological patterns change during the resolution phase, when the deposits become larger and more scattered and often are detected only with C3 [6, 32, 42, 60, 64, 93]. During the acute phase, the characteristic electron microscopic finding is the subepithelial humplike deposit.

Membranous nephropathy (Fig. 16–5) is the most common lesion in the idiopathic nephrotic syndrome in adults but is seldom found in children and adolescents [22, 36, 37, 60]. There is diffuse and generalized discrete granular IgG, together with C3 and the variable presence of IgM, IgA, C1q, C4, and properdin. This picture is the most consistent of the immunofluorescence patterns except in the very late stages of the disease [51, 120]. The morphological lesion is consistent and recognizable through several stages. Typically, there is

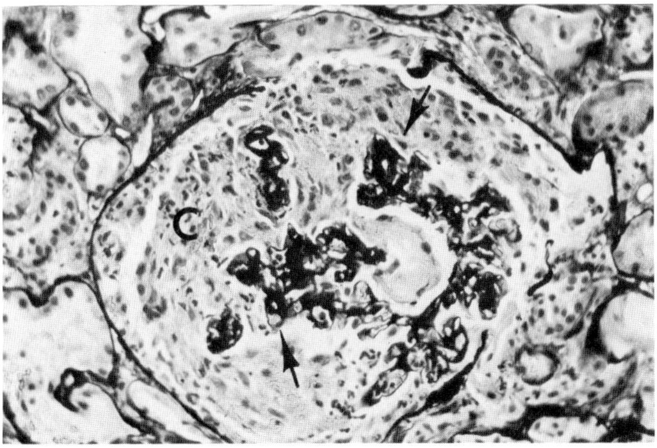

A

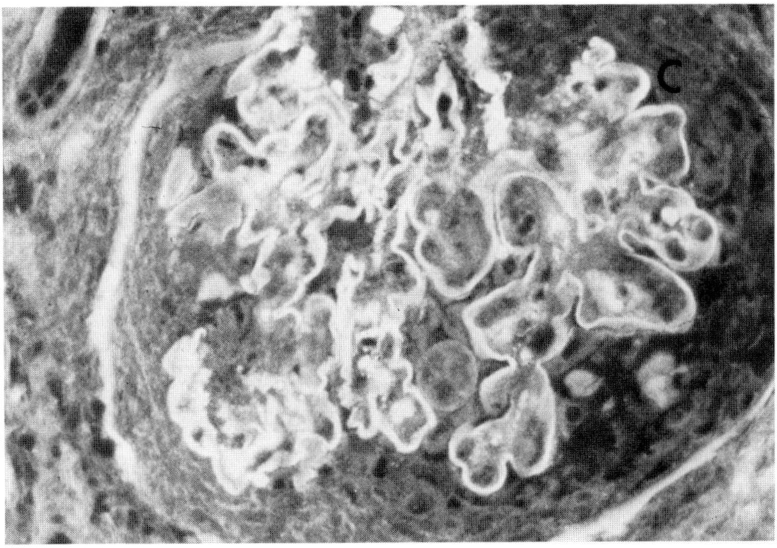

B

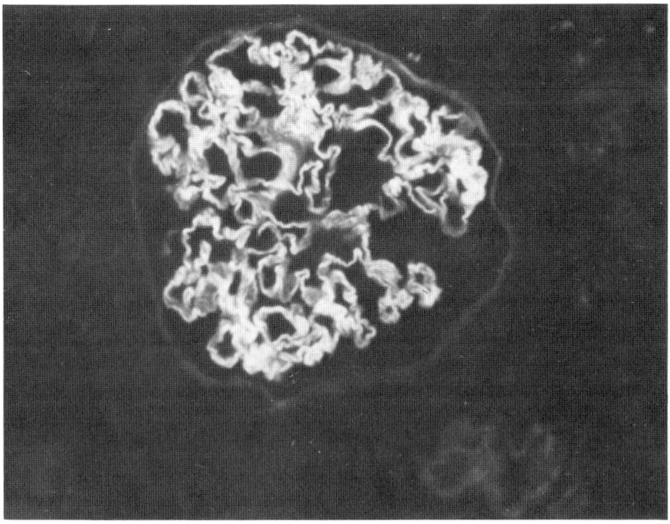

C

Figure 16–3
Anti-GBM disease. (A) Light microscopy shows extensive crescent formation (*C*) (extracapillary proliferation), with compression of the glomerular tuft (*arrows*). (Methenamine silver stain; 250X.) (B) Immunofluorescence microscopy reveals diffuse linear staining of GBM with antihuman IgG, which has been compressed by crescent formation (*C*). Note that some granular features appear as the disease progresses and distorts the glomerulus. (250X.) (C) Demonstration of anti-GBM antibodies in the serum of a patient with Goodpasture's syndrome by indirect immunofluorescence. Normal kidney tissue was incubated with the patient's serum and subsequently with labeled antihuman IgG. Note the diffuse linear staining of the normal glomerulus. (250X.) (A and B reprinted, by permission, from R. D. Wagoner and K. E. Holley, Parenchymal Renal Disease: Clinical and Pathologic Features. In F. G. Knox (Ed.), *Textbook of Renal Pathophysiology*. Hagerstown, Md.: Harper & Row, 1978.)

diffuse and uniform thickening of the capillary wall without appreciable cell proliferation [22, 36, 60]. Silver impregnation techniques usually demonstrate the presence of characteristic "spikes" [36, 66]. Most frequently, this type of pattern corresponds to the so-called idiopathic membranous nephropathy. One important exception is the membranous type of lupus, an infrequent presentation of this disease when no other important morphological features are present. Electron microscopy confirms the presence of subepithelial immune deposits. The findings are variable and depend on the evolutionary stage of the disease. Basement membrane-like material that corresponds to the silver spikes is deposited around the immune deposits [22, 36, 134].

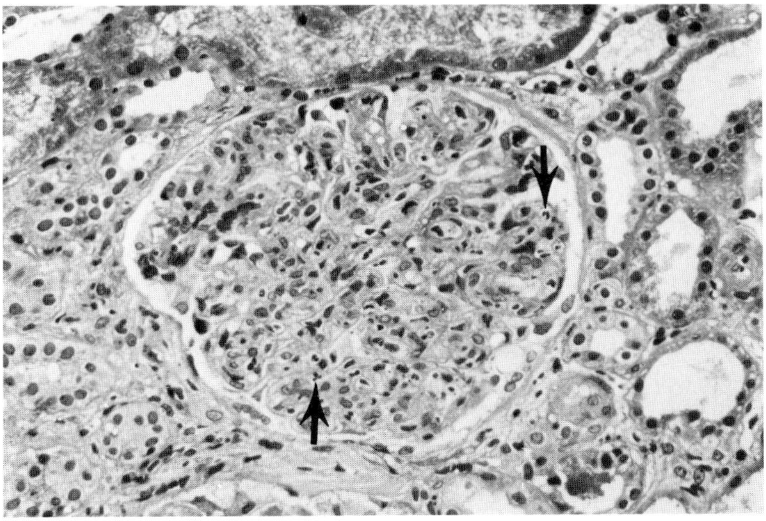

A

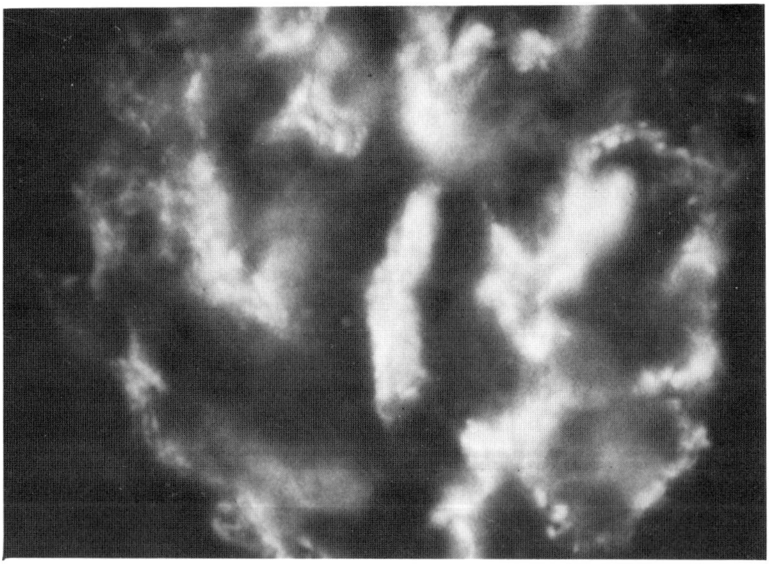

B

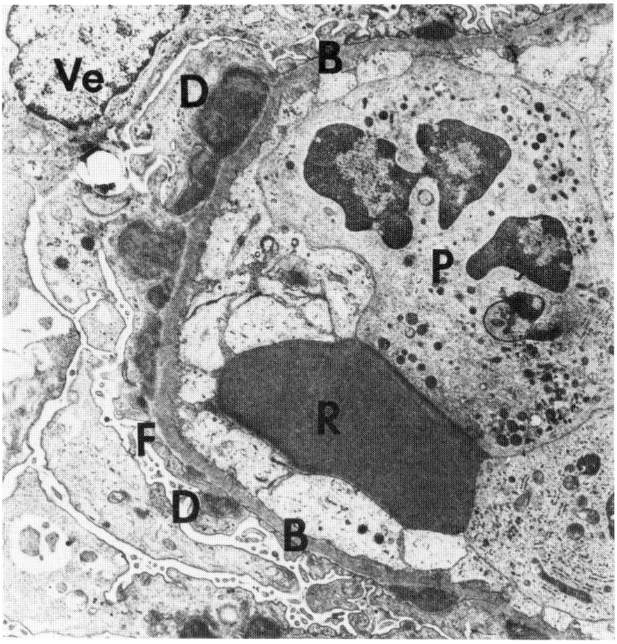

C

Figure 16–4
Poststreptococcal glomerulonephritis. (A) Light microscopy shows diffuse endocapillary cellular increase. Polymorphonuclear leukocytes are prominent (*arrows*) in nearly obliterated capillary lumina. (Hematoxylin and eosin; 250X.) (B) Immunofluorescence microscopy reveals granular staining along the capillary wall with antihuman IgG. (400X.) (C) Electron microscopy discloses subepithelial deposits (*D*), no thickening of basement membrane (*B*), and substantial narrowing of capillary lumina. *R* = red cell; *P* = polymorphonuclear leukocyte; *Ve* = visceral epithelial cell; *F* = fused visceral epithelial foot processes. (C reprinted, by permission, from R. D. Wagoner and K. E. Holley, Parenchymal Renal Disease: Clinical and Pathologic Features. In F. G. Knox (Ed.), *Textbook of Renal Pathophysiology*. Hagerstown, Md.: Harper & Row, 1978.)

SUBENDOTHELIAL-MESANGIAL DEPOSITS. There are two types of membranoproliferative (mesangiocapillary) glomerulonephritis: type I (Fig. 16–6) and type II (Fig. 16–7). The immunofluorescence pattern has consistently demonstrated a coarse, peripheral, lobular deposition of C3 and properdin, frequently associated with IgG and IgM. C1q and C4 are present in about half of the cases and IgA in one-fifth [44, 120, 167]. In type II MPGN, C3 is found in the mesangium and along the glomerular and tubular basement membranes [44]. Morphologically, thickening of the capillary wall and mesangial proliferation are present. By electron microscopy, type I MPGN shows subendothelial deposits and mesangial cell deposition between the basement membrane and the capillary

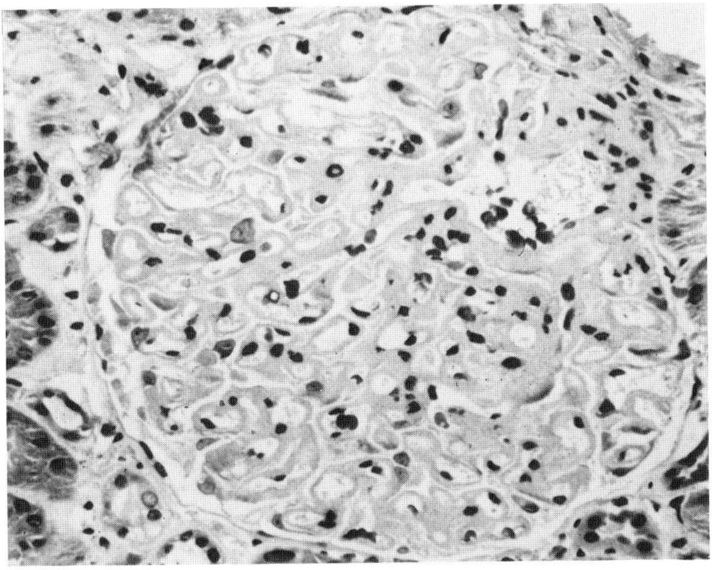

A

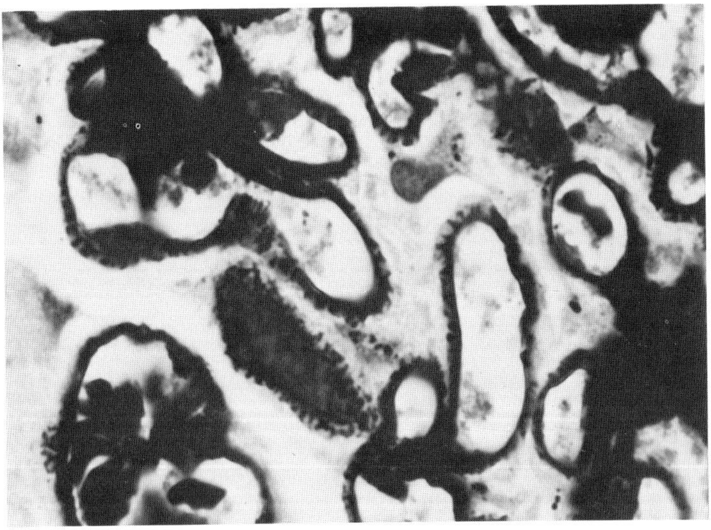

B

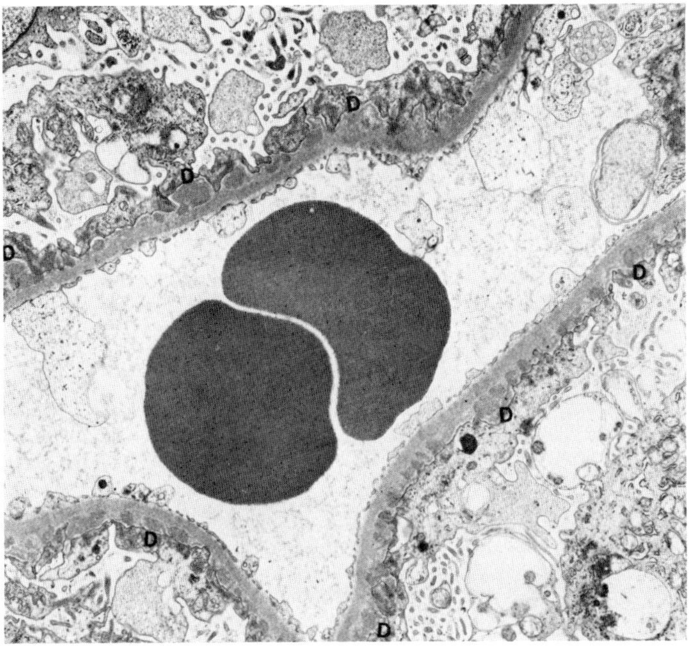

C

Figure 16–5
Membranous nephropathy. (A) Diffuse thickening of the capillary walls, with no cellular proliferation. (Hematoxylin and eosin; 400X.) (B) Note projections ("spiking") of basement membrane along subepithelial margin of GBM. Deposits are located between spikes. (Methenamine silver stain; 1370X.) (C) Electron microscopy shows individual capillary loop with numerous subepithelial electron-dense deposits (*D*). (7500X.) (B reprinted, by permission, from R. D. Wagoner and K. E. Holley, Parenchymal Renal Disease: Clinical and Pathologic Features. In F. G. Knox (Ed.), *Textbook of Renal Pathophysiology*. Hagerstown, Md.: Harper & Row, 1978.)

endothelium [19, 55, 60]. Mesangial deposits are usually abundant. In type II MPGN, the electron-dense deposits are present within the basement membrane [15, 44].

IgA nephropathy (Fig. 16–8) is an immunopathological diagnosis in patients with the clinical syndrome of recurrent hematuria and, less frequently, in patients with mild-to-moderate proteinuria associated with microscopic hematuria [14, 90, 95, 111, 121]. It has a typical and consistent immunofluorescence pattern: generalized and diffuse granular deposition of IgA, C3, properdin, and, in most but not all cases, IgG. The first presentation is most common in children, whereas the second is most prevalent in adults. The microscopic picture is also variable: the glomeruli may be normal or may show focal segmental or

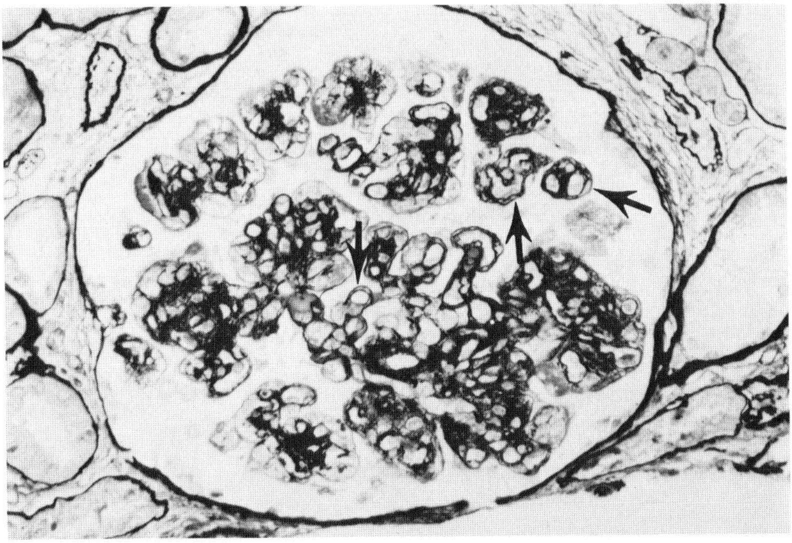

A

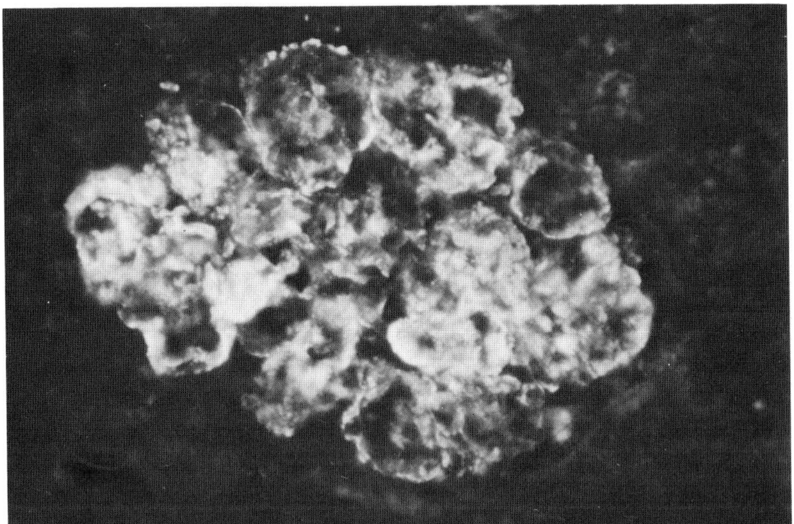

B

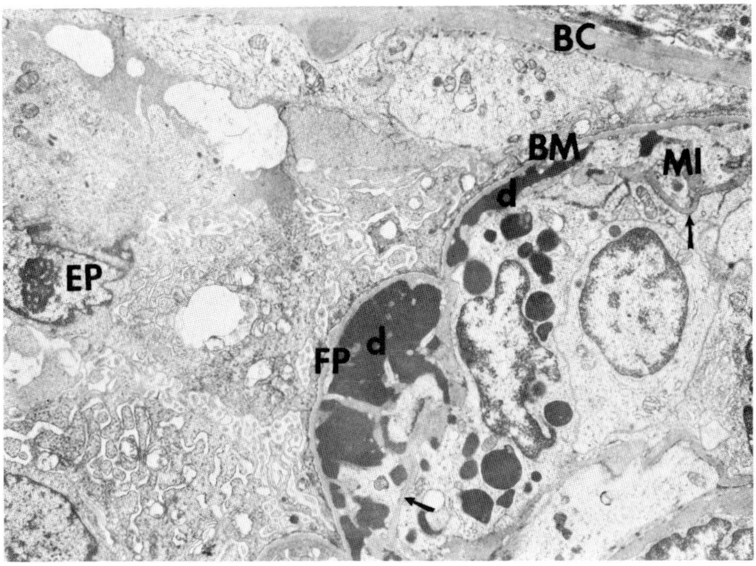

C

Figure 16–6
Membranoproliferative glomerulonephritis. Type I. Light microscopy (A) shows diffuse endocapillary proliferation, with prominent circumferential mesangial interposition. Note "split" reduplicated basement membrane (*arrows*). (Methenamine silver stain; 250X.) Immunofluorescence microscopy (B) reveals granular staining of the capillary walls and mesangial region with antihuman IgG. Note the lobular pattern. (250X.) Electron microscopy (C) shows subendothelial deposits (*d*), reduplicated basement membrane-like material (*arrows*), epithelial cell (*EP*), mesangial interposition (*MI*), and fused epithelial cell foot processes (*FP*). *BM* = basement membrane; *BC* = Bowman's capsule. (10,000X.) (Portion (C) reprinted, by permission, from R. D. Wagoner and K. E. Holley, Parenchymal Renal Disease: Clinical and Pathologic Features. In F. G. Knox (Ed.), *Textbook of Renal Pathophysiology*. Hagerstown, Md.: Harper & Row, 1978.)

more generalized, diffuse mesangial proliferation. There may be diffuse or segmental glomerulosclerosis, or both, and occasionally small crescents.

In focal (mesangiopathic) glomerulonephritis, there are two well-characterized conditions. Schönlein-Henoch purpura is usually recognized both by clinical examination and by immunofluorescence and microscopic findings. Immunofluorescence studies show generalized, diffuse, granular mesangial deposition of IgG, IgA, C3, and properdin. The presence of fibrin is variable [38, 56, 151]. The morphological picture is also variable and usually parallels the clinical status. There is a wide range of findings: normal, focal increase of mesangial cells only, focal segmental glomerulonephritis, or generalized and diffuse glomerulonephritis with necrotizing features, with or without crescent formation [56, 60, 115]. By electron microscopy, the main abnormalities are in the

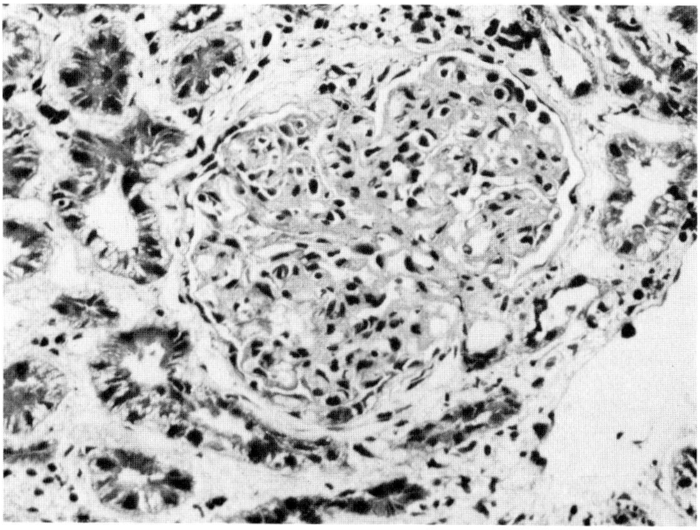

A

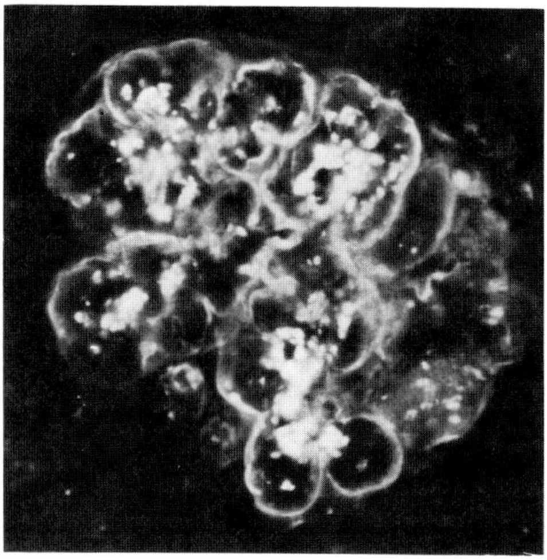

B

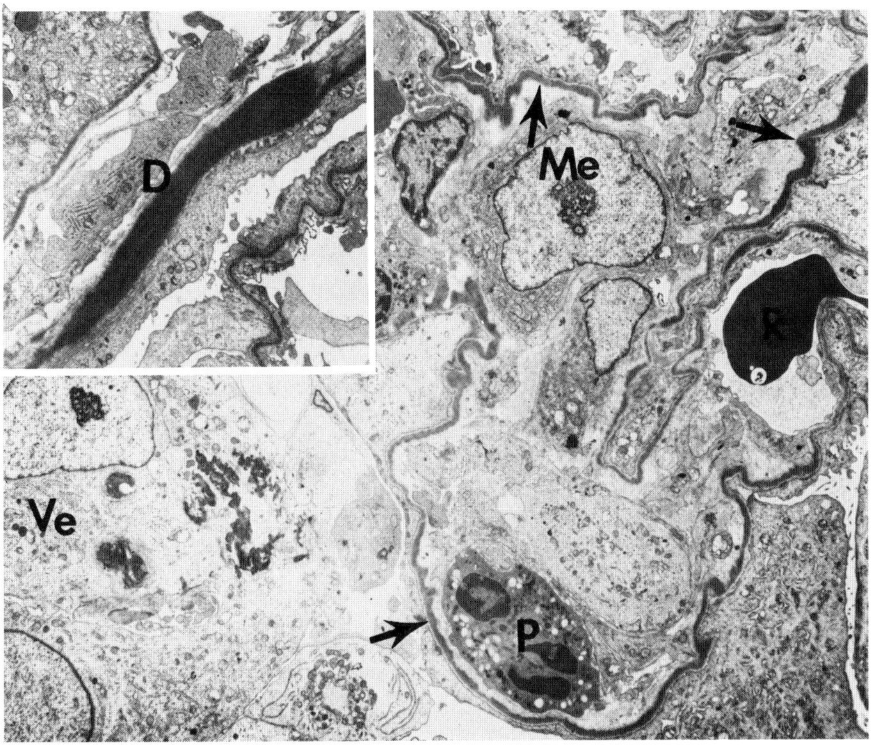

C

Figure 16–7
Membranoproliferative glomerulonephritis. Type II. Light microscopy (A) shows minimal cellularity and thickened capillary walls. (Hematoxylin and eosin; 250X.) Immunofluorescence microscopy (B) reveals linear staining of the capillary walls and Bowman's capsule with antihuman C3 complement. No positive staining was obtained for immunoglobulins. (250X.) Electron microscopy (C) discloses intramembranous electron-dense deposits on capillary walls (*arrows*). Inset shows deposit (*D*) within the basement membrane of Bowman's capsule. *Me* = mesangial cell; *R* = red cell; *P* = polymorphonuclear leukocyte; *Ve* = visceral epithelial cell. (5000X.) (Portions A and C reprinted, by permission, from R. D. Wagoner and K. E. Holley, Parenchymal Renal Disease: Clinical and Pathologic Features. In F. G. Knox (Ed.), *Textbook of Renal Pathophysiology*. Hagerstown, Md.: Harper & Row, 1978.)

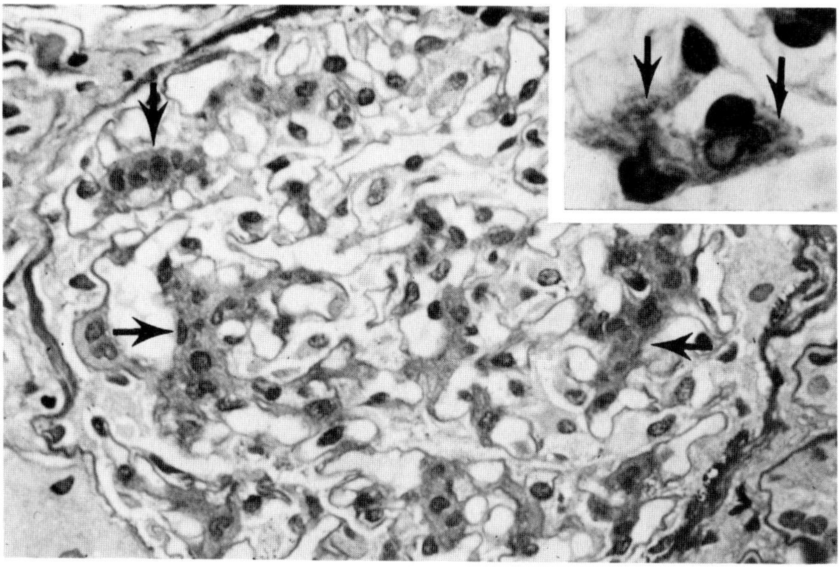

A

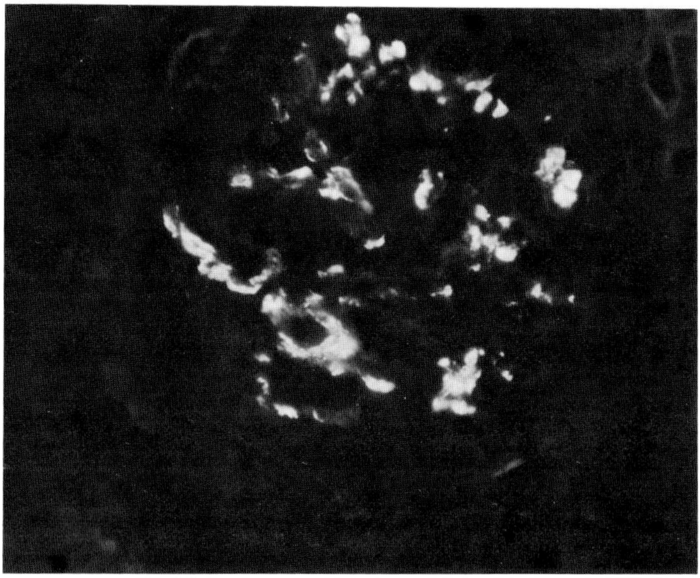

B

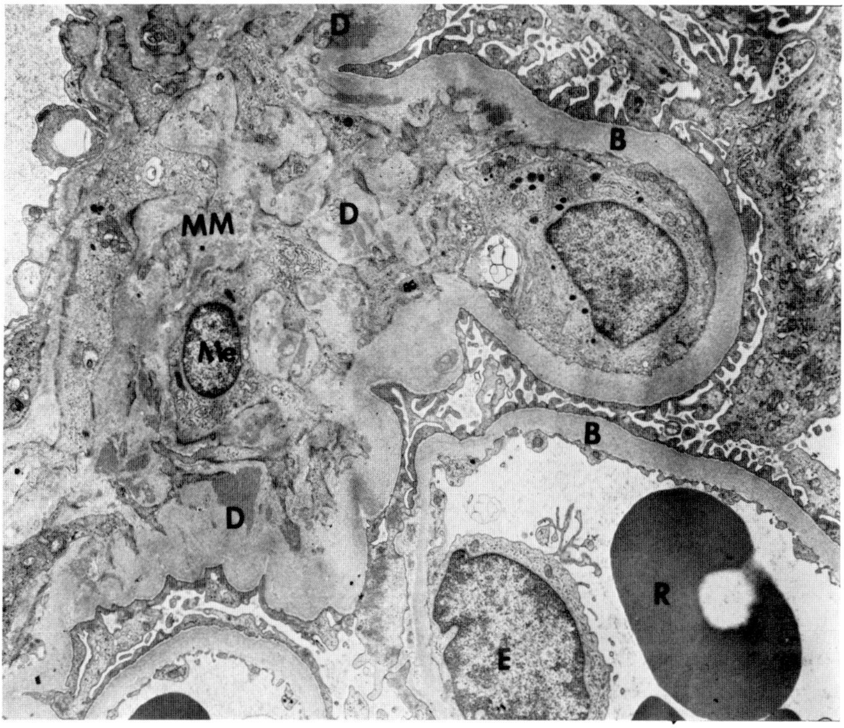

C

Figure 16–8
IgA nephropathy. (A) Light microscopy reveals mesangial cellular and matrix increase (*arrows*). (Periodic acid–Schiff; 250X.) In inset, note mesangial granular deposits (*arrows*). (Periodic acid–Schiff; 1000X.) (B) Immunofluorescence microscopy shows diffuse mesangial granular staining with antihuman IgA. (250X.) (C) Electron microscopy reveals mesangial electron-dense deposits (*D*). *Me* = mesangial cell; *MM* = mesangial matrix; *E* = endothelial cell; *R* = red cell; *B* = basement membrane. (7500X.) (B reprinted, by permission, from R. D. Wagoner and K. E. Holley, Parenchymal Renal Disease: Clinical and Pathologic Features. In F. G. Knox (Ed.), *Textbook of Renal Pathophysiology*. Hagerstown, Md.: Harper & Row, 1978.)

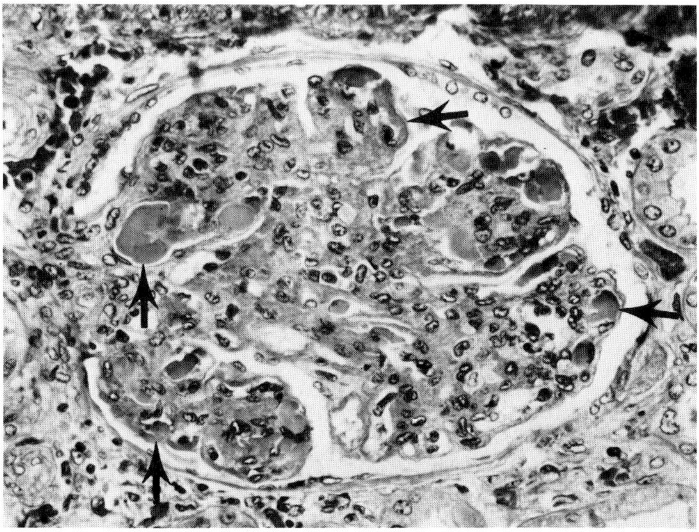

A

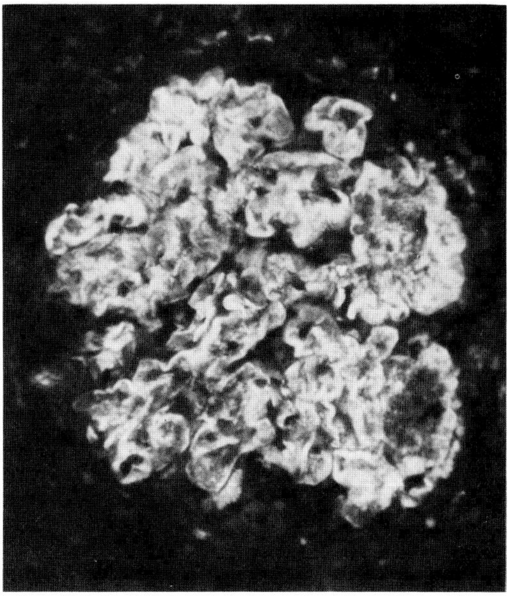

B

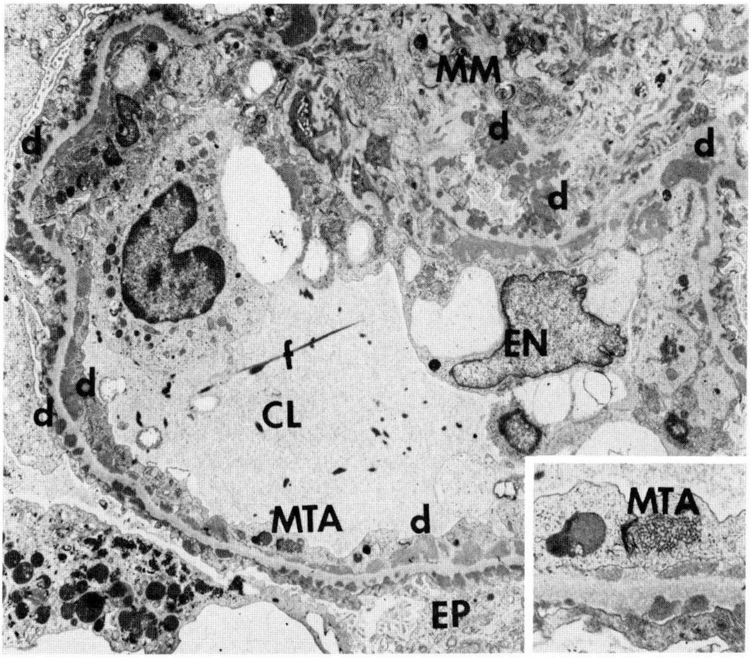

C

Figure 16–9
Lupus nephritis. (A) Light microscopy shows diffuse endocapillary cellular proliferation. Note fibrinoid (*arrows*) along inside of capillary wall, which results in thickening. Some material appears to be detached within capillary lumina (hyaline or fibrinoid thrombi). (Hematoxylin and eosin; 400X.) (B) Immunofluorescence microscopy reveals diffuse granular and lumpy staining for IgG along the capillary walls and mesangium. (250X.) (C) Electron microscopy shows electron-dense deposits (*d*) present in the mesangium and on both sides of the basement membrane. *EN* = endothelial cells; *MTA* = microtubular arrays; *CL* = capillary lumen; *f* = fibrin; *MM* = mesangial matrix; *EP* = epithelial cell. (7500X.) (A and C reprinted, by permission, from R. D. Wagoner and K. E. Holley, Parenchymal Renal Disease: Clinical and Pathologic Features. In F. G. Knox (Ed.), *Textbook of Renal Pathophysiology*. Hagerstown, Md.: Harper & Row, 1978.)

mesangium—namely increases in mesangial matrix and electron-dense deposits [151].

Lupus Glomerulonephritis

Renal involvement is a common and serious manifestation of systemic lupus erythematosus. Morphological classifications of the renal disease are based primarily on the glomerular changes [8, 28, 104, 131, 132, 135]. Subgroups include mesangial proliferative, focal proliferative, diffuse proliferative, and membranous glomerulonephritis. In all subgroups, immune complexes and complement components are deposited in the glomeruli in various amounts. These deposits are located in the mesangium, along the capillary basement membrane (subendothelial, subepithelial), and within the basement membrane proper (intramembranous). Immunohistologically, IgG and IgM are frequently demonstrated, and some cases show prominent IgA. C3 and C4 are most commonly demonstrated, and C1q, fibrinogen, and properdin are also frequently demonstrated. In the mesangial type of involvement, the pattern is generally homogeneous or finely granular. In both the focal and diffuse proliferative types, fine to coarse granular and lumpy deposits are seen along the capillary basement membrane in addition to mesangial staining [2, 3, 48, 73, 74]. The glomerular response is generally proliferative in nature, either segmental (localized) or diffuse and involving primarily mesangial cells with lesser degrees of endothelial and epithelial cell increase. Frequently there are areas of karyorrhexis and necrosis, with partial or complete obliteration of individual capillary lumina, lobules, or glomeruli.

The lupus mesangial proliferative lesion is characterized by mesangial hypercellularity associated with immune complexes that are generally confined to the mesangium. The membranous form of the disease is similar to that described in membranous glomerulonephropathy, with primarily subepithelial deposits. Usually there is some degree of mesangial hypercellularity, and immune complexes can be demonstrated in the mesangium. In many instances, the presence of immunoglobulins and complement component can be demonstrated along segments of tubular basement membrane. Similar findings may also be noted within the walls of small vessels (arteries and veins).

In some instances, large subendothelial deposits (hyaline or fibrinoid thrombi) will compromise the capillary lumen. Electron microscopic studies confirm the presence of electron-dense deposits in the regions of staining noted on immunofluorescence examination (Fig. 16–9).

Nephropathies Without Known Primary Immune Injury

There are two important primary renal diseases for which no immune mechanism has been satisfactorily demonstrated: minimal-lesion nephrotic syndrome and steroid-resistant nephrotic syndrome with focal sclerosis. The first disease shows no immunoprotein deposition [20, 33, 54, 60]; the second shows immunofluorescence findings, usually IgM, C3, and properdin, restricted to glomeruli undergoing sclerosis. Normal or completely fibrosed glomeruli are negative [61, 120, 154]. These findings are common in other diseases [153].

Acknowledgment

The authors would like to thank Sharri L. Hackbarth for assistance in preparation of the manuscript.

References

1. Agnello, V., Koffler, D., Eisenberg, J. W., et al. C1q precipitins in the sera of patients with systemic lupus erythematosus and other hypocomplementemic states: Characterization of high and low molecular weight types. *J. Exp. Med.* 134:228s, 1971.
2. Agnello, V., Koffler, D., and Kunkel, H. G. Immune complex systems in the nephritis of systemic lupus erythematosus. *Kidney Int.* 3:90, 1973.
3. Andres, G. A., Accinni, L., Beiser, S. M., et al. Localization of fluorescein-labeled antinucleoside antibodies in glomeruli of patients with active systemic lupus erythematosus nephritis. *J. Clin. Invest.* 49:2106, 1970.
4. Andres, G. A., and McCluskey, R. T. Tubular and interstitial renal disease due to immunologic mechanisms. *Kidney Int.* 7:271, 1975.
5. Austen, K. F. Hageman-factor-dependent coagulation, fibrinolysis, and kinin generation. *Transplant. Proc.* 6:39, 1974.
6. Baldwin, D. S., Gluck, M. C., Schacht, R. G., et al. The long-term course of poststreptococcal glomerulonephritis. *Ann. Intern. Med.* 80:342, 1974.
7. Baldwin, D. S., Levine, B. B., McCluskey, R. T., et al. Renal failure and interstitial nephritis due to penicillin and methicillin. *N. Engl. J. Med.* 279:1245, 1968.
8. Baldwin, D. S., Lowenstein, J., Rothfield, N. F., et al. The clinical course of the proliferative and membranous forms of lupus nephritis. *Ann. Intern. Med.* 73:929, 1970.
9. Bardana, E. J., Jr., Harbeck, R. J., Hoffman, A. A., et al. The prognostic and therapeutic implications of DNA:anti-DNA immune complexes in systemic lupus erythematosus (SLE). *Am. J. Med.* 59:515, 1975.
10. Beirne, G. J., and Brennan, J. T. Glomerulonephritis associated with hydrocarbon solvents: Mediated by antiglomerular basement membrane antibody. *Arch. Environ. Health* 25:365, 1972.
11. Beirne, G. J., Octaviano, G. N., Kopp, W. L., et al. Immunohistology of the lung in Goodpasture's syndrome. *Ann. Intern. Med.* 69:1207, 1968.
12. Benacerraf, B., McCluskey, R. T., and Patras, D. Localization of colloidal substances in vascular endothelium: A mechanism of tissue damage: I. Factors causing the pathologic deposition of colloidal carbon. *Am. J. Pathol.* 35:75, 1959.
13. Benoit, F. L., Rulon, D. B., Theil, G. B., et al. Goodpasture's syndrome: A clinicopathologic entity. *Am. J. Med.* 37:424, 1964.
14. Berger, J. IgA glomerular deposits in renal disease. *Transplant. Proc.* 1:939, 1969.
15. Berger, J., and Galle, P. Dépôts denses au sein des membranes basales du rein: Étude en microscopies optique et électronique. *Presse Med.* 71:2351, 1963.
16. Berger, J., Noel, L.-H., and Yanerva, H. Complement deposition in the kidney. *Adv. Nephrol.* 4:37, 1974.
17. Border, W. A., Lehman, D. H., Egan, J. D., et al. Antitubular basement-

membrane antibodies in methicillin-associated interstitial nephritis. *N. Engl. J. Med.* 291:381, 1974.
18. Brentjens, J. R., Sepulveda, M., Baliah, T., et al. Interstitial immune complex nephritis in patients with systemic lupus erythematosus. *Kidney Int.* 7:342, 1975.
19. Burkholder, P. M., Marchand, A., and Krueger, R. P. Mixed membranous and proliferative glomerulonephritis: A correlative light, immunofluorescence, and electron microscopic study. *Lab. Invest.* 23:459, 1970.
20. Cameron, J. S., Turner, D. R., Ogg, C. S., et al. The nephrotic syndrome in adults with "minimal change" glomerular lesions. *Q. J. Med.* (new series) 43:461, 1974.
21. Chang, R. L. S., Deen, W. M., Robertson, C. R., et al. Permselectivity of the glomerular capillary wall: Studies of experimental glomerulonephritis in the rat using neutral dextran. *J. Clin. Invest.* 57:1272, 1976.
22. Churg, J., and Ehrenreich, T. Membranous Nephropathy. In P. Kincaid-Smith, T. H. Mathew, and E. L. Becker (Eds.), *Glomerulonephritis: Morphology, Natural History, and Treatment, Part I.* New York: Wiley, 1973.
23. Cochrane, C. G. Immunologic tissue injury mediated by neutrophilic leukocytes. *Adv. Immunol.* 9:97, 1968.
24. Cochrane, C. G. Mechanisms involved in the deposition of immune complexes in tissues. *J. Exp. Med.* 134:75s, 1971.
25. Cochrane, C. G., and Hawkins, D. Studies on circulating immune complexes: III. Factors governing the ability of circulating complexes to localize in blood vessels. *J. Exp. Med.* 127:137, 1968.
26. Cochrane, C. G., and Janoff, A. The Arthus Reaction: A Model of Neutrophil and Complement-Mediated Injury. In B. W. Zweifach, L. Grant, and R. T. McCluskey (Eds.), *The Inflammatory Process* (2nd ed.), Vol. 3. New York: Academic, 1974.
27. Cochrane, C. G., and Koffler, D. Immune complex disease in experimental animals and man. *Adv. Immunol.* 16:185, 1973.
28. Comerford, F. R., and Cohen, A. S. The nephropathy of systemic lupus erythematosus: An assessment by clinical, light and electron microscopic criteria. *Medicine (Baltimore)* 46:425, 1967.
29. Couser, W. G., Wagonfeld, J. B., Spargo, B. H., et al. Glomerular deposition of tumor antigen in membranous nephropathy associated with colonic carcinoma. *Am. J. Med.* 57:962, 1974.
30. Day, N. K., Geiger, H., McLean, R., et al. The association of respiratory infection, recurrent hematuria, and focal glomerulonephritis with activation of the complement system in the cold. *J. Clin. Invest.* 52:1698, 1973.
31. Dixon, F. J. The role of antigen-antibody complexes in disease. *Harvey Lect.* 58:21, 1963.
32. Dodge, W. F., Spargo, B. H., Travis, L. B., et al. Poststreptococcal glomerulonephritis: A prospective study in children. *N. Engl. J. Med.* 286:273, 1972.
33. Drummond, K. N., Michael, A. F., Good, R. A., et al. The nephrotic syndrome of childhood: Immunologic, clinical, and pathologic correlations. *J. Clin. Invest.* 45:620, 1966.
34. Duncan, D. A., Drummond, K. N., Michael, A. F., et al. Pulmonary hemorrhage and glomerulonephritis: Report of six cases and study of the renal lesion by the fluorescent antibody technique and electron microscopy. *Ann. Intern. Med.* 62:920, 1965.
35. Dupont, E., Mendès da Costa, C. R., and Dupuis, F. Linear deposits of immunoglobulins on glomerular basement membrane of human stored kidneys. *Transplantation* 18:458, 1974.

36. Ehrenreich, T., and Churg, J. Pathology of membranous nephropathy. *Pathol. Annu.* 3:145, 1968.
37. Erwin, D. T., Donadio, J. V., Jr., and Holley, K. E. The clinical course of idiopathic membranous nephropathy. *Mayo Clin. Proc.* 48:697, 1973.
38. Evans, D. J., Williams, D. G., Peters, D. K., et al. Glomerular deposition of properdin in Henoch-Schönlein syndrome and idiopathic focal nephritis. *Br. Med. J.* 3:326, 1973.
39. Farquhar, M. G., and Palade, G. E. Functional evidence for the existence of a third cell type in the renal glomerulus: Phagocytosis of filtration residues by a distinctive "third" cell. *J. Cell Biol.* 13:55, 1962.
40. Fearon, D. T., Ruddy, S., Knostman, J. D., et al. The functional significance of complement. *Adv. Nephrol.* 4:15, 1974.
41. Feltkamp, T. E. W., and Boode, J. H. Elution of antibodies from biopsy tissue. *J. Clin. Pathol.* 23:629, 1970.
42. Fish, A. J., Herdman, R. C., Michael, A. F., et al. Epidemic acute glomerulonephritis associated with type 49 streptococcal pyoderma: II. Correlative study of light, immunofluorescent and electron microscopic findings. *Am. J. Med.* 48:28, 1970.
43. Fisher, E. R., and Bark, J. Effect of hypertension on vascular and other lesions of serum sickness. *Am. J. Pathol.* 39:665, 1961.
44. Galle, P., and Mahieu, P. Electron dense alteration of kidney basement membranes: A renal lesion specific of a systemic disease. *Am. J. Med.* 58:749, 1975.
45. Gamble, C. N., and Reardan, J. B. Immunopathogenesis of syphilitic glomerulonephritis: Elution of antitreponemal antibody from glomerular immune-complex deposits. *N. Engl. J. Med.* 292:449, 1975.
46. Germuth, F. G., Jr., Kelemen, W. A., and Pollack, A. D. Immune complex disease: II. The role of circulatory dynamics and glomerular filtration in the development of experimental glomerulonephritis. *Johns Hopkins Med. J.* 120: 252, 1967.
47. Germuth, F. G., Jr., and Rodriguez, E. *Immunopathology of the Renal Glomerulus: Immune Complex Deposit and Antibasement Membrane Disease.* Boston: Little, Brown, 1973.
48. Germuth, F. G., Jr., and Rodriguez, E. *Immunopathology of the Renal Glomerulus: Immune Complex Deposit and Antibasement Membrane Disease.* Boston: Little, Brown, 1973. Pp. 113–145.
49. Gewurz, H., Pickering, R. J., Mergenhagen, S. E., et al. The complement profile in acute glomerulonephritis systemic lupus erythematosus and hypocomplementemic chronic glomerulonephritis: Contrasts and experimental correlations. *Int. Arch. Allergy Appl. Immunol.* 34:556, 1968.
50. Gewurz, H., Shin, H. S., and Mergenhagen, S. E. Interactions of the complement system with endotoxic lipopolysaccharide: Consumption of each of the six terminal complement components. *J. Exp. Med.* 128:1049, 1968.
51. Gluck, M. C., Gallo, G., Lowenstein, J., et al. Membranous glomerulonephritis: Evolution of clinical and pathologic features. *Ann. Intern. Med.* 78:1, 1973.
52. Götze, O., and Müller-Eberhard, H. J. The C3-activator system: An alternate pathway of complement activation. *J. Exp. Med.* 134:90s, 1971.
53. Götze, O., and Müller-Eberhard, H. J. The role of properdin in the alternate pathway of complement activation. *J. Exp. Med.* 139:44, 1974.
54. Habib, R., Kleinknecht, C., and Gubler, M. C. The Nephrotic Syndrome. In P. Royer, R. Habib, H. Mathieu, et al. (Eds.), *Pediatric Nephrology.* Philadelphia: Saunders, 1974.

55. Habib, R., Kleinknecht, C., Gubler, M. C., et al. Idiopathic membranoproliferative glomerulonephritis in children: Report of 105 cases. *Clin. Nephrol.* 1:194, 1973.
56. Habib, R., and Levy, M. Anaphylactoid purpura nephritis: Observations with sixty childhood cases. *Clin. Pediatr.* 12:445, 1973.
57. Henson, P. M. The adherence of leucocytes and platelets induced by fixed IgG antibody or complement. *Immunology* 16:107, 1969.
58. Henson, P. M. Release of Biologically Active Constituents From Blood Cells and Its Role in Antibody-Mediated Tissue Injury. In B. Amos (Ed.), *Progress in Immunology*. New York: Academic, 1971.
59. Henson, P. M. Pathologic mechanisms in neutrophil-mediated injury. *Am. J. Pathol.* 68:593, 1972.
60. Heptinstall, R. H. *Pathology of the Kidney* (2nd ed.). Boston: Little, Brown, 1974.
61. Hyman, L. R., and Burkholder, P. M. Focal sclerosing glomerulonephropathy with segmental hyalinosis: A clinicopathologic analysis. *Lab. Invest.* 28:533, 1973.
62. Hyman, L. R., Wagnild, J. P., Beirne, G. J., et al. Immunoglobulin-A distribution in glomerular disease: Analysis of immunofluorescence localization and pathogenetic significance. *Kidney Int.* 3:397, 1973.
63. Izui, S., Lambert, P.-H., and Miescher, P. A. In vitro demonstration of a particular affinity of glomerular basement membrane and collagen for DNA: A possible basis for a local formation of DNA-anti-DNA complexes in systemic lupus erythematosus. *J. Exp. Med.* 144:428, 1976.
64. Jennings, R. B., and Earle, D. P. Post-streptococcal glomerulonephritis: Histopathologic and clinical studies of the acute, subsiding acute and early chronic latent phases. *J. Clin. Invest.* 40:1525, 1961.
65. Johnson, G. D., and Holborow, E. J. Immunofluorescence. In D. M. Weir (Ed.), *Handbook of Experimental Immunology* (2nd ed.), Vol. 1. Oxford: Blackwell, 1973.
66. Jones, D. B. Nephrotic glomerulonephritis. *Am. J. Pathol.* 33:313, 1957.
67. Kincaid-Smith, P. Coagulation and renal disease. *Kidney Int.* 2:183, 1972.
68. Klassen, J., Andres, G. A., Brennan, J. C., et al. An immunologic renal tubular lesion in man. *Clin. Immunol. Immunopathol.* 1:69, 1972.
69. Klassen, J., Elwood, C., Grossberg, A. L., et al. Evolution of membranous nephropathy into anti-glomerular-basement-membrane glomerulonephritis. *N. Engl. J. Med.* 290:1340, 1974.
70. Klassen, J., Kano, K., Milgrom, F., et al. Tubular lesions produced by autoantibodies to tubular basement membrane in human renal allografts. *Int. Arch. Allergy Appl. Immunol.* 45:675, 1973.
71. Kniker, W. T., and Cochrane, C. G. Pathogenic factors in vascular lesions of experimental serum sickness. *J. Exp. Med.* 122:83, 1965.
72. Kniker, W. T., and Cochrane, C. G. The localization of circulating immune complexes in experimental serum sickness: The role of vasoactive amines and hydrodynamic forces. *J. Exp. Med.* 127:119, 1968.
73. Koffler, D., Agnello, V., Carr, R. I., et al. Variable patterns of immunoglobulin and complement deposition in the kidneys of patients with systemic lupus erythematosus. *Am. J. Pathol.* 56:305, 1969.
74. Koffler, D., Agnello, V., Thoburn, R., et al. Systemic lupus erythematosus: Prototype of immune complex nephritis in man. *J. Exp. Med.* 134:169s, 1971.
75. Koffler, D., and Paronetto, F. Immunofluorescent localization of immunoglobulins, complement, and fibrinogen in human diseases: II. Acute, subacute, and chronic glomerulonephritis. *J. Clin. Invest.* 44:1665, 1965.

76. Koffler, D., Sandson, J., Carr, R., et al. Immunologic studies concerning the pulmonary lesions in Goodpasture's syndrome. *Am. J. Pathol.* 54:293, 1969.
77. Koffler, D., Sandson, J., and Kunkel, H. G. Elution studies on tissues from patients with Goodpasture's syndrome and other forms of subacute glomerulonephritis (abstract). *J. Clin. Invest.* 47:55a, 1968.
78. Koffler, D., Schur, P. H., and Kunkel, H. G. Immunological studies concerning the nephritis of systemic lupus erythematosus. *J. Exp. Med.* 126:607, 1967.
79. Krishnan, C., and Kaplan, M. H. Immunopathologic studies of systemic lupus erythematosus: II. Antinuclear reaction of γ-globulin eluted from homogenates and isolated glomeruli of kidneys from patients with lupus nephritis. *J. Clin. Invest.* 46:569, 1967.
80. Lambert, P. H., Bricteux, N., Salmon, J., et al. Dynamics of immune complex nephritis during antibody excess. *Int. Arch. Allergy Appl. Immunol.* 45: 185, 1973.
81. Lambert, P. H., Perrin, L. H., Mahieu, P., et al. Activation of complement in human nephritis. *Adv. Nephrol.* 4:79, 1974.
82. Leber, P. D., and McCluskey, R. T. Complement and the immunohistology of renal disease. *Transplant. Proc.* 6:67, 1974.
83. Lehman, D. H., Marquardt, H., Wilson, C. B., et al. Specificity of autoantibodies to tubular and glomerular basement membranes induced in guinea pigs. *J. Immunol.* 112:241, 1974.
84. Lehman, D. H., Wilson, C. B., and Dixon, F. J. Interstitial nephritis in rats immunized with heterologous tubular basement membrane. *Kidney Int.* 5:187, 1974.
85. Lehman, D. H., Wilson, C. B., and Dixon, F. J. Extraglomerular immunoglobulin deposits in human nephritis. *Am. J. Med.* 58:765, 1975.
86. Lerner, R. A., and Dixon, F. J. Transfer of ovine experimental allergic glomerulonephritis (EAG) with serum. *J. Exp. Med.* 124:431, 1966.
87. Lerner, R. A., and Dixon, F. J. The induction of acute glomerulonephritis in rabbits with soluble antigens isolated from normal homologous and autologous urine. *J. Immunol.* 100:1277, 1968.
88. Lerner, R. A., Glassock, R. J., and Dixon, F. J. The role of antiglomerular basement membrane antibody in the pathogenesis of human glomerulonephritis. *J. Exp. Med.* 126:989, 1967.
89. Levinsky, R. J., Cameron, J. S., and Soothill, J. F. Serum immune complexes and disease activity in lupus nephritis. *Lancet* 1:564, 1977.
90. Levy, M., Beaufils, H., Gubler, M. C., et al. Idiopathic recurrent macroscopic hematuria and mesangial IgA-IgG deposits in children (Berger's disease). *Clin. Nephrol.* 1:63, 1973.
91. Lewis, E. J., Cavallo, T., Harrington, J. T., et al. An immunopathologic study of rapidly progressive glomerulonephritis in the adult. *Hum. Pathol.* 2:185, 1971.
92. Lewis, M. G., Loughridge, L. W., and Phillips, T. M. Immunological studies in nephrotic syndrome associated with extrarenal malignant disease. *Lancet* 2:134, 1971.
93. Lewy, J. E., Salinas-Madrigal, L., Herdson, P. B., et al. Clinico-pathologic correlations in acute poststreptococcal glomerulonephritis: A correlation between renal functions, morphologic damage and clinical course of 46 children with acute poststreptococcal glomerulonephritis. *Medicine (Baltimore)* 50:453, 1971.
94. Lightfoot, R. W., Jr., Drusin, R. E., and Christian, C. L. Properties of soluble immune complexes. *J. Immunol.* 105:1493, 1970.
95. Lowance, D. C., Mullins, J. D., and McPhaul, J. J., Jr. Immunoglobulin A (IgA) associated glomerulonephritis. *Kidney Int.* 3:167, 1973.

96. Luna, G. *Manual of Histologic Staining Methods of the Armed Forces Institute of Pathology* (3rd ed.). New York: McGraw-Hill, 1968.
97. Luthra, H. S., McDuffie, F. C., Hunder, G. G., et al. Immune complexes in sera and synovial fluids of patients with rheumatoid arthritis: Radioimmunoassay with monoclonal rheumatoid factor. *J. Clin. Invest.* 56:458, 1975.
98. Mahieu, P., Lambert, P. H., and Miescher, P. A. Detection of anti-glomerular basement membrane antibodies by a radioimmunological technique: Clinical application in human nephropathies. *J. Clin. Invest.* 54:128, 1974.
99. Marder, V. J. Fibrinogen and fibrin degradation products: Physicochemical and physiological considerations. *Thromb. Diath. Haemorrh.* [Suppl.] 47:85, 1971.
100. Marquardt, H., Wilson, C. B., and Dixon, F. J. Isolation and immunological characterization of human glomerular basement membrane antigens. *Kidney Int.* 3:57, 1973.
101. Mauer, S. M., Fish, A. J., Blau, E. B., et al. The glomerular mesangium: I. Kinetic studies of macromolecular uptake in normal and nephrotic rats. *J. Clin. Invest.* 51:1092, 1972.
102. Mauer, S. M., Michael, A. F., Fish, A. J., et al. Spontaneous immunoglobulin and complement deposition in glomeruli of diabetic rats. *Lab. Invest.* 27:488, 1972.
103. Mauer, S. M., Sutherland, D. E. R., Howard, R. J., et al. The glomerular mesangium: III. Acute immune mesangial injury: A new model of glomerulonephritis. *J. Exp. Med.* 137:553, 1973.
104. McCluskey, R. T. Lupus nephritis. *Pathol. Annu.* 5:125, 1970.
105. McCluskey, R. T. The value of immunofluorescence in the study of human renal disease. *J. Exp. Med.* 134:242s, 1971.
106. McCluskey, R. T., and Klassen, J. Immunologically mediated glomerular, tubular and interstitial renal disease. *N. Engl. J. Med.* 288:564, 1973.
107. McIntosh, R. M., Kihara, H., Kulvinskas, C., et al. Chemical and immunological characterization of a basement membrane-like glycoprotein in the rat. *Ann. Rheum. Dis.* 30:631, 1971.
108. McIntosh, R. M., Tinglof, B., Kaufman, D., et al. Immunohistology in renal disease: Diagnostic, prognostic, therapeutic, and etiologic value and limitations. *Q. J. Med.* (new series) 40:385, 1971.
109. McLean, R. H., and Michael, A. F. Properdin and C3 proactivator: Alternate pathway components in human glomerulonephritis. *J. Clin. Invest.* 52:634, 1973.
110. McLean, R. H., and Michael, A. F. Activation of the Complement System in Renal Conditions in Animals and Man. In L. Brent and J. Holborow (Eds.), *Progress in Immunology II.* Amsterdam: North-Holland, 1974. Vol. 5, pp. 69–79.
111. McPhaul, J. J., Jr. IgA-associated glomerulonephritis. *Annu. Rev. Med.* 28: 37, 1977.
112. McPhaul, J. J., Jr., and Dixon, F. J. The presence of anti-glomerular basement membrane antibodies in peripheral blood. *J. Immunol.* 103:1168, 1969.
113. McPhaul, J. J., Jr., and Dixon, F. J. Characterization of human anti-glomerular basement membrane antibodies eluted from glomerulonephritic kidneys. *J. Clin. Invest.* 49:308, 1970.
114. McPhaul, J. J., Jr., and Dixon, F. J. Characterization of immunoglobulin G anti-glomerular basement membrane antibodies eluted from kidneys of patients with glomerulonephritis: II. IgG subtypes and *in vitro* complement fixation. *J. Immunol.* 107:678, 1971.

115. Meadow, S. R., Glasgow, E. F., White, R. H. R., et al. Schönlein-Henoch nephritis. *Q. J. Med.* (new series) 41:241, 1972.
116. Michael, A. F., Fish, A. J., and Good, R. A. Glomerular localization and transport of aggregated proteins in mice. *Lab. Invest.* 17:14, 1967.
117. Michael, A. F., and McLean, R. H. Evidence for activation of the alternate pathway in glomerulonephritis. *Adv. Nephrol.* 4:49, 1974.
118. Michael, A. F., Jr., Drummond, K. N., Good, R. A., et al. Acute poststreptococcal glomerulonephritis: Immune deposit disease. *J. Clin. Invest.* 45:237, 1966.
119. Morel-Maroger, L., Kourilsky, O., Mignon, F., et al. Antitubular basement membrane antibodies in rapidly progressive poststreptococcal glomerulonephritis: Report of a case. *Clin. Immunol. Immunopathol.* 2:185, 1974.
120. Morel-Maroger, L., Leathem, A., and Richet, G. Glomerular abnormalities in nonsystemic diseases: Relationship between findings by light microscopy and immunofluorescence in 433 renal biopsy specimens. *Am. J. Med.* 53:170, 1972.
121. Morel-Maroger, L., Mery, J. P., Robert, C. L., et al. Mesangial IgA Deposits. In P. Kincaid-Smith, T. H. Mathew, and E. L. Becker (Eds.), *Glomerulonephritis: Morphology, Natural History, and Treatment, Part I.* New York: Wiley, 1973.
122. Müller-Eberhard, H. J. Biochemistry of Complement. In B. Amos (Ed.), *Progress in Immunology.* New York: Academic, 1971.
123. Müller-Eberhard, H. J. The molecular basis of the biological activities of complement. *Harvey Lect.* 66:75, 1972.
124. Naruse, T., Kitamura, K., Miyakawa, Y., et al. Deposition of renal tubular epithelial antigen along the glomerular capillary walls of patients with membranous glomerulonephritis. *J. Immunol.* 110:1163, 1973.
125. Nydegger, U. E., Lambert, P. H., Gerber, H., et al. Circulating immune complexes in the serum in systemic lupus erythematosus and in carriers of hepatitis B antigen: Quantitation by binding to radiolabeled C1q. *J. Clin. Invest.* 54:297, 1974.
126. Ooi, Y. M., Vallota, E. H., and West, C. D. Classical complement pathway activation in membranoproliferative glomerulonephritis. *Kidney Int.* 9:46, 1976.
127. Paronetto, F., and Koffler, D. Immunofluorescent localization of immunoglobulins, complement, and fibrinogen in human diseases: I. Systemic lupus erythematosus. *J. Clin. Invest.* 44:1657, 1965.
128. Perrin, L. H., Lambert, P. H., and Miescher, P. A. Properdin levels in systemic lupus erythematosus and membranoproliferative glomerulonephritis. *Clin. Exp. Immunol.* 16:575, 1974.
129. Pickering, R. J., Michael, A. F., Jr., Herdman, R. C., et al. The complement system in chronic glomerulonephritis: Three newly associated aberrations. *J. Pediatr.* 78:30, 1971.
130. Pillemer, L., Schoenberg, M. D., Blum, L., et al. Properdin system and immunity: II. Interaction of the properdin system with polysaccharides. *Science* 122:545, 1955.
131. Pirani, C. L., and Manaligod, J. R. The kidneys in collagen diseases. *Monogr. Pathol.* (*Int. Acad. Pathol.*) No. 6, 147, 1966.
132. Pollak, V. E., Pirani, C. L., and Schwartz, F. D. The natural history of the renal manifestations of systemic lupus erythematosus. *J. Lab. Clin. Med.* 63:537, 1964.
133. Proskey, A. J., Weatherbee, L., Easterling, R. E., et al. Goodpasture's syndrome: A report of five cases and review of the literature. *Am. J. Med.* 48:162, 1970.

134. Rosen, S. Membranous glomerulonephritis: Current status. *Hum. Pathol.* 2:209, 1971.
135. Rothfield, N. F., McCluskey, R. T., and Baldwin, D. S. Renal disease in systemic lupus erythematosus. *N. Engl. J. Med.* 269:537, 1963.
136. Ruddy, S., Gigli, I., and Austen, K. F. The complement system of man. *N. Engl. J. Med.* 287:489; 545; 592; 642, 1972.
137. Scheer, R. L., and Grossman, M. A. Immune aspects of the glomerulonephritis associated with pulmonary hemorrhage. *Ann. Intern. Med.* 60:1009, 1964.
138. Schreiber, R. D., Medicus, R. G., Götze, O., et al. Properdin- and nephritic factor-dependent C3 convertases: Requirement of native C3 for enzyme formation and the function of bound C3b as properdin receptor. *J. Exp. Med.* 142:760, 1975.
139. Siqueira, M., and Nelson, R. A., Jr. Platelet agglutination by immune complexes and its possible role in hypersensitivity. *J. Immunol.* 86:516, 1961.
140. Soothill, J. F., and Steward, M. W. The immunopathological significance of the heterogeneity of antibody affinity. *Clin. Exp. Immunol.* 9:193, 1971.
141. Steblay, R. W. Glomerulonephritis induced in sheep by injections of heterologous glomerular basement membrane and Freund's complete adjuvant. *J. Exp. Med.* 116:253, 1962.
142. Steblay, R. W. Glomerulonephritis induced in sheep by injections of homologous sheep glomerular basement membrane (SGBM) and Freund's adjuvant (FA) (abstract). *Fed. Proc.* 24:693, 1965.
143. Steblay, R. W. Some immunologic properties of human glomerular basement membrane: IV. Immediate or delayed nephritis induced in rabbits by sheep anti-human glomerular basement membrane sera. *J. Immunol.* 95:517, 1965.
144. Steblay, R. W., and Rudofsky, U. Renal tubular disease and autoantibodies against tubular basement membrane induced in guinea pigs. *J. Immunol.* 107:589, 1971.
145. Strauss, J., Pardo, V., Koss, M. N., et al. Nephropathy associated with sickle cell anemia: An autologous immune complex nephritis: I. Studies on nature of glomerular-bound antibody and antigen identification in a patient with sickle cell disease and immune deposit glomerulonephritis. *Am. J. Med.* 58:382, 1975.
146. Sugisaki, T., Klassen, J., Milgrom, F., et al. Immunopathologic study of an autoimmune tubular and interstitial renal disease in Brown Norway rats. *Lab. Invest.* 28:658, 1973.
147. Theofilopoulos, A. N., Wilson, C. B., and Dixon, F. J. The Raji cell radioimmune assay for detecting immune complexes in human sera. *J. Clin. Invest.* 57:169, 1976.
148. Tung, K. S. K., and Black, W. C. Association of renal glomerular and tubular immune complex disease and antitubular basement membrane antibody. *Lab. Invest.* 32:696, 1975.
149. Unanue, E. R., and Dixon, F. J. Experimental glomerulonephritis: V. Studies on the interaction of nephrotoxic antibodies with tissues of the rat. *J. Exp. Med.* 121:697, 1965.
150. Unanue, E. R., and Dixon, F. J. Experimental allergic glomerulonephritis induced in the rabbit with heterologous renal antigens. *J. Exp. Med.* 125:149, 1967.
151. Urizar, R. E., Michael, A., Sisson, S., et al. Anaphylactoid purpura: II. Immunofluorescent and electron microscopic studies of the glomerular lesions. *Lab. Invest.* 19:437, 1968.
152. Vallota, E. H., Götze, O., Spiegelberg, H. L., et al. A serum factor in chronic hypocomplementemic nephritis distinct from immunoglobulins and activating the alternate pathway of complement. *J. Exp. Med.* 139:1249, 1974.

153. Velosa, J., Miller, K., and Michael, A. F. Immunopathology of the end-stage kidney: Immunoglobulin and complement component deposition in nonimmune disease. *Am. J. Pathol.* 84:149, 1976.
154. Velosa, J. A., Donadio, J. V., Jr., and Holley, K. E. Focal sclerosing glomerulonephropathy: A clinicopathologic study. *Mayo Clin. Proc.* 50:121, 1975.
155. Velosa, J. A., Glasser, R. J., Nevins, T. E., et al. Experimental model of focal sclerosis: II. Correlation with immunopathologic changes, macromolecular kinetics, and polyanion loss. *Lab. Invest.* 36:527, 1977.
156. Vernier, R. L., Mauer, S. M., Fish, A. J., et al. The mesangial cell in glomerulonephritis. *Adv. Nephrol.* 1:31, 1971.
157. Verroust, P. J., Wilson, C. B., Cooper, N. R., et al. Glomerular complement components in human glomerulonephritis. *J. Clin. Invest.* 53:77, 1974.
158. Wardle, E. N. Fibrin in renal disease: Functional considerations. *Clin. Nephrol.* 2:85, 1974.
159. Weigle, W. O. Fate and biological action of antigen-antibody complexes. *Adv. Immunol.* 1:283, 1961.
160. Westberg, N. G., and Michael, A. F. Immunohistopathology of diabetic glomerulosclerosis. *Diabetes* 21:163, 1972.
161. Westberg, N. G., Naff, G. B., Boyer, J. T., et al. Glomerular deposition of properdin in acute and chronic glomerulonephritis with hypocomplementemia. *J. Clin. Invest.* 50:642, 1971.
162. Williams, D. G., Peters, D. K., Fallows, J., et al. Studies of serum complement in the hypocomplementaemic nephritides. *Clin. Exp. Immunol.* 18:391, 1974.
163. Wilson, C. B. Immunohistopathology of the Kidney. In N. R. Rose and H. Friedman (Eds.), *Manual of Clinical Immunology.* Washington, D.C.: American Society for Microbiology, 1976.
164. Wilson, C. B., and Dixon, F. J. Antigen quantitation in experimental immune complex glomerulonephritis: I. Acute serum sickness. *J. Immunol.* 105:279, 1970.
165. Wilson, C. B., and Dixon, F. J. Quantitation of acute and chronic serum sickness in the rabbit. *J. Exp. Med.* 134:7s, 1971.
166. Wilson, C. B., and Dixon, F. J. Anti-glomerular basement membrane antibody-induced glomerulonephritis. *Kidney Int.* 3:74, 1973.
167. Wilson, C. B., and Dixon, F. J. Diagnosis of immunopathologic renal disease (editorial). *Kidney Int.* 5:389, 1974.
168. Wilson, C. B., and Dixon, F. J. The Renal Response to Immunological Injury. In B. M. Brenner and F. C. Rector, Jr. (Eds.), *The Kidney,* Vol. 2. Philadelphia: Saunders, 1976.
169. Wilson, C. B., Marquardt, H., and Dixon, F. J. Radioimmunoassay (RIA) for circulating antiglomerular basement membrane (GBM) antibodies (abstract). *Kidney Int.* 6:114a, 1974.
170. Wilson, C. B., and Smith, R. C. Goodpasture's syndrome associated with influenza A2 virus infection. *Ann. Intern. Med.* 76:91, 1972.
171. Winfield, J. B., Faiferman, I., and Koffler, D. Avidity of anti-DNA antibodies in serum and IgG glomerular eluates from patients with systemic lupus erythematosus: Association of high avidity antinative DNA antibody with glomerulonephritis. *J. Clin. Invest.* 59:90, 1977.
172. Wood, B. T., Thompson, S. H., and Goldstein, G. Fluorescent antibody staining: III. Preparation of fluorescein-isothiocyanate-labeled antibodies. *J. Immunol.* 95:225, 1965.
173. Zimmerman, T. S., and Müller-Eberhard, H. J. Blood coagulation initiation by a complement-mediated pathway. *J. Exp. Med.* 134:1601, 1971.

Index